D1093118

WITH
FRO

BRITISH MEDICAL ASSOCIATION

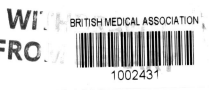

1002431

Pathology of the Prostate

An Algorithmic Approach

Pathology of the Prostate

An Algorithmic Approach

Antonio Lopez-Beltran
Cordoba University Medical School, Cordoba, Spain

Liang Cheng
Indiana University School of Medicine, USA

Maria Rosaria Raspollini
University Hospital Careggi, Florence, Italy

Rodolfo Montironi
Polytechnic University of the Marche Region, School of Medicine, United Hospitals, Ancona, Italy

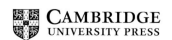

CAMBRIDGE
UNIVERSITY PRESS

WITHDRAWN FROM LIBRARY

BMA LIBRARY
BRITISH MEDICAL ASSOCIATION

CAMBRIDGE
UNIVERSITY PRESS

University Printing House, Cambridge CB2 8BS, United Kingdom

One Liberty Plaza, 20th Floor, New York, NY 10006, USA

477 Williamstown Road, Port Melbourne, VIC 3207, Australia

4843/24, 2nd Floor, Ansari Road, Daryaganj, Delhi – 110002, India

79 Anson Road, #06–04/06, Singapore 079906

Cambridge University Press is part of the University of Cambridge.

It furthers the University's mission by disseminating knowledge in the pursuit of education, learning, and research at the highest international levels of excellence.

www.cambridge.org
Information on this title: www.cambridge.org/9781108185653
DOI: 10.1017/9781108695947

© Cambridge University Press 2017

This publication is in copyright. Subject to statutory exception and to the provisions of relevant collective licensing agreements, no reproduction of any part may take place without the written permission of Cambridge University Press.

First published 2017

Printed in the United Kingdom by Clays, St Ives plc

A catalogue record for this publication is available from the British Library.

ISBN: 978-1-108-18565-3 Mixed Media
ISBN: 978-1-108-41564-4 Hardback
ISBN: 978-1-108-69594-7 Cambridge Core

Cambridge University Press has no responsibility for the persistence or accuracy of URLs for external or third-party internet websites referred to in this publication and does not guarantee that any content on such websites is, or will remain, accurate or appropriate.

....

Every effort has been made in preparing this book to provide accurate and up-to-date information which is in accord with accepted standards and practice at the time of publication. Although case histories are drawn from actual cases, every effort has been made to disguise the identities of the individuals involved. Nevertheless, the authors, editors and publishers can make no warranties that the information contained herein is totally free from error, not least because clinical standards are constantly changing through research and regulation. The authors, editors and publishers therefore disclaim all liability for direct or consequential damages resulting from the use of material contained in this book. Readers are strongly advised to pay careful attention to information provided by the manufacturer of any drugs or equipment that they plan to use.

Contents

Preface

The prostate is subject to a unique and extraordinarily diverse array of diseases including congenital, inflammatory, metaplastic or neoplastic abnormalities. Frequently in clinical practice, non-neoplastic diseases may present as tumor-like entities. The objective of *Pathology of the Prostate: An Algorithmic Approach* is to provide contemporary, comprehensive and evidence-based information for pathologists, urologists and medical oncologists. The text describes and illustrates the full spectrum of pathologic conditions that afflict the prostate. Also, it incorporates separate chapters with up-to-date information on the pathology of the seminal vesicles and prostatic urethra.

This book is aimed for the practicing pathologist with an emphasis on diagnostic criteria and differential diagnoses based on light microscopic and immunohistochemical examination of prostatic specimens. Particularly helpful is the inclusion of a full set of selected images to guide the diagnostic process. A set of diagnostic algorithms should help the reader more easily achieve this. It is our hope that this book will aid in the pathologist's recognition, understanding and accurate interpretation of the findings in the specimens of the prostate, seminal vesicles and the prostatic urethra.

In this text, we strive to provide a comprehensive resource for practicing surgical pathologists and their clinical colleagues so that they might better meet the daily demands and challenges in this ever-evolving field.

Antonio Lopez-Beltran, MD
Liang Cheng, MD
Maria Raspollini, MD
Rodolfo Montironi, MD

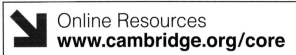

Online Resources
www.cambridge.org/core

↘ Fully searchable HTML text of the whole book
↘ Expandable figures and tables

Basic Anatomy and Histology of the Prostate

1.1 Basic Anatomy and Histology of the Prostate

- The adult prostate surrounds the urethra and is located posterior to the inferior symphysis pubis, superior to the urogenital diaphragm, and anterior to the rectum. It measures 5 cm x 4 cm x 3 cm and weighs 20 gr through ages 20 to 50 years, then there is an increase to 30 gr from ages of 60 to 80 years. Hyperplasia frequently occurs at later ages with larger prostates >30 gr. Table 1.1
- The three-zone model defines the central zone, the transition zone, and the peripheral zone. Fig 1.1

- Cancer tends to arise in the peripheral zone (20% do arise in the transition zone), and BPH typically arises in the transition zone. The central zone is more resistant to disease. The prostatic urethra exits the prostate at the apex where it is continuous with the membranous urethra. Transition zone cells typically express estrogen receptors, and peripheral zone cells typically express both androgen and estrogen receptors. Figs 1.2–1.7
- The paired ejaculatory ducts run through the central zone from the seminal vesicles to their exit at the posterior urethral protuberance, known as the verumontanum. Within the verumontanum is the prostatic utricle, located between the ejaculatory ducts. After puberty, the utricle shows a complicated and variable architecture.

Table 1.1 Types of Epithelial Cells in the Normal Prostate

Secretory (luminal cells)
Basal cells
Neuroendocrine cells
Urothelial cells (central ducts)
Ejaculatory duct cells including basal and luminal cells

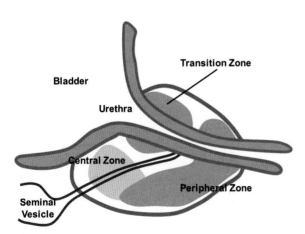

Fig 1.1 The three-zone model defines the central zone, the transition zone, and the peripheral zone.

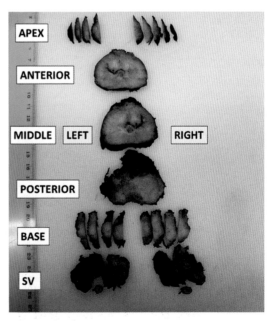

Fig 1.2 Partial sampling of the prostate after radical prostatectomy allows one to obtain information on the presence of cancer at different anatomic regions of the organ and to state laterality.

1

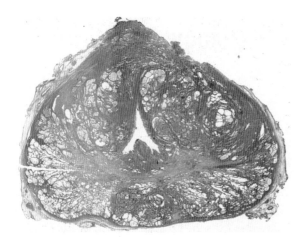

Fig 1.3 This macro-section of the prostate shows the transition zone (periurethral) and the peripheral zone.

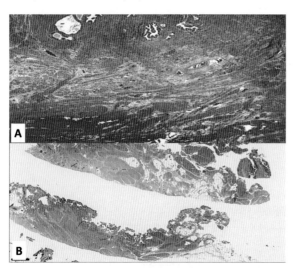

Fig 1.5 Different views (A and B) of base and posterior prostate (100x).

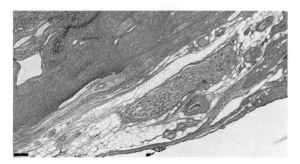

Fig 1.7 Transition between external connective tissue (so called prostate capsule) and periprostatic soft tissues with fat, vessels and nerves. The prostate tissue margin is highlighted by black ink.

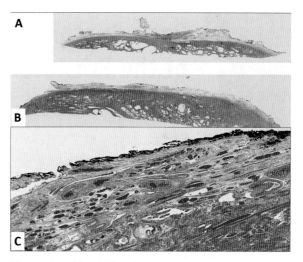

Fig 1.4 Apex (A) and (B), and anterior (C) prostate (100x).

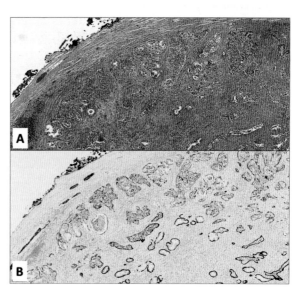

Fig 1.6 Occasionally, one may see prostate glands and acini with extensive apoptotic change on H&E (A) and with anti-cytockeratin 5/6 which highlights basal cells (B) (x100).

- Squamous cell metaplasia and urothelial metaplasia involving the prostatic utricle have been observed occasionally in patients treated with various forms of androgen manipulation therapies for Pca and benign prostatic hyperplasia. Similar morphologic findings are also seen in the periurethral ducts. Fig 1.10
- Orifices of the prostatic ducts are located in the area of the verumontanum, separately from the utricle and ejaculatory ducts. The ducts are lined by a bilayered prostatic epithelium histologically

The epithelium no longer differs from that of the prostate glands, both morphologically and immunohistochemically. Figs 1.8–1.9

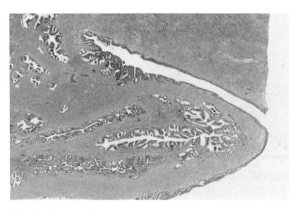

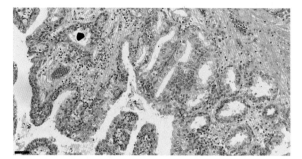

Fig 1.9 Close up view of the covering epithelium at the verumontanum (200x).

Fig 1.8 The paired ejaculatory ducts exit at the verumontanum. The prostatic utricle is seen located between the ejaculatory ducts. After puberty, the utricle shows an epithelium that no longer differs from the prostate glands.

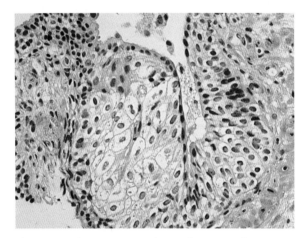

Fig 1.10 Focal squamous metaplasia in the prostate duct.

identical to that seen in the ducts and acini away from the urethra.
- The opening of the ejaculatory ducts is lateral to the prostatic utricle. The epithelial lining includes a basal cell layer and a luminal cell layer. The former are morphologically and immunohistochemically similar to those of the prostate. The luminal cells show acidophilic abundant cytoplasm with a variable amount of yellow pigment, whereas the nuclei show condensed chromatin and size variation.
- Occasionally, large epithelial cells with hyperchromatic nuclei can be seen. This epithelium is similar to that of the seminal vesicles. There is no morphological equivalent in the lower female genital tract.

- Intraductal and invasive neoplasms originating from the periurethral ducts can grow within the urethral lumen or infiltrate the prostatic utricle. In particular, intraductal carcinoma of the prostate and prostatic ductal adenocarcinomas can be seen in the periurethral prostatic ducts. The former is similar morphologically to the counterpart duct carcinoma in situ in the female breast and the latter shows similarities with the endometrioid carcinoma of the female genital tract.
- The anterior fibromuscular stroma is present anteriorly over the prostate and extends from the bladder neck to the apex of the prostate.
- The adult prostate gland is a branching duct-acinar embedded in a fibromuscular stroma. The epithelium has two cell layers: the luminal/secretory and the basal layer with some neuroendocrine cells in the epithelium. The cytoplasm of secretory cells is clear and occasionally may exhibit yellow-brown pigment (lipofuscin). Figs 1.11–1.20
- Secretory cells are positive for CKAE1/AE3, CK 8–18, PSA, PAP, PSMA, p501S (prostein) and NKX3-1. P504S (racemase) may show a focal non-circumferential positivity in normal secretory cells.
- Basal cells have a dense cytoplasm and small hyperchromatic nuclei. They react with p63, p40, CK5/6 and high molecular weight CK clone 34βE12 (CK903). Fig 1.21
- Neuroendocrine cells are less frequent and show an immunohistochemical profile more similar to secretory cells with variable androgen receptors and PSA/PAP expression. They express

3

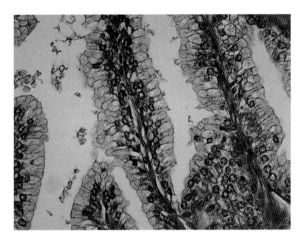

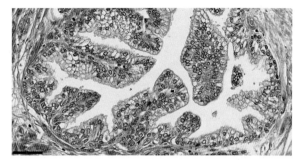

Fig 1.12 Prostate glands show secretory and basal cells surrounded by fibromuscular stroma.

Fig 1.11 Prostate glands show basal cell layer and the secretory cells towards the lumen.

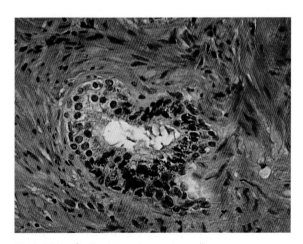

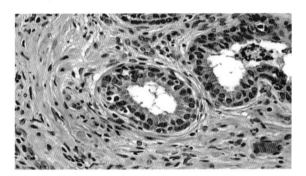

Fig 1.14 Neuroendocrine cells are present within the basal cells, but may extend to luminal surface of the gland (Anti-cromogranin antibody) (200x).

Fig 1.13 Paneth-like neuroendocrine cells may be seen in prostate glands.

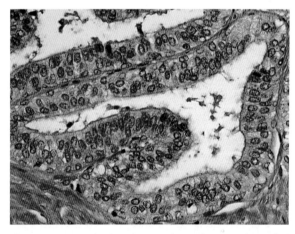

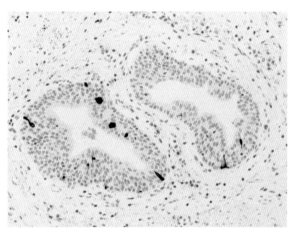

Fig 1.16 Prostate glands in the central zone show pseudostratified nuclei.

Fig 1.15 Lipofucsin pigment in secretory cells.

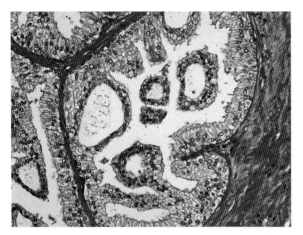

Fig 1.17 Prostate glands seen in the central zone with occasional roman-bridge structures.

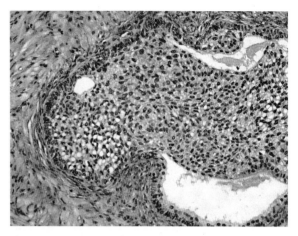

Fig 1.18 Urothelial metaplasia is focally seen in some prostate glands.

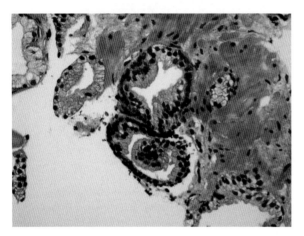

Fig 1.19 "Telescoping" is occasionally seen in some normal prostate glands, a finding not to be mistaken as glomeruloid pattern of carcinoma.

a number of immunohistochemical markers, including chromogranin, synaptophysin, neuron-specific enolase, CD56 and many other active peptides.

- Urothelium is also normally present in the prostate, sometimes showing a clear cytoplasm. It is PSA negative and p63, p40, GATA3 positive.
- Intraluminal contents of normal prostate glands include degenerated epithelial cells, corpora amylacea and calculi. Rarely, it may contain focal blue-tinged mucin, pink amorphous acellular secretions and crystalloids. Figs 1.22–1.23

- The prostatic stroma, including fibroblasts, smooth muscle, vasculature and nerves, and rarely adipocytes (carcinoma in fat should be viewed as extraprostatic extension). There are zonal differences in prostatic fibromuscular stroma density. Figs 1.24–1.27
- The prostate does not have a true capsule. The so called outer prostatic "capsule" is a band of concentrically placed fibromuscular and vascular tissue that is inseparable from prostatic stroma and surrounding fascia. This is absent in the apex. Figs 1.4; 1.7
- Histologically, nerves are seen in the periprostatic neurovascular bundle, in the outer fibromuscular band, and in the prostate itself. Paraganglia (clear cells that should not be mistaken as carcinoma) are usually adjacent to neurovascular bundles, but may be seen deeper. Posterolateral prostate shows abundant adipose tissue together with neurovascular bundles. Figs 1.7; 1.28–1.29
- Bulbourethral Cowper glands are extrinsic to the prostate, but eventually may be seen in prostate biopsies. Histologically, they are tubule-alveolar glands with lobules of acini, admixed with excretory ducts and ductuli. Frequently, they are associated with skeletal muscle fibers. The cells are cuboidal to columnar, pale-staining mucinous cytoplasm and small, bland, basally located nuclei. A basal cell layer is not readily apparent with H&E. Immunohistochemistry shows 34β

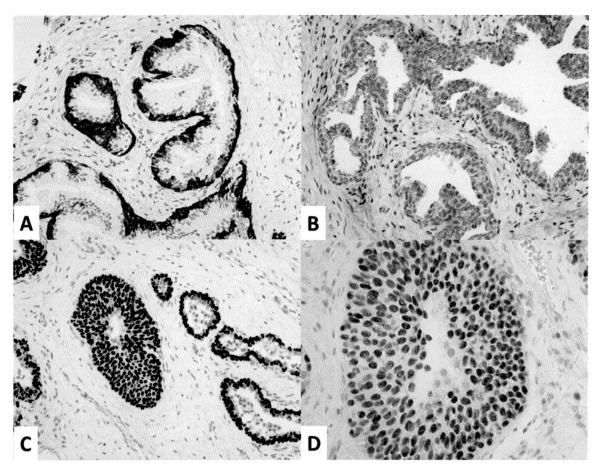

Fig 1.20 Immunohistochemistry of the prostate glands and acini. Basal cells highlighted by 34βE12 antibody (A). Secretory cells showing weak racemase expression toward the lumen (B). Basal cells highlighted by p63 (C). GATA3 decorates urothelial metaplasia in the prostate.

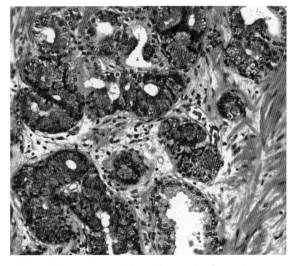

Fig 1.21 Mucinous metaplasia may be occasionally seen in prostate glands.

Fig 1.22 Corpora amylacea may be present in the lumen of prostate glands.

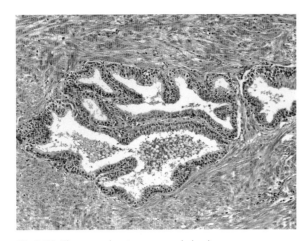

Fig 1.23 Fibromuscular stroma around glands.

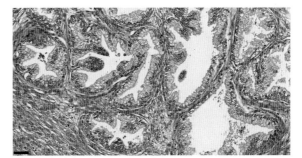

Fig 1.24 Fibromuscular stroma around glands (closer view).

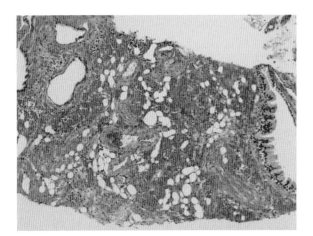

Fig 1.25 Fat may be seen rarely in the prostate stroma (100x).

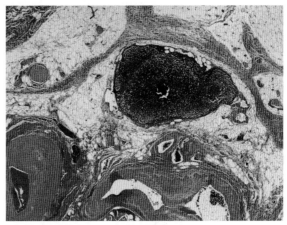

Fig 1.26 Small lymph nodes may be seen in the soft tissues around the prostate.

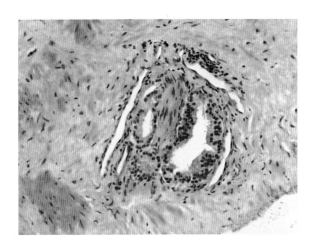

Fig 1.27 Benign glands encircling a nerve.

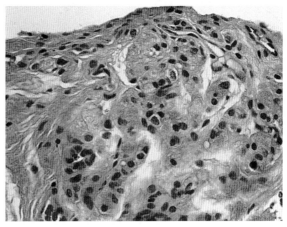

Fig 1.28 Paraganglia may be seen in needle prostate biopsies.

E12+/p63+ basal cells and PSA-/racemase-secretory-type cells. Figs 1.30–1.31

- Other rare findings related to the prostate include distorted colorectal epithelium seen as

a component of prostate biopsy that can potentially be confused with prostatic adenocarcinoma since they are negative for basal cell markers 34βE12 and p63 and positive with racemase. Mesonephric remnants may also rarely occur in the prostate and become hyperplastic, a finding that should not be misdiagnosed as carcinoma (see Chapter 2). Ectopic prostatic tissue has been reported in a number of extraprostatic locations, including epididymis and testes, urinary bladder, penile urethra, seminal vesicle and many others. In females, ectopic prostate may be seen in the cervix, ovaries, vagina, or urethra. In some cases, it may form polyploid structures typically PSA+. Paraurethral Skene glands are also PSA+.

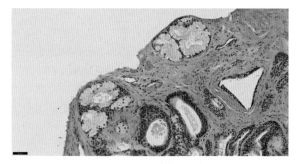

Fig 1.29 Cowper gland as seen in a needle prostate biopsy.

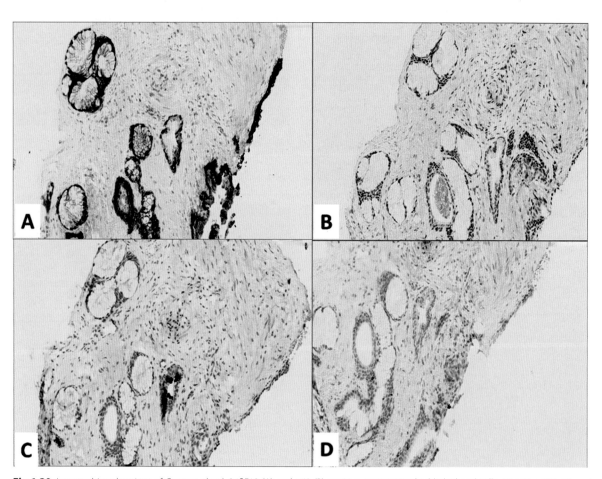

Fig 1.30 Immunohistochemistry of Cowper gland. 34βE12 (A) and p63 (B) positive expressions highlight basal cells. Negative PSA (C) and racemase (D).

Table 1.2 Potential Tumor-like Conditions of the Prostate Likely to Be Misdiagnosed as Carcinoma

Atypical adenomatous hyperplasia (adenosis)

Atrophy

Cribriform hyperplasia

Basal cell hyperplasia

Nephrogenic metaplasia (nephrogenic adenoma)

Verumontanum mucosal gland hyperplasia

Squamous metaplasia

Urothelial metaplasia

Radiation atypia

Xanthogranulomatois prostatitis and other prostatitis

Malacoplakia

Extramedullary hematopoiesis

Endometriosis (rarity in men receiving estrogen therapy)

Atypical stromal cells related to BPH

Postoperative spindle cell nodule

Cowper glands

Paraganglia

Benign glands adjacent to nerves and skeletal muscle

Crowded benign acini

Signet ring cell change in stromal nodule

Seminal vesicle/ejaculatory duct epithelium

Suggested Reading

Cheng L, MacLennan GT, Abdul-Karim FW, Lopez-Beltran A, Montironi R. Eosinophilic Metaplasia of the Prostate: A Newly Described Lesion Distinct from Other Eosinophilic Changes in Prostatic Epithelium. Anal Quant Cytol Histol. 2008 Aug; 30(4): 226–30.

McNeal JE. Normal and pathologic anatomy of prostate. Urology. 1981; 17: 11–16

Fine SW, Al-Ahmadie HA, Gopalan A, et al. Anatomy of the Anterior Prostate and Extraprostatic Space. A Contemporary Surgical Pathology Analysis. Adv Anat Pathol. 2007; 14: 401–07.

Brennick JB, O, Connell JX, Dickersin GR, et al. Lipofucsin Pigmentation (So-called Melanosis) of the Prostate. Am J Surg Pathol 1994; 18: 446–54.

Yossepowitch O, Briganti A, Eastham JA, Epstein J, Graefen M, Montironi R, Touijer K. Positive Surgical Margins after Radical Prostatectomy: A Systematic Review and Contemporary Update. Eur Urol. 2014 Feb; 65(2): 303–13.

Cheng L, MacLennan GT, Lopez-Beltran A, Montironi R. Anatomic, Morphologic and Genetic Heterogeneity of Prostate Cancer: Implications for Clinical Practice. Expert Rev Anticancer Ther. 2012 Nov; 12(11): 1371–74.

Quick Charles M. MDa, Gokden Neriman MDa, Sangoi Ankur R. MDb, Brooks James D. MDc, McKenney Jesse K. MDa, The Distribution of PAX-2 Immunoreactivity in the Prostate Gland, Seminal Vesicle, and Ejaculatory Duct: Comparison with Prostatic Adenocarcinoma and Discussion of Prostatic Zonal Embryogenesis. Human Pathology. (2010) 41: 1145–49.

Montironi R, Lopez-Beltran A, Scarpelli M, Mazzucchelli R, Cheng L. Handling of Radical Prostatectomy Specimens: Total Embedding with Whole Mounts, with Special Reference to the Ancona Experience (Letter). Histopathology. 2011 Nov; 59(5): 1006–10.

Lopez-Beltran A, Cheng L, Blanca A, Montironi R. Cell Proliferation and Apoptosis in Prostate Needle Biopsies with Adenocarcinoma Gleason Score 6 or 7. Anal Quant Cytol Histol. 2012 Apr; 34(2): 61–65.

De Marzo AM, Platz EA, Epstein JI, Ali T, Billis A, Chan TY, Cheng L, Datta M, Egevad L, Ertoy-Baydar D, Farre X, Fine SW, Iczkowski KA, Ittmann M, Knudsen BS, Loda M, Lopez-Beltran A, Magi-Galluzzi C, Mikuz G, Montironi R, Pikarsky E, Pizov G, Rubin MA, Samaratunga H, Sebo T, Sesterhenn IA, Shah RB, Signoretti S, Simko J, Thomas G, Troncoso P, Tsuzuki TT, van Leenders GJ, Yang XJ, Zhou M, Figg WD, Hoque A, Lucia MS. A Working Group Classification of Focal Prostate Atrophy Lesions. Am J Surg Pathol. 2006 Oct; 30(10): 1281–89.

Aaron L, Franco OE, Hayward SW. Review of Prostate Anatomy and Embryology and the Etiology of Benign Prostatic Hyperplasia. Urol Clin North Am. 2016 Aug; 43(3): 279–88.

Chapter 2

Inflammatory and Tumor-like Conditions of the Prostate

2.1 Background

- Inflammation and infection of the prostate is common, but the presence of histologic inflammation within the prostate samples does not correlate with clinical symptoms and therefore it is not supportive of clinical "prostatitis." Accordingly, the pathologist should not make the diagnosis of prostatitis in these samples.
- Instead, the pathologist should report "inflammatory, chronic or acute changes present." Some authors include a somewhat extent, focal or non-focal extension or even notice tissular distribution, as stromal, peri-glandular or intra-glandular followed by the type chronic/acute inflammation present. Infective agents are uncommonly seen in prostatic biopsies.
- A number of other entities such atrophy, metaplastic or hyperplastic lesions and conditions may be considered within the context of cancer diagnosis, and therefore are considered tumor-like conditions. Table 2.1; Fig 2.1 More relevant inflammatory and tumor-like conditions will be reviewed along this chapter.

2.2 Acute and Chronic Inflammation

- Acute inflammatory cell infiltrates made up of neutrophils are a common finding in the prostate, and may be seen in patients presenting symptoms of prostatitis or seen as incidental histologic finding in patients showing no symptoms.
- Microscopically, the acute inflammation may be intraluminal and varies in extent from a few scattered neutrophils to micro-abscesses. Often, this is associated with necrotic debris, mild reactive epithelial atypia, or duct rupture. Basal cells, as seen by p63 or 34βE12 immunostains, remain present in cases of histologic acute inflammation. Figs 2.2–2.3

- Chronic inflammatory cell infiltrates consisting of histiocytes, plasma cells and lymphocytes are a common observation in most prostate samples.
- Microscopically, lymphocytic and plasma cell chronic inflammatory infiltrates tend to be stroma-based and peri-glandular. Lymphoid follicle formation may also be seen.
- Acute and/or chronic inflammation is frequently seen in association with atrophy. Macrophages, eosinophils or mast cells can also be identified in the prostate frequently admixed with other inflammatory cells. Inflammation rarely involves PIN or carcinoma foci. Minor foci of chronic inflammatory cells may eventually be seen with prostatic cancer acini occasionally.
- Rarely, benign lymphocytes may be mistaken as carcinoma (Gleason pattern 4 or 5) due to arrangements of lymphocytes in cords, sheets or

Table 2.1 Potential Tumor-like Conditions of the Prostate Likely to Be Misdiagnosed as Carcinoma

Atypical adenomatous hyperplasia (adenosis)
Atrophy
Cribriform hyperplasia
Basal cell hyperplasia
Nephrogenic metaplasia (nephrogenic adenoma)
Verumontanum mucosal gland hyperplasia
Squamous metaplasia
Urothelial metaplasia
Radiation atypia
Xanthogranulomatous prostatitis and other prostatitis
Malacoplakia
Extramedullary hematopoiesis
Endometriosis (a rarity in men receiving estrogen therapy)
Atypical stromal cells related to BPH
Postoperative spindle cell nodule
Cowper glands
Paraganglia
Benign glands adjacent to nerves and skeletal muscle
Crowded benign acini
Signet ring cell change in stromal nodule
Seminal vesicle/ejaculatory duct epithelium

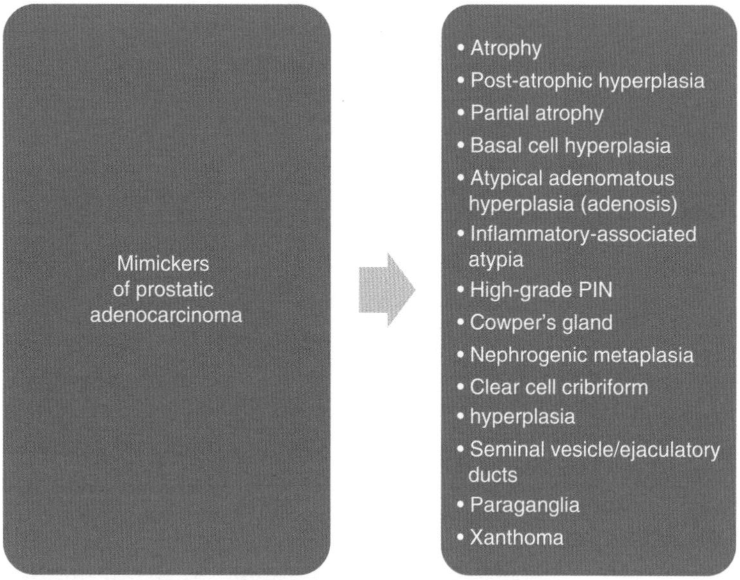

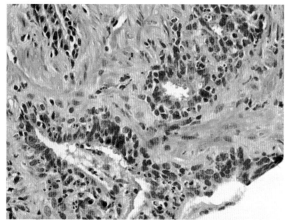

Mimickers of prostatic adenocarcinoma →

- Atrophy
- Post-atrophic hyperplasia
- Partial atrophy
- Basal cell hyperplasia
- Atypical adenomatous hyperplasia (adenosis)
- Inflammatory-associated atypia
- High-grade PIN
- Cowper's gland
- Nephrogenic metaplasia
- Clear cell cribriform
- hyperplasia
- Seminal vesicle/ejaculatory ducts
- Paraganglia
- Xanthoma

Fig 2.1 Lesions that can simulate prostate cancer in biopsy.

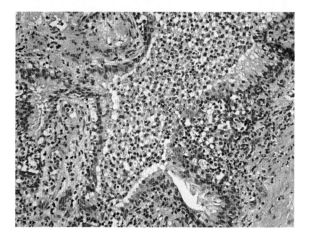

Fig 2.2 Acute inflammation with abscess formation.

Fig 2.3 Focal acute inflammation.

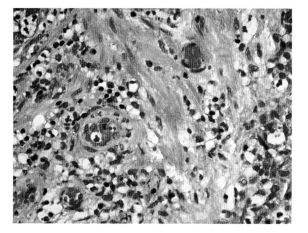

Fig 2.4 Signet ring-like lymphocytes and eosinophils seen in the prostate.

linear arrays. Signet-ring cell change due to thermal artifact has also been described in the prostate mimicking signet-ring cell adenocarcinoma. Fig 2.4

2.3 Granulomatous Prostatitis

- Is a distinctive form of prostatitis with potential of being misdiagnosed as cancer, clinically or at histopathological level; it may be seen in about 1% of prostatic biopsies of patients and present with altered digital rectal examination (indurated fixed prostate), hypoechoic lesions on ultrasound examination and elevated PSA levels.

11

Table 2.2 Etiologic Classification of Granulomatous Prostatitis

1   Non-specific granulomatous prostatitis due to duct-acinar rupture
    -   Granulomatous prostatitis usual type
    -   Xanthogranulomatous prostatitis
    -   Xanthoma
2   Infectious
    -   Bacterial (tuberculosis, brucellosis, BCG-related)
    -   Spirochetal (syphilis)
    -   Fungal (candidiasis, aspergillosis, histoplasmosis, blastomycosis, cryptococosis, coccidiomycosis, paracoccidiomycosis)
    -   Viral (herpes zoster)
    -   Parasitic (schistosomiasis)
3   Post-biopsy/resection
4   Malacoplakia
5   Systemic granulomatous disease (allergic/eosinophilic, sarcoidosis, Wegener granulomatosis)
6   Foreign body (teflon, others)

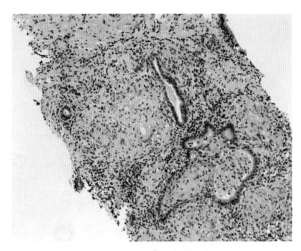

Fig 2.5 Non-caseating granulomatous inflammatory cell infiltrate in a prostate biopsy.

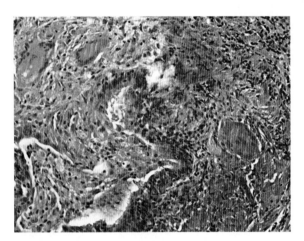

Fig 2.6 Multinucleate giant cells are present in granulomatous prostatitis.

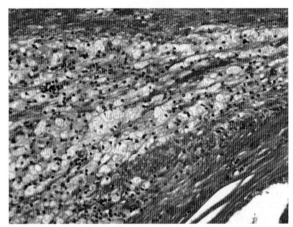

Fig 2.7 Xanthogranulomatous prostatitis.

-   Current etiologic classification of granulomatous prostatitis is presented in Table 2.2. Non-specific granulomatous prostatitis seen in over 70% of cases is the most common form followed by those cases related to previous biopsy or resection or of infectious origin.

2.3.1 Non-specific Granulomatous Prostatitis

-   Foreign body-type granulomatous response to prostatic secretions associated with ductal/acinar rupture. Grossly, appears as firm and small yellow nodules. Microscopically, is a non-caseating granulomatous inflammatory cell infiltrate centered on ducts/glands with variable degree of obstruction. Necrosis is not usually present.

-   Mixed cellularity may include epithelioid histiocytes, lymphocytes, plasma cells, neutrophils and occasionally eosinophils. Multinucleate giant cells, when present, can be of Touton, Langhans or foreign body types. Figs 2.5–2.6
-   The morphologic spectrum seen in non-specific granulomatous prostatitis also includes prostatic xanthoma or Xanthogranulomatous prostatitis characterized by histiocytes with clear cytoplasm. The term xanthoma applies when a localized lesion is lacking relevant inflammation other than histiocytes, but when there is an evident inflammatory component some authors apply the term xanthogranulomatous prostatitis. Fig 2.7

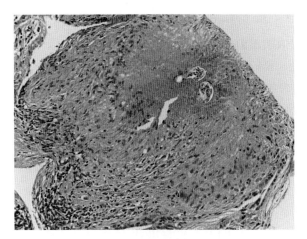

Fig 2.8 Schistosoma related granulomatous prostatitis.

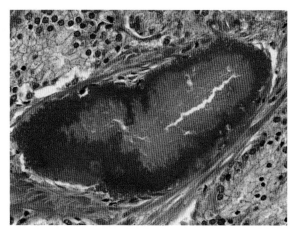

Fig 2.9 Actinomycosis in a background of prostate adenocarcinoma.

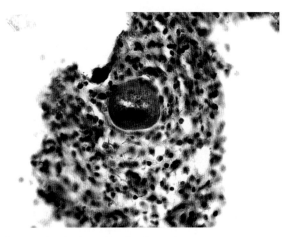

Fig 2.10 Cocidioides imitis related granulomatous prostatitis.

- A more problematic lesion is the so-called nodular histiocytic prostatitis, which is characterized by a proliferation of epithelioid histiocytes with virtually absent giant cells and other inflammatory cells, therefore raising concern on the diagnosis of high grade solid prostate cancer.
- A limited marker panel of immunostains usually solves these cases since histiocytes/macrophages are CD68+ and PSA-, PSAP-, or pan-cytokeratin-.

2.3.2 BCG Granulomatous Prostatitis

- Is the most common type of infectious granulomatous prostatitis, and it is due to BCG (Bacillus Calmette-Guerin) treatment for urothelial bladder carcinoma. Grossly, the prostate shows multiple white to yellowish-gray nodules which may present central caseation or rarely abscess formation.
- Microscopically, the granulomas are of the caseating tuberculoid type. Smaller granulomas are usually epithelioid granulomas lacking caseating necrosis. Giant cell may or not be present. In some cases, Ziehl-Neelsen stain for acid-fast organism demonstrates mycobacteria in the granulomas.

2.3.3 Other Infectious Granulomatous Prostatitis

- Table 2.2 shows more common infectious granulomas that can be seen in the prostate. Hematogenous dissemination of tuberculosis (usually from lung) to the prostate is rare. Fungal, parasitic or viral granulomatous prostatitis is also rare, but may occasionally be seen in immunosuppressed or diabetic patients. Figs 2.8–2.10

2.3.4 Post-resection/Biopsy Granulomatous Prostatitis

- Microscopically, the granulomas may appear as elongated, stellate or ovoid, typically showing fibrinoid central necrosis and surrounding palisaded epithelioid histiocytes and fibroblasts. A rim of lymphocytes, plasma cells and occasionally eosinophils may be present outside the palisaded cell layer. Multinucleated giant cells, usually of foreign body-type, may be present in some cases.

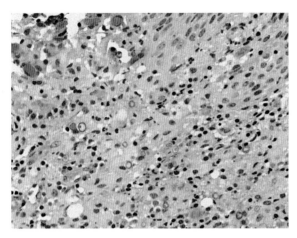

Fig 2.11 Malakoplakia.

2.3.5 Malakoplakia

- Is a form of granulomatous prostatitis that may simulate carcinoma. Usually there is history of urinary infection with *Escherichia Coli*. Grossly appears as soft yellow nodules or chips if TURP. Microscopically, there are sheets of macrophages admixed with variable number of lymphocytes, plasma cells, neutrophils and eosinophils. The macrophages contain basophilic, round intracytoplasmic inclusions 2–10 μm in diameter. These represent calcified bacterial debris within phagolysosomes and are known as Michaelis-Gutmann bodies. Fig 2.11 As mentioned earlier, histiocytes in malakoplakia are CD68+ and pan-cytockeratin-, PSA-, or PSAP-.

2.3.6 Systemic Granulomatous Disease Affecting the Prostate

- Virtually all systemic granulomatous diseases may be rarely seen in the prostate. Allergic/eosinophilic granulomatous prostatitis must be differentiated from other prostatic granulomas with eosinophils. Typically have central fibrinoid necrosis, palisaded histiocytes, and numerous eosinophils on microscopic evaluation.
- Rare cases of sarcoidosis (non-caseating epithelioid granulomas) and Wegener granulomatosis (vasculitis and necrotizing granulomas) have been described in the prostate.

2.3.7 Foreign Body-type Granulomatous Prostatitis

- Teflon (polytetrafluoroethylene) granulomas have been described in the prostate secondary to its injection during treatment of urinary incontinence. It produces a foreign body-type reaction. Teflon is highly birefringent with polarized light, a diagnostically useful fact. Fig 2.12 Hair granulomas seeds into the prostate via catheter or perineal prostate biopsy are on record.

2.3.8 Prostatic Vasculitis

- Vasculitis in the prostate may be localized or be part of a systemic disease. Localized vasculitis includes vasculitis in post-TURP granulomatous prostatitis, giant cell arteritis and lymphocytic vasculitis of the prostatic transition zone (Beltran-Cheng-Montironi vasculitis). Figs 2.13–2.14
- This is essentially a non-fibrinoid, isolated or multicentric lymphocytic vasculitis, showing mainly CD3-positive T-cells infiltrating through the vessel wall typically seen in the transition zone of patients with BPH. Reported evidences suggest that the presence of Beltran-Cheng-Montironi vasculitis in prostate samples could identify patients at risk of prostatic infarction and acute urinary retention.
- Systemic vasculitis that may be seen in the prostate include rare cases of Wegener granulomatosis, allergic/eosinophilic granulomatous prostatitis and poly-arteritis nodosa.

2.4 Atrophy

- Atrophy is a common, age-related, benign lesion that may be misdiagnosed as carcinoma in biopsies, where it is most commonly seen in peripheral zone samples. In radical prostatectomies, it is also more common in the peripheral zone. Morphologic types of atrophy are presented in Table 2.3, with frequent mixed cases. Fig 2.14
- To know the subtypes of prostatic atrophy is considered worthy, mainly in routine differential diagnosis of prostatic biopsies. Likewise, it is not essential to subtype any atrophic lesion due to the lack of clinical relevance of such activity.

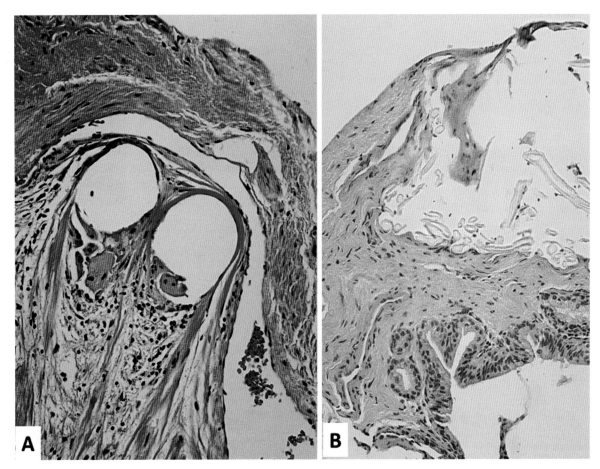

Fig 2.12 Foreign body-type granulomatous prostatitis (A and B).

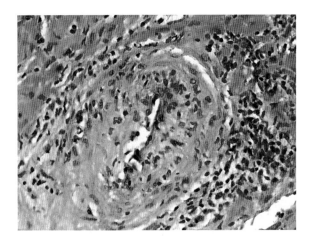

Fig 2.13 Lymphocytic vasculitis of the prostatic transition zone.

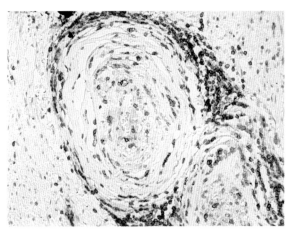

Fig 2.14 CD3 positive immunohistochemistry in lymphocytic vasculitis of the prostatic transition zone.

Table 2.3 Current Classification of Atrophy of the Prostate

Simple atrophy
Simple cystic atrophy
Sclerotic atrophy
Partial atrophy
Post-atrophic hyperplasia
Proliferative inflammatory atrophy (PIA)

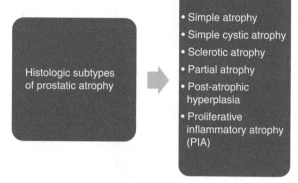

Histologic subtypes of prostatic atrophy ➡

- Simple atrophy
- Simple cystic atrophy
- Sclerotic atrophy
- Partial atrophy
- Post-atrophic hyperplasia
- Proliferative inflammatory atrophy (PIA)

Fig 2.15 Classification of atrophy of the prostate.

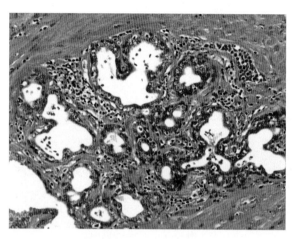

Fig 2.16 Simple acinar atrophy.

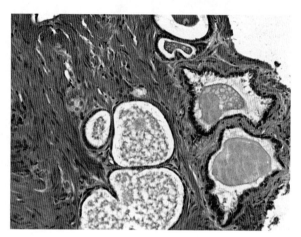

Fig 2.17 Simple acinar atrophy with cysts.

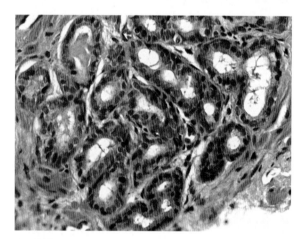

Fig 2.18 Post-atrophic hyperplasia.

Therefore, reporting atrophy is not necessary. Figs 2.15–2.20

- Luminal mucin may be focally seen in any subtype of atrophy, but is not a salient feature.
- Any subtype of atrophy shows basal cells, but their detection in some of the biopsies may be difficult. Some acini lack any basal cell on H&E examination and even with basal cell immunohistochemistry. Fig 2.21

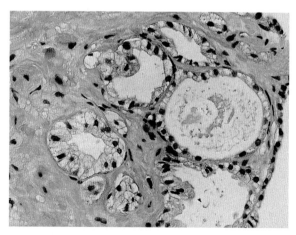

Fig 2.19 Partial atrophy.

- Immunohistochemistry for basal cells based on p63 and 34βE12 basal cell markers shows a frequently fragmented basal cell layer, with some acini completely negative for these commonly

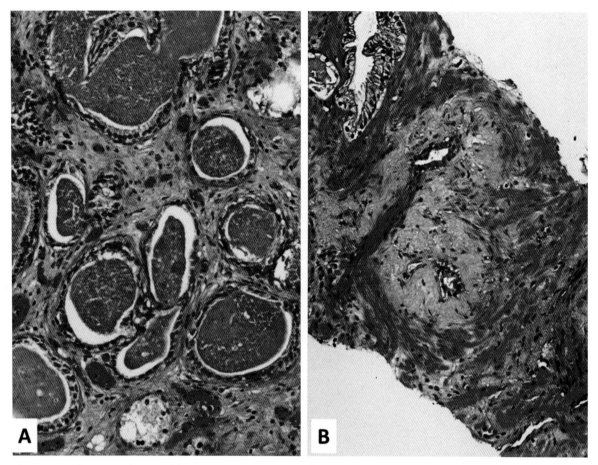

Fig 2.20 Atrophic acini with eosinophilic proteinaceous material (A) and atrophy-related hyaline stroma (B).

used markers (seen in about 20% of cases). Racemase can be positive in some atrophy samples and is frequently positive in partial atrophy cases showing a cancer-like immunophenotype (p63-, 34βE12-, racemase+) in up to 25%. Fig 2.22

- Differential diagnosis of benign atrophy vs. prostatic adenocarcinoma is a common relevant exercise in daily practice; it is mainly based on the demonstration of basal cells and knowing the potential pitfall of immunohistochemistry as presented in the above paragraph. Also, there is an atrophic variant of prostate adenocarcinoma showing typical features of carcinoma, including loss of basal cells.

2.4.1 Simple Atrophy and Simple Cystic Atrophy

- Microscopically, is the most common subtype of atrophy and presents as localized or diffuse lesion. Acini are rounded-to-angular, small and dark. The stroma in the lobule shows frequent pale fibrosis. Mixed inflammation is variably present in simple atrophy. The epithelial lining of the glands is atrophic cuboidal or flattened. The nuclei show deep staining. Nuclear atypia and prominent nucleoli is a rare observation and when present is usually focal. Cystic change is common in simple atrophy with mild dilatation to larger cysts.

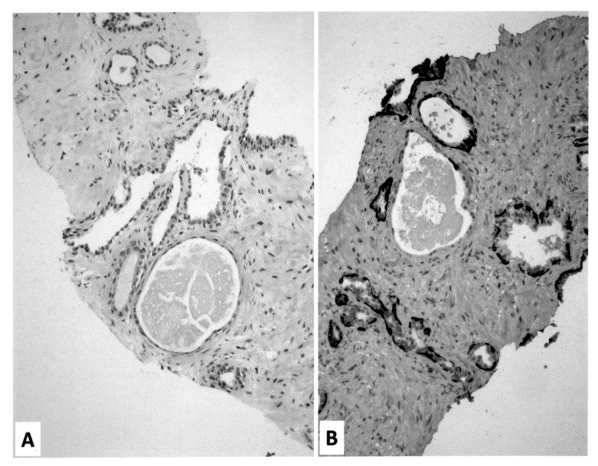

Fig 2.21 Atrophy in a prostate biopsy (A) with discontinuous basal cell staining by anti-34βE12 antibody (B).

2.4.2 Sclerotic Atrophy

- Is a frequently seen lesion admixed with other types of atrophy. The hallmark is exuberant fibrosis with lobular disarray. Accompanying inflammation is typically present. A pseudo-infiltrative growth is also common in this type of atrophy, a finding that should not be misdiagnosed as malignancy. In support is the fact that the lining cells are bland with rare focal atypia.

2.4.3 Partial Atrophy

- This is a morphologic variant of atrophy in which glands appear crowded, lacking stromal fibrosis and inflammation, and lining cells show scant pale cytoplasm. Morphology of acini shows typically variable sized with occasional stellate shape. The nuclei of the cells are typically enlarged and may be elongated. The nucleoli may be prominent, but does not have the size seen in carcinoma. Macro-nucleoli (seen at 10X magnification) are not present.

2.4.4 Post-atrophic Hyperplasia

- Post-atrophic hyperplasia is seen in about 4% of prostatic biopsies, but is a common finding in other prostatic tissue samples, and it is more frequently seen in peripheral zone of the prostate.
- Microscopically has lobular outline with a central duct surrounded by small, regular,

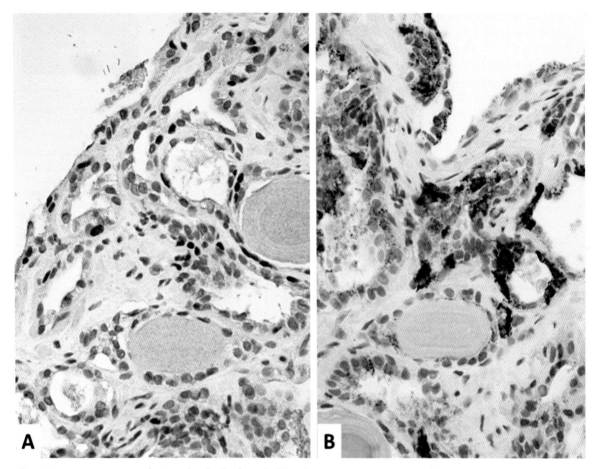

Fig 2.22 Immuno-expression of p63+ in basal cells of atrophy (A) and racemase expression in atrophic acini.

closely packed acini with slight variability in shape and size. The epithelium of the acini is usually cuboidal with mildly enlarged nuclei showing small nucleoli. Prominent nucleoli can be seen in some cases focally. Occasionally, the central duct is cystic and lined by low cuboidal to flat atrophic epithelium.

- Stromal changes range from smooth muscle atrophy to fibrosis and sclerosis or elastosis. Associated chronic inflammation may be present.
- Like in other subtypes of atrophy, basal cells are present, but their detection may be difficult. Some acini lack any basal cell on H&E even with basal cell immunohistochemistry. Mucin may be present in some acini just like in any other subtype of atrophy.
- In limited biopsies when the characteristic lobular appearance is lost, post-atrophic hyperplasia may be misdiagnosed as adenocarcinoma.

2.4.5 Proliferative Atrophy (PA)/ Proliferative Inflammatory Atrophy (PIA)

- These terms refer to different forms of atrophy with an increased proliferation index (Ki67/MIB1 immunostaining) when compared to normal epithelium. PIA has been suggested as precursor or PIN.
- Reporting of isolated PA or PIA in routine biopsies or other prostate samples is not recommended due to the lack of prediction for the subsequent detection of carcinoma.

2.5 Metaplasia

- Metaplastic changes in the prostate are usually secondary to inflammation, ischemia, hormonal alterations or as a result of therapy. Occasionally,

19

metaplastic changes are within the differential of carcinoma of the prostate, and therefore, are considered tumor-like lesions. Four major categories of metaplasia may be seen in the prostate: squamous metaplasia, urothelial metaplasia, mucinous metaplasia and Paneth cell-like/eosinophilic metaplasia. Nephrogenic metaplasia (adenoma) may also be present in prostatic samples.

- Squamous metaplasia may be morphologically quite atypical, showing high mitotic count, nuclear enlargement and prominent nucleoli, in particular, when seen adjacent to a prostatic infarction. In this situation, basal cells can be demonstrated by 34βE12 or other basal cell markers.

- Urothelial metaplasia may also be seen adjacent to infarction or cryotherapy, after hormonal therapy or being related to inflammation, and therefore may be present with cellular atypia or cytoplasmic clearing. The main differential diagnosis is PIN, or early prostatic primary, or secondary urothelial carcinoma.

- Mucinous metaplasia is defined as the replacement of benign luminal epithelium by benign mucin-secreting PAS+ (after diastase digestion)/Alcian blue+(pH2.5) cells. These glands present a preserved basal cell layer, but mucinous cells are PSA-. Mucinous metaplasia is uncommon and seen most frequently in a background of atrophy and inflammation. Mucinous metaplasia may simulate Cowper glands.

- Eosinophilic metaplasia and Paneth cell-like change is characterized by the presence of large cytoplasmic eosinophilic granules. In benign epithelium, the granules are considered exocrine-related lysosome-like granules (eosinophilic metaplasia). In PIN and carcinoma, the granules are related to neuroendocrine differentiation (Paneth cell-like). These eosinophilic granules are unrelated to lipofuscin pigment.

- Nephrogenic metaplasia (nephrogenic adenoma) arising in the prostatic urethra may extend into smooth muscle and the prostate in some cases. Classic patterns of growth are tubular, tubulocystic and papillary/polypoid. Cases with atypia including prominent nucleolus present show typically no mitotic features, negative to very low Ki67 expression and negative p53. Some

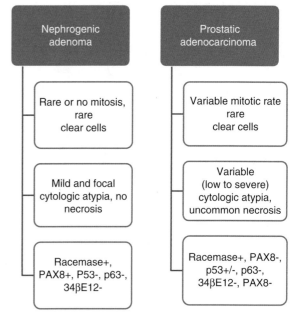

Fig 2.23 Main differential characteristics of nephrogenic metaplasia vs. well-differentiated adenocarcinoma.

overlapping features with carcinoma include basal cell markers loss with expression of racemase. Immunohistochemical approach to diagnosis includes PSA (negative to weak), PAX2/PAX8 positive, CK7+, p63- and 34βE12- in nephrogenic metaplasia (adenoma). Fig 2.23

- A rare case of cartilaginous stromal metaplasia has been described in a 69-year-old man with BPH treated by TURP.

2.6 Hyperplasia

2.6.1 Benign Prostatic Hyperplasia (BPH)

- Is one of the common diseases to occur in men and is strongly related with patient's age. It is not common in men under the age of 40 years, but may be present in about 90% of men over 80 years. BPH is one of the causes of the clinical situation collectively known as lower urinary tract symptoms.

- In BPH, a number of nodules develop in the transition zone, producing variable urethral obstruction. BPH may be seen in all types of prostate samples but is rare in needle biopsies since in this case the procedure tends to sample peripheral zone. However, when present, it may

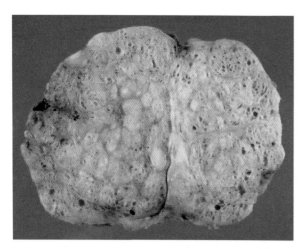

Fig 2.24 Gross features of BPH. This simple prostatectomy specimen weighted over 200 gr.

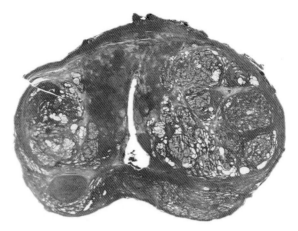

Fig 2.25 Macro-section showing BPH nodules at low power.

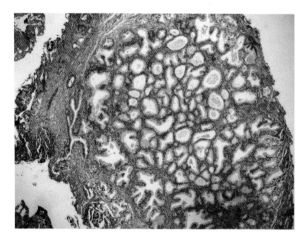

Fig 2.26 BPH nodule in TURP.

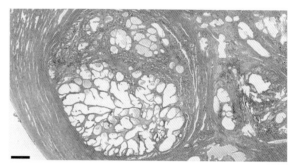

Fig 2.27 BPH nodules with cystic atrophy in RP specimen.

be recognized by the presence of partially sampled nodules. If this is the case, then the pathologist can make a diagnosis of BPH in needle biopsies, although it is not considered a necessary diagnosis giving the fact that BPH diagnosis and its derived therapy is defined by clinical means and not by histology.

- Grossly, formation of nodules can be recognized mainly in TURPs, simple prostatectomy, radical prostatectomy or in the prostate at time of cysto-prostatectomy, mainly in the transition zone (periurethral) tissues. Figs 2.24–2.25
- Microscopically, nodules may be pure stromal (myxoid, fibrosis-type, smooth-muscle type or

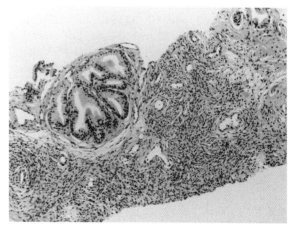

Fig 2.28 BPH stromal nodule in prostate biopsy.

mixtures thereof), glandular nodules with prominent glandular component and less fibromuscular stroma or mixed glandular and stromal nodules. Figs 2.26–2.30

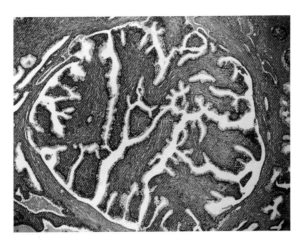

Fig 2.29 BPH nodule of fibroadenoma type.

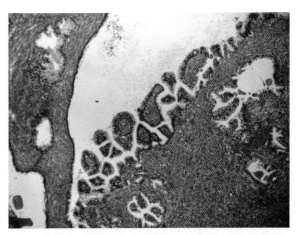

Fig 2.30 BPH nodule partially cystic with papillary projections.

2.6.2 Basal Cell Hyperplasia

- It is an uncommon, frequently multifocal lesion defined as an increase in the number of benign basal cells. Microscopically, the acini typically shows two or more cell layers that may look infiltrative between benign glands (pseudo-infiltrative growth), and frequently form tubular, cribriform or solid structures. Occasionally, some basal cells may show prominent nucleoli, but not macro-nucleoli of the type seen in cancer. Rare cases may show luminal mucin. Characteristically, basal cell markers (p63, p40, CK 34βE12, or Ck5/6) are positive in basal cell hyperplasia, but racemase is negative. Likewise, racemase and PSA may positive in the secretory luminal rim of cells present in many of hyperplastic acini. Typically, basal cell hyperplasia is negative for BCL-2 and shows low proliferation (<20%), findings that may be used to differentiate from prostatic carcinoma or basaloid type carcinoma rising in the prostate. Figs 2.31–2.32

2.6.3 Cribriform Hyperplasia (Clear Cell Cribriform Hyperplasia)

- Histologically, is more frequently seen in the transition zone of the prostate and may be seen in all types of specimens. Cells are homogeneous with bland nuclei, inconspicuous nucleoli and clear cytoplasm. Basal cells are present. (Table 2.4; Figs 2.33–2.35)

2.6.4 Mesonephric Remnant Hyperplasia

- Is rare in the prostate and peri-prostatic tissues and its importance resides in the fact that it can be misdiagnosed as prostatic adenocarcinoma. Microscopically, it shows a vaguely lobular or infiltrative growth of small tubules with cuboidal lining epithelium. Occasionally, eosinophilic luminal secretion may be present. The lesion shows bland cytology with no evidence or nuclear enlargement or prominent nucleoli. Typically, the lesion is negative with PSA or PSAP and does not highlight basal cells with 34βE12; however, some cases may show focal 34βE12 stain in lining epithelial cells. Figs 2.36–2.38

2.6.5 Verumontanum Mucosal Gland Hyperplasia

- A benign micro-acinar proliferation seen in the verumontanum and adjacent posterior urethra defines the lesion. Its importance resides in the fact that it can mimic carcinoma in the rare cases in which the lesion is seen in needle biopsy. Basal cells are present, as well as corpora amylacea, but mucin and crystalloids are rare. Luminal cells express PSA and basal cells can be highlighted by basal cell markers. Fig 2.39

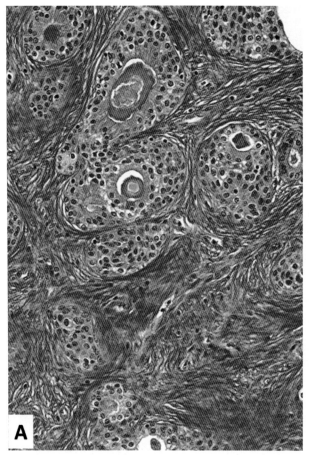 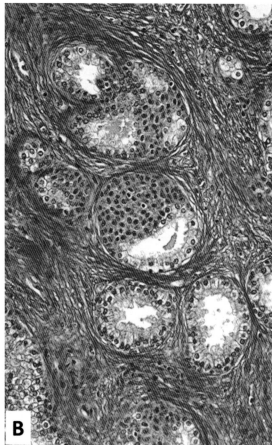

Fig 2.31 Basal cell hyperplasia (A and B).

2.6.6 Atypical Adenomatous Hyperplasia (AAH; Adenosis)

- It has been defined as a localized small glandular proliferation within the prostate with potential of being misdiagnosed as carcinoma. It may be seen in all types of prostate samples, but is rare in needle biopsies. Microscopically, AAH is typically a well-circumscribed lesion composed of small, densely packed pale acini, which merges with larger, more complex glands.
- The most important immunohistochemical markers are those basally related (p63, 34βE12, CK5/6, p40) that typically highlight basal cell. An important potential pitfall, however, is the fact that some AAH cases have an extremely low number of basal cell even with immunohistochemistry, and therefore diagnosis might need immunohistochemistry on deeper sections. In addition, it is well-known that racemase stains <20% of AAH cases (see chapter 3).

2.6.7 Sclerosing Adenosis

- It is defined as compact small gland proliferation embedded in a spindle cell background, most frequently seen in a background of BPH. Rare cases may be seen in needle biopsy samples. An atypical form of sclerosing adenosis has been reported to show nuclear atypia and prominent nucleoli. It is characteristic of these lesions to show myoepithelial differentiation in addition to basal cells, therefore, S100 may be at least focally positive in addition of positivity for basal cell markers. Other markers of myoepithelial differentiation are positive. Racemase is negative. Fig 2.40

2.7 Other Rare Lesions and Tumor-like Conditions

- Rare examples of melanosis, blue nevus and Ochronosis have been reported as benign lesions to occur in the prostate. Melanosis is defined by the presence of melanin in the glandular epithelium, but occasionally may also be seen in the stroma. It should not be mistaken as lipofuscin, another pigment that may occasionally be present in glandular epithelium.

- Blue nevus is similar to its counterpart in the dermis, and is characterized by the presence of stromal melanin-laden spindle cells. It should not be mistaken as hemosiderin-laden macrophages and malignant melanoma.

- Cysts seen in the prostate may be classified as utricular (endodermal origin) most probably originating from the urogenital sinus, or müllerian duct cysts (mesodermal origin). Both types are rare and may be associated to symptoms such as hematospermia, infertility, pelvic pain, dysuria and other symptoms in patients below 40 years. Race cysts seen at the opening of the ejaculatory ducts are on record. A malignancy may rarely develop in the cystic lesions with examples of ductal carcinoma, clear cell müllerian carcinoma or squamous cell carcinoma.

Table 2.4 Cribriform Lesions Seen in the Prostate

Normal central zone glands
Basal cell hyperplasia
Cribriform PIN
Clear cell cribriform hyperplasia
Intraductal carcinoma
Acinar carcinoma
Ductal carcinoma

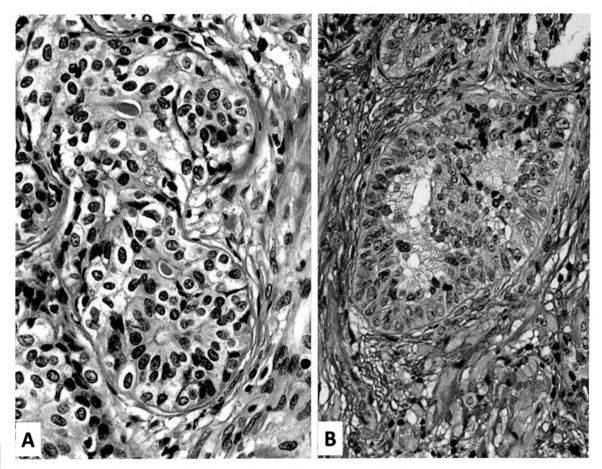

Fig 2.32 Atypical basal cell hyperplasia (A and B) with slightly variable nuclear size and visible nucleoli.

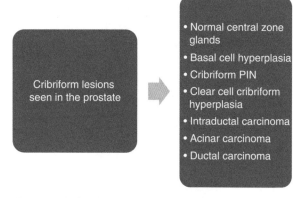

Cribriform lesions seen in the prostate ➡

- Normal central zone glands
- Basal cell hyperplasia
- Cribriform PIN
- Clear cell cribriform hyperplasia
- Intraductal carcinoma
- Acinar carcinoma
- Ductal carcinoma

Fig 2.33 Cribriform lesions seen in the prostate.

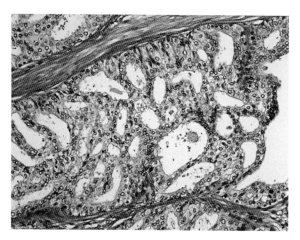

Fig 2.34 Cribriform hyperplasia of the prostate.

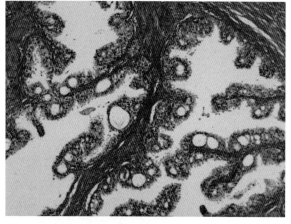

Fig 2.35 The presence of Roman-Bridge morphology in the central zone should not be mistaken as cribriform hyperplasia.

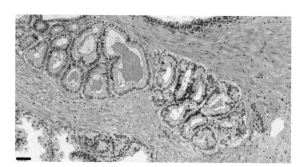

Fig 2.36 Mesonephric remnant hyperplasia. This particular case was mistaken as well-differentiated adenocarcinoma of the transition zone.

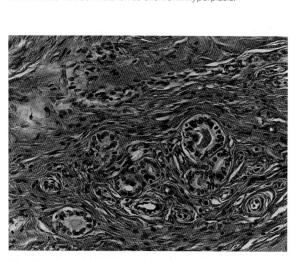

Fig 2.37 Mesonephric remnant hyperplasia with pseudo-infiltrative appearance.

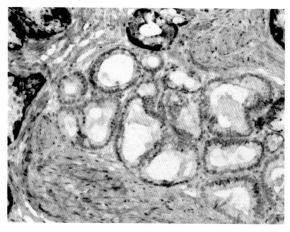

Fig 2.38 Mesonephric remnant hyperplasia typically shows negative PSA and 34βE12 expressions, but a focal positivity of 34βE12 may be seen in secretory cells.

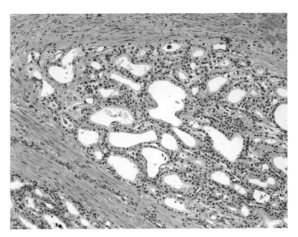

Fig 2.39 Verumontanum mucosal gland hyperplasia.

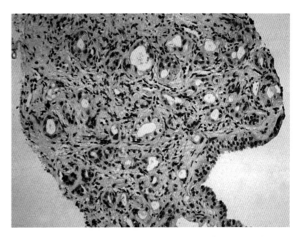

Fig 2.40 Sclerosing adenosis may simulate malignancy in limited prostate biopsies.

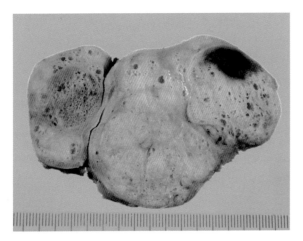

Fig 2.41 Gross features of prostatic infarction.

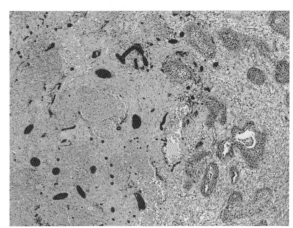

Fig 2.42 Histology of prostatic infarction (low power).

- Prostatic infarction may induce atypical squamous metaplasia within prostate glands, a finding that should not be mistaken as malignancy, in particular in prostate limited biopsies. Figs 2.41–2.43
- Cistadenoma has also been described in the prostate. Figs 2.44–2.45
- Other rarities in the prostate may include amyloid deposits, endometriosis in association with estrogen therapy, extramedullary hematopoiesis or vasculitis. Ochronosis is extremely rare in the prostate and is related to a hereditary metabolic disorder with alkaptonuria.

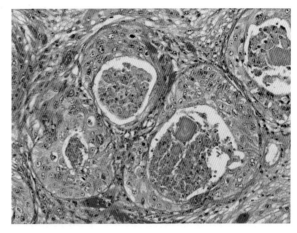

Fig 2.43 Histology of prostatic infarction (200x) showing atypical squamous epithelium.

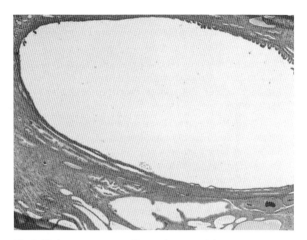

Fig 2.44 Low power view of cystadenoma of the prostate.

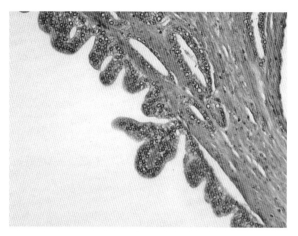

Fig 2.45 High power view of case in Fig 2.44 showing bland cytologic features of the covering epithelium with focal papillary formation.

Suggested Reading

Montironi R, Lopez-Beltran A, Cheng L, Galosi AB, Montorsi F, Scarpelli M. Seminal Vesicle Intraepithelial Neoplasia versus Basal Cell Hyperplasia in a Seminal Vesicle. Eur Urol. 2014 Oct; **66**(4): 623–27.

Brennick JB, O, Connell JX, Dickersin GR, et al. Lipofucsin Pigmentation (So-called Melanosis) of the Prostate. Am J Surg Pathol. 1994; **18**: 446–54.

Cheng L, MacLennan GT, Lopez-Beltran A, Montironi R Anatomic. Morphologic and Genetic Heterogeneity of Prostate Cancer: Implications for Clinical Practice. Expert Rev Anticancer Ther. 2012 Nov; **12**(11): 1371–74.

Quick, Charles M. MDa, Neriman Gokden MDa, Sangoi Ankur R. MDb, Brooks James D. MDc, McKenney Jesse K. MDa. The Distribution of PAX-2 Immunoreactivity in the Prostate Gland, Seminal Vesicle, and Ejaculatory Duct: Comparison with Prostatic Adenocarcinoma and Discussion of Prostatic Zonal Embryogenesis. Human Pathology. 2010; **41**: 1145–49.

De Marzo AM, Platz EA, Epstein JI, Ali T, Billis A, Chan TY, Cheng L, Datta M, Egevad L, Ertoy-Baydar D, Farre X, Fine SW, Iczkowski KA, Ittmann M, Knudsen BS, Loda M, Lopez-Beltran A, Magi-Galluzzi C, Mikuz G, Montironi R, Pikarsky E, Pizov G, Rubin MA, Samaratunga H, Sebo T, Sesterhenn IA, Shah RB, Signoretti S, Simko J, Thomas G, Troncoso P, Tsuzuki TT, van Leenders GJ, Yang XJ, Zhou M, Figg WD, Hoque A, Lucia MS. A Working Group Classification of Focal Prostate Atrophy Lesions. Am J Surg Pathol. 2006 Oct; **30**(10): 1281–89.

Montironi R, Vela Navarrete R, Lopez-Beltran A, Mazzucchelli R, Mikuz G, Bono AV. Histopathology Reporting of Prostate Needle Biopsies. 2005 Update. Virchows Arch. 2006; **449**(1): 1–13.

Lopez-Beltran A, Vidal A, Montironi R, Kirkali Z, Muñoz E, Blanca A, Cheng L. Lymphocytic Vasculitis of the Prostate Transition Zone. BJU Int. 2012 Mar 30. doi: 10.1111/j.1464-410X.2012.11079.x.

Cheng L, Davidson DD, Maclennan GT, Lopez-Beltran A, Montironi R, Wang M, Tan PH, Baldridge LA, Zhang S. Atypical Adenomatous Hyperplasia of Prostate Lacks TMPRSS2-ERG Gene Fusion. Am J Surg Pathol. 2013 Oct; **37**(10): 1550–54. doi: 10.1097/PAS.0b013e318294e9bc.

Montironi R, Lopez-Beltran A, Cheng L, Scarpelli M. Cervical-type Squamous Metaplasia and Myoepithelial Cell Differentiation in Stromal Tumor of the Prostate. Am J Surg Pathol. 2011 Nov; **35**(11): 1752–54. No abstract available

Lopez-Beltran A, Qian Junqi, Montironi Rodolfo, Luque Rafael J., and Bostwick David G. Atypical Adenomatous Hyperplasia (Adenosis) of the Prostate: DNA Ploidy Analysis and Immunophenotype. Int J Surgical Pathology. 2005; **13**: 167–73

Luque RJ, Lopez-Beltran A, Perez-Seoane C, Suzigan S. Sclerosing Adenosis of the Prostate. Histologic Features in Needle Biopsy Specimens. Arch Pathol Lab Med. 2003 Jan; **127**(1): e14–16.

Harik LR, O'Toole KM. Nonneoplastic Lesions of the Prostate and Bladder. Arch Pathol Lab Med. 2012 Jul; **136**(7): 721–34.

Chen YB, Fine SW, Epstein JI. Mesonephric Remnant Hyperplasia Involving Prostate and Periprostatic Tissue: Findings at Radical Prostatectomy. Am J Surg Pathol. 2011 Jul; **35**(7): 1054–61.

Cheng L, Bostwick DG. Atypical Sclerosing Adenosis of the Prostate: A Rare Mimic of Adenocarcinoma. Histopathology. 2010 Apr; **56**(5): 627–31.

Berney DM, Fisher G, Kattan MW, Oliver RT, Møller H, Fearn P, Eastham J, Scardino P, Cuzick J, Reuter VE, Foster CS. Trans-Atlantic Prostate Group. Pitfalls in the Diagnosis of Prostatic Cancer: Retrospective Review of 1791 Cases with Clinical Outcome. Histopathology. 2007 Oct; **51**(4): 452–57.

Kumbar R, Dravid N, Nikumbh D, Patil A, Nagappa KG. Clinicopathological Overview of Granulomatous Prostatitis: An Appraisal. J Clin Diagn Res. 2016 Jan; **10**(1): EC20–23.

Alba MA, Moreno-Palacios J, Beça S, Cid MC. Urologic and Male Genital Manifestations of Granulomatosis with Polyangiitis. Autoimmun Rev. 2015 Oct; **14**(10): 897–902.

Epstein JI, Egevad L, Humphrey PA, Montironi R. Members of the ISUP Immunohistochemistry in Diagnostic Urologic Pathology Group. Best Practices Recommendations in the Application of Immunohistochemistry in the Prostate: Report from the International Society of Urologic Pathology Consensus Conference. Am J Surg Pathol. 2014 Aug; **38**(8): e6–e19.

Muezzinoglu B, Erdamar S, Chakraborty S, Wheeler TM. Verumontanum Mucosal Gland Hyperplasia Is Associated with Atypical Adenomatous Hyperplasia of the Prostate. Arch Pathol Lab Med. 2001 Mar; **125**(3): 358–60.

Gagucas RJ, Brown RW, Wheeler TM. Verumontanum Mucosal Gland Hyperplasia. Am J Surg Pathol. 1995 Jan; **19**(1): 30–36.

Bachurska SY, Staykov DG, Ivanov GP, Belovezhdov VT. Lack of ERG-Antibody in Benign Mimickers of Prostate Cancer. Folia Med (Plovdiv). 2016 Mar 1; **58**(1): 48–53.

Chen S, Patil PA, Lepe M, Lombardo KA, Amin A, Matoso A. Retrospective Analysis of Atypical Glands Suspicious for Carcinoma in Transurethral Resection of Prostate. Appl Immunohistochem Mol Morphol. 2016 Jun 13. [Epub ahead of print]

Arista-Nasr J, Martinez-Benitez B, Bornstein-Quevedo L, Aguilar-Ayala E, Aleman-Sanchez CN. Ortiz-Bautista R Low Grade Urothelial Carcinoma Mimicking Basal Cell Hyperplasia and Transitional Metaplasia in Needle Prostate Biopsy. Int Braz J Urol. 2016 Mar–Apr; **42**(2): 247–52.

Dikov D, Bachurska S, Staikov D, Sarafian V. Intraepithelial Lymphocytes in Relation to NIH Category IV Prostatitis in Autopsy Prostate. Prostate. 2015 Jul 1; **75**(10): 1074–84.

Garg M, Kaur G, Malhotra V, Garg R. Histopathological Spectrum of 364 Prostatic Specimens Including Immunohistochemistry with Special Reference to Grey Zone Lesions. Prostate Int. 2013; **1**(4): 146–51.

Preneoplastic Lesions and Conditions of the Prostate

3.1 Prostatic Intraepithelial Neoplasia

- Prostatic intraepithelial neoplasia (PIN) refers to the preinvasive end of the continuum of cellular proliferations within the lining of prostatic ducts, ductuli, and acini. It is recommended compression of the PIN classification into two grades: low grade (formerly PIN grade l) or high grade PIN (formerly PIN grades 2 and 3).
- PIN is an important prostatic lesion that can be mistaken as carcinoma mainly in evaluating prostate biopsies. Fig 3.1

3.2 Diagnostic Criteria for High Grade Prostatic Intraepithelial Neoplasia (HGPIN)

- The classification of PIN into low grade and high grade is chiefly based on the cytological characteristics of the cells. The nuclei of cells composing low grade PIN are enlarged, vary in size, have slightly increased chromatin content, and possess small or inconspicuous nucleoli. Fig 3.2
- HGPIN is characterized by cells with large nuclei of relatively uniform size, an increased chromatin content, which may be irregularly distributed, and prominent nucleoli that are similar to those of carcinoma cells. The basal cell layer is intact or rarely interrupted in low grade PIN, but may have frequent disruptions in high grade lesions. Figs 3.3–3.8
- There are four main patterns of HGPIN: tufting, micropapillary, cribriform and flat. Fig 3.9 The tufting pattern is the most common, present in 97% of cases, although most cases have admixed patterns. There are no known clinically important differences between the architectural patterns of HGPIN, and their recognition appears to be only of diagnostic utility. Other unusual patterns of HGPIN include the signet ring-cell pattern, small

Mimickers of prostatic adenocarcinoma

- Atrophy
- Post-atrophic hyperplasia
- Partial atrophy
- Basal cell hyperplasia
- Atypical adenomatous hyperplasia (adenosis)
- Inflammatory-associated atypia
- High-grade PIN
- Cowper's gland
- Nephrogenic metaplasia
- Ciear cell cribriform
- hyperplasia
- Seminal vesicle/ejaculatory ducts
- Paraganglia
- Xanthoma

Fig 3.1 Main lesions that can mimic prostate carcinoma.

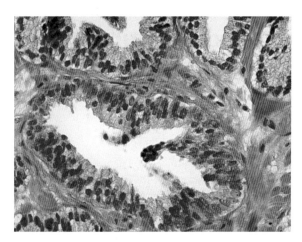

Fig 3.2 Low grade PIN.

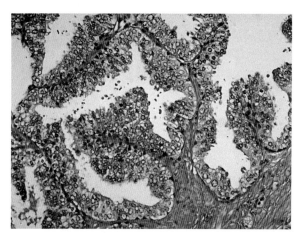

Fig 3.3 Low power view of high grade PIN.

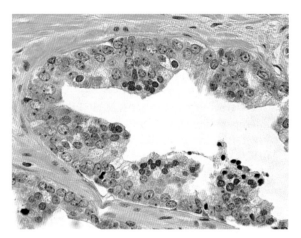

Fig 3.4 High power view of high grade PIN.

cell neuroendocrine pattern, mucinous pattern, inverted-type, squamous-type and foamy pattern. Figs 3.10–3.18

- HGPIN is multicentric in 70% of radical prostatectomies with cancer, including 65% of those involving the non-transition zone and 7% of those involving the transition zone; 2% of cases have concomitant single foci in all zones.
- The peripheral zone of the prostate, the area in which the majority of prostatic carcinomas occur (70%), is also the most common location for HGPIN, where it is frequently multicentric.
- Early stromal invasion (PIN with microinvasion), the earliest evidence of carcinoma, occurs at sites

of acinar outpouching and basal cell disruption in acini with HGPIN. Such microinvasion is present in about 2% of high power microscopic fields of HGPIN, and is seen with equal frequency with all architectural patterns.

- Evidence linking HGPIN and prostate cancer has been found in morphological, immunohistochemical, morphometric, molecular and genetic studies. Virtually all such studies have indicated that HGPIN is related more closely to prostate cancer than to benign epithelium. HGPIN was more extensive in small cancers than in larger cancers, presumably due to "overgrowth" or obliteration of HGPIN by larger cancers.
- Discrepancies in the diagnosis of HGPIN were greatest between HGPIN with cribriform proliferations. Fig 3.19
- When the small atypical acini are too numerous and too crowded to be outpouchings or simply tangential sections, then cancer can be diagnosed. Immunohistochemical stains for the basal cell markers are of value in selected cases. Fig 3.20
- HGPIN shows a discontinuous basal cell layer when labeled with the antibody to high-molecular-weight keratin or p63. HGPIN is considered nowadays the most frequent cause of misdiagnosis of Pca in needle prostate biopsies.
- HGPIN has a limited predictive value as a marker of adenocarcinoma in subsequent biopsies when single and unilateral. Bilateral and multifocal

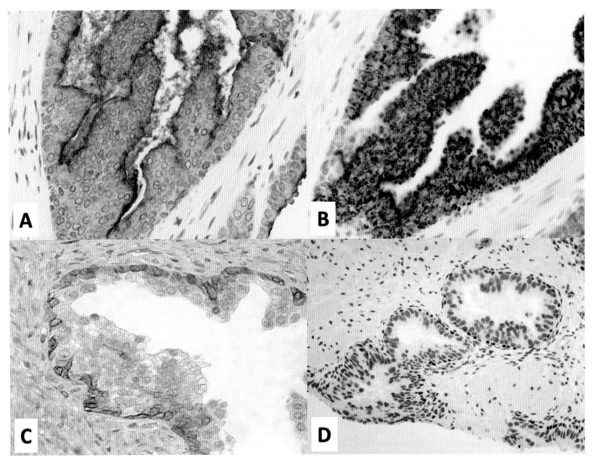

Fig 3.5 Immunohistochemistry of high grade PIN. PSA (A), racemase (B), 34βE12 (C), p63 (D).

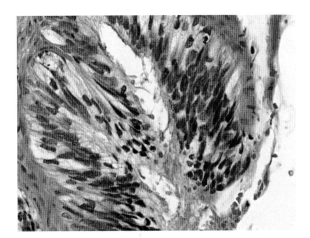

Fig 3.6 High grade PIN with pseudostratified nuclei and focal mucin production.

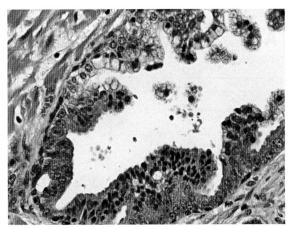

Fig 3.7 High grade PIN cells may colonize prostatic ducts and acini.

31

HGPIN increases likelihood of Pca being diagnosed in up to 10%.

- Cancer detection rate in patients with low grade PIN is identical to that in patients who

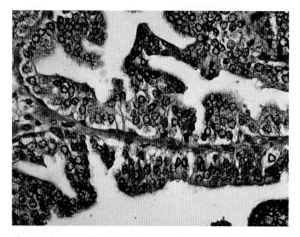

Fig 3.8 Occasionally, high grade PIN may have lipofuscin pigment.

underwent repeat biopsies for persistent elevated serum PSA or because of an abnormal digital rectal examination.

- High grade PIN needs to be differentiated from intraductal carcinoma (see Chapter 5) Figs 3.21–3.22

3.3 Atypical Adenomatous Hyperplasia

- Atypical adenomatous hyperplasia (AAH, adenosis) is characterized by a circumscribed proliferation of closely packed small glands that, rather than appearing invasive, tend to merge with the surrounding histologically benign glands.
- Microscopically, AAH is typically well circumscribed lesion composed of small, densely packed, pale acini, which merges with larger more complex glands. The most important

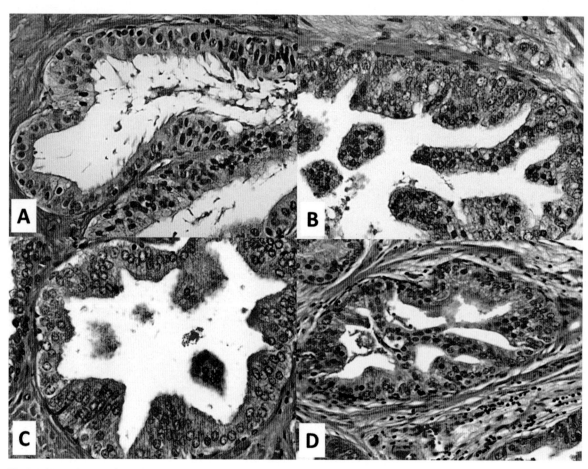

Fig 3.9 Main subtypes of PIN. Flat (A), micropapillary (B), tufting (C) and cribriform (D).

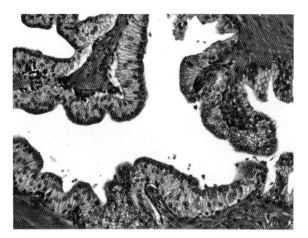

Fig 3.10 Inverted type high grade PIN.

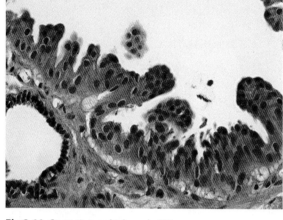

Fig 3.11 Oncoytic type high grade PIN.

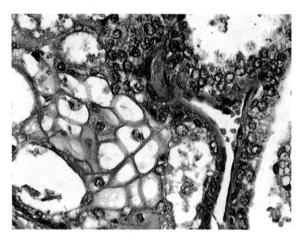

Fig 3.12 Squamous type high grade PIN.

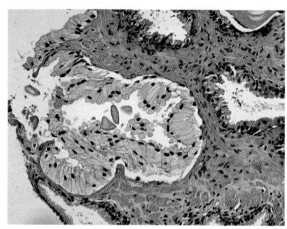

Fig 3.13 Foamy type high grade PIN.

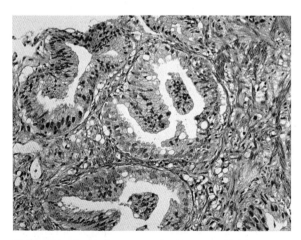

Fig 3.14 Small cytoplasmic vacuoles (signet ring-like) high grade PIN.

immunohistochemical markers are those basally related (p63, 34βE12, CK5/6, p40) that typically highlight basal cell. Figs 3.23–3.25

- An important potential pitfall, however, is the fact that some AAH cases have an extremely low number of basal cells even with immunohistochemistry, and therefore diagnosis might need immunohistochemistry on deeper sections. Table 3.1

- AAH frequently demonstrates budding acini from adjacent foci of benign hyperplastic glands, and the cells have clear cytoplasm with variable intraluminal secretions. Architecturally, AAH resembles well-differentiated adenocarcinoma of low Gleason score, and most cases of Gleason primary pattern 1 cancer are now considered

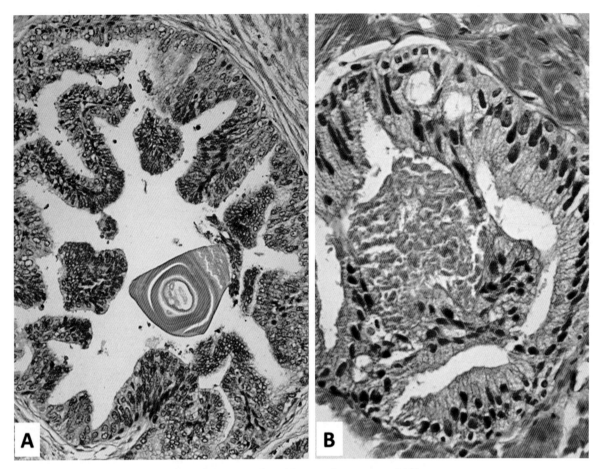

Fig 3.15 High grade PIN may present luminal corpora amylacea (A) or proteinaceous material (B).

within the spectrum of AAH. Recognition of the basal cell layer excludes the diagnosis of carcinoma.

- Unfortunately, identification of the basal epithelium is often difficult, as it is usually attenuated and may be discontinuous in AAH, and this may be the rule in needle biopsy specimens.
- Recognition of the basal cell layer may be facilitated by use of an antibody to p63 or to high-molecular-weight cytokeratin. An additional compelling feature is the observed positive immunoreactivity of AAH foci with racemase (P504S) in about 20% of the cases. AAH lacks TMPRSS2-ERG gene fusion, as recently demonstrated.

- Nuclear and nucleolar morphology is the key differentiating feature between AAH and carcinoma, but this has less power than the presence of basal cells after immunohistochemistry. About 85% of cases of AAH are located in the transition zone. The incidence of AAH in prostate specimens is largely variable in reported series (range 2% to 23%).

3.4 Post-inflammatory Atrophy (PIA)

- Recent reports suggest that post-inflammatory atrophy may be causally linked to PIN and therefore to prostate adenocarcinoma. This hypothesis is based upon recognition of increased proliferative activity, albeit low, in

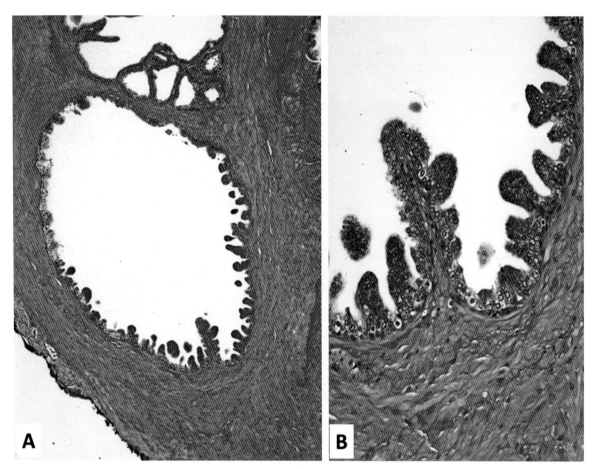

Fig 3.16 Cystic type high grade PIN.

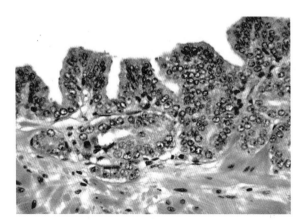

Fig 3.17 High grade PIN may present focal microinvasion, occasionally.

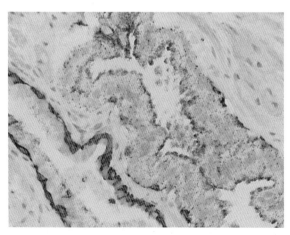

Fig 3.18 Double immunostaining of racemase (brown) and 34βE12 for basal cells (red) shows intense luminal racemase expression in high grade PIN and disrupted basal cell layer.

the secretory cells that persist within atrophic acini. Fig 3.26

- Reporting of isolated PIA in routine biopsies or other prostate samples is not recommended due to the lack of prediction for the subsequent detection of carcinoma.

3.5 Atypical Small Acinar Proliferation Suspicious for but Not Diagnostic of Malignancy

- Atypical focus suspicious but not diagnostic of malignancy (ASAP), also referred to as atypical small acinar proliferation suspicious for but not diagnostic of malignancy or just atypical prostate glands (ATYP), is not a preneoplastic lesion. Fig 3.27 It is descriptive diagnostic terminology used in the pathology report of a needle biopsy containing a small group of glands suspicious for adenocarcinoma, but with insufficient cytological and/or architectural atypia to establish a definitive diagnosis. In some cases (16% to 31%), the

Cribriform lesions seen in the prostate →

- Normal central zone glands
- Basal cell hyperplasia
- Cribriform PIN
- Clear cell cribriform hyperplasia
- Intraductal carcinoma
- Acinar carcinoma
- Ductal carcinoma

Fig 3.19 Cribriform lesion seen in the prostate.

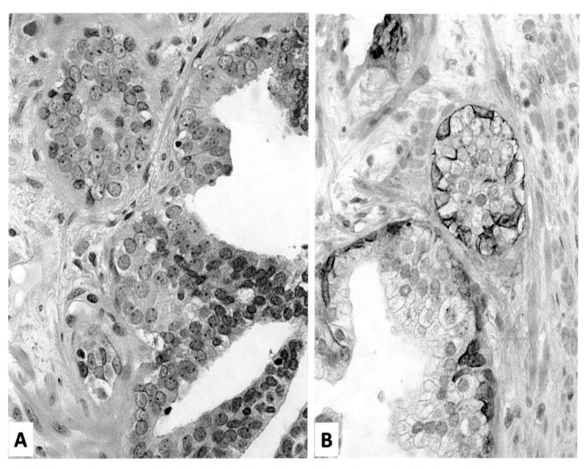

A **B**

Fig 3.20 Outpouchings or tangential sections should not be misdiagnosed as carcinoma or atypical acinar proliferation.

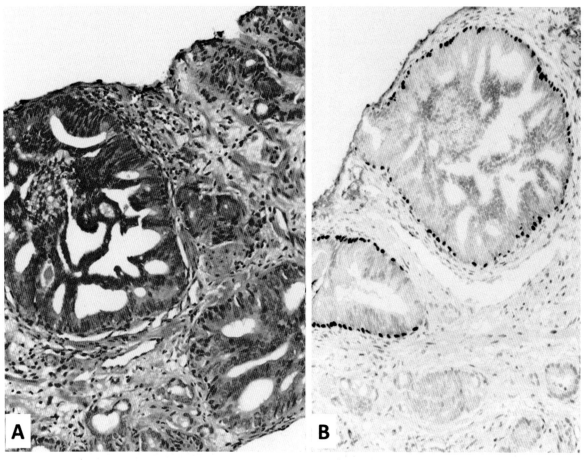

Fig 3.21 Intraductal carcinoma of the prostate and associated invasive acinar carcinoma (A) with persistent basal cells (anti-p63) (B).

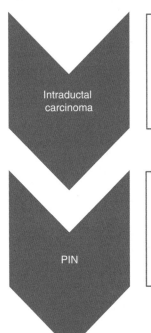

Intraductal carcinoma

- Expanded ductal/lobular unit, >2 times size of normal glands, comedonecrosis may be present

- Micropapillary, solid, cribriform, lumen-spanning cell mass, basal cells present

PIN

- Preserved ductal/lobular unit, normal gland size, no comedonecrosis, basal cells present

- Micropapillary, Cribriform (loose), Tufting, Flat, lumen-spanning cell mass in Cribriform subtype only

Fig 3.22 Differential diagnosis between high grade PIN and intraductal carcinoma of the prostate.

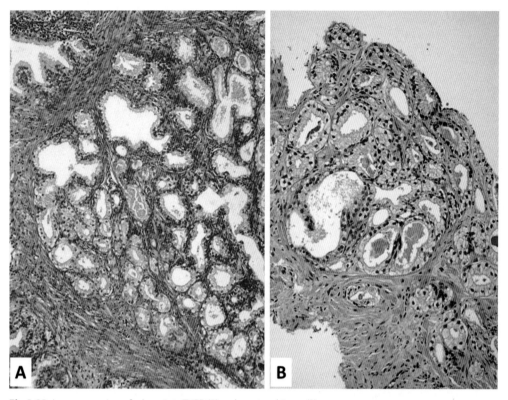

Fig 3.23 Low power view of adenosis in TURP (A) and prostate biopsy (B).

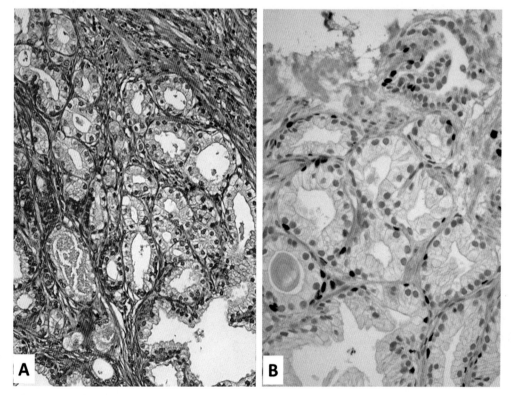

Fig 3.24 High power view of adenosis in TURP (A) and low number of basal cells highlighted by anti-p63 immunohistochemistry (B).

lesion is associated with PIN (PIN ASAP or PIN ATYP). Figs 3.28–3.33

- It is a broad diagnostic category that encompasses benign lesions mimicking malignant glandular proliferations and under sampled, small foci of carcinoma that harbor some, but not all, of the features needed for a definitive diagnosis of malignancy. It is not

Table 3.1 Differential Diagnoses of Prostate Adenocarcinoma

Common:

- Atrophy
- Post-atrophic hyperplasia
- Partial atrophy
- Basal cell hyperplasia
- Atypical adenomatous hyperplasia (adenosis)
- Inflammatory-associated atypia
- High grade PIN

Less Common:

- Cowper's gland
- Nephrogenic metaplasia
- Clear cell cribriform hyperplasia
- Seminal vesicle/ejaculatory ducts
- Paraganglia
- Xanthoma

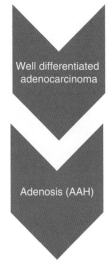

Well differentiated adenocarcinoma

- No basal cells present (p63-, p40-, 34βE12-), Racemase (P504S)+, ERG may be positive or negative

Adenosis (AAH)

- Basal cells+(may be focally present only), (p63+, p40+, 34βE12+), Racemase (P504S)+, ERG- (rarely positive)

Fig 3.25 Differential diagnosis between adenosis and well differentiated adenocarcinoma.

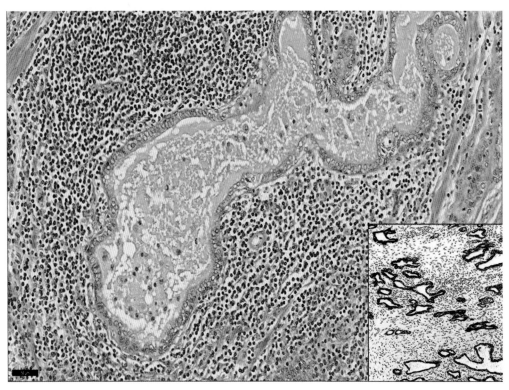

Fig 3.26 Prostate inflammatory atypia (PIA) with presence of basal cells (anti-34βE12) (Inset).

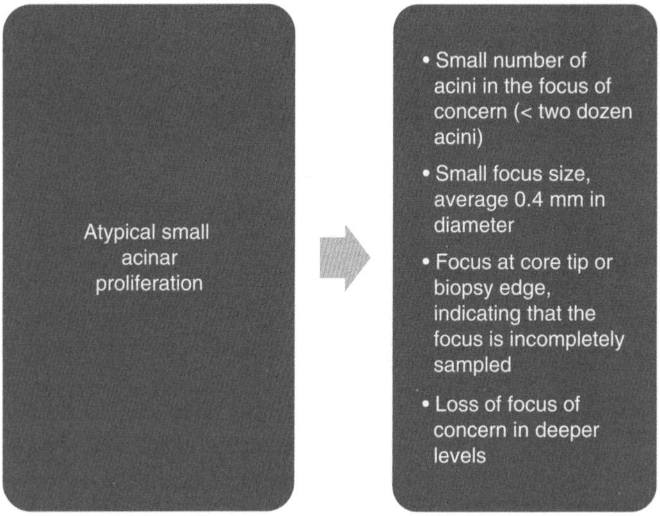

Fig 3.27 Defining criteria of ASAP.

Atypical small acinar proliferation →

- Small number of acini in the focus of concern (< two dozen acini)
- Small focus size, average 0.4 mm in diameter
- Focus at core tip or biopsy edge, indicating that the focus is incompletely sampled
- Loss of focus of concern in deeper levels

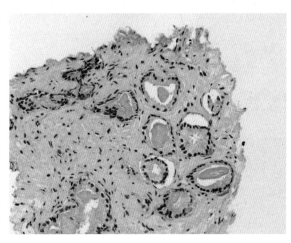

Fig 3.28 Architecturally atypical acini on H&E suspicious for carcinoma.

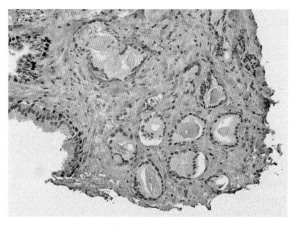

Fig 3.29 The absence of basal cell on immunohistochemistry with anti-p63 support diagnosis of malignancy (same case as in Fig 3.28).

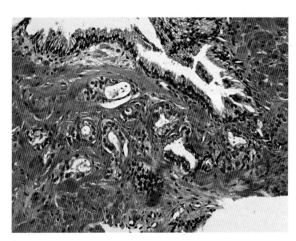

Fig 3.30 Architecturally atypical acini on H&E suspicious for carcinoma.

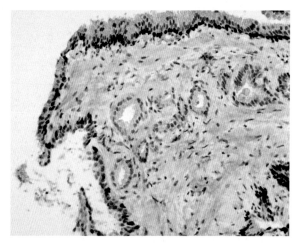

Fig 3.31 The presence of basal cell focally on immunohistochemistry with anti-p40 support benign lesion (same case as in Fig 3.30).

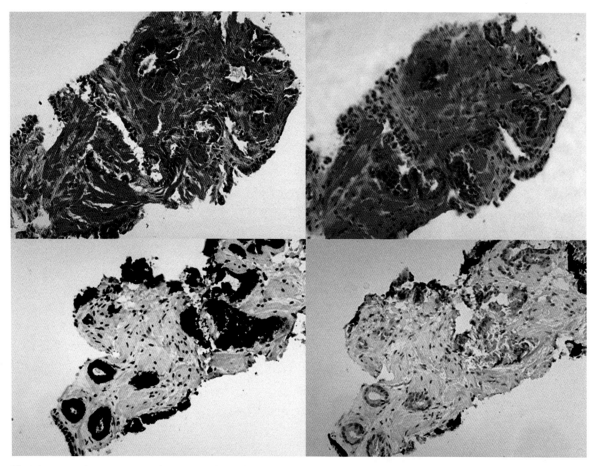

Fig 3.32 Atypical acini on prostate biopsy seen also in deeper sections (upper panel), intense positive expression of racemase (lower left) and lacking of basal cells with anti-34βE12 immunohistochemistry (lower right) supports malignancy.

a diagnostic entity and is not synonymous with high grade prostatic intraepithelial neoplasia. Table 3.2

- The widespread use of basal cell immunohistochemistry using antibodies against p63 or 34βE12 or the use of racemase (P504S) has made the use of the diagnostic term ASAP uncommon nowadays. Figs 3.34–3.36

Suggested Reading

Montironi R, Lopez-Beltran A, Cheng L, Galosi AB, Montorsi F, Scarpelli M. Seminal Vesicle Intraepithelial Neoplasia versus Basal Cell Hyperplasia in a Seminal Vesicle. Eur Urol. 2014 Mar 4; **pii:** S0302–2838 (14): 00183–83.

Montironi R, Cheng L, Lopez-Beltran A, Montironi MA, Galosi AB, Scarpelli M. A Low Grade PIN-like Neoplasm of the Transition Zone Immunohistochemically Negative for Basal Cell Markers: A Possible Example of Low Grade Adenocarcinoma with Stratified Epithelium. Pathology. 2014 Jan; **46**(1): 88–91. doi: 10.1097/PAT.0000000000000036.

Cheng L, Davidson DD, Maclennan GT, Lopez-Beltran A, Montironi R, Wang M, Tan PH, Baldridge LA, Zhang S. A Typical Adenomatous Hyperplasia of Prostate Lacks TMPRSS2-ERG Gene Fusion. Am J Surg Pathol. 2013 Oct; **37**(10): 1550–54. doi: 10.1097/PAS.0b013e318294e9bc.

Montironi R, Lopez-Beltran A, Cheng L, Montorsi F, Scarpelli M. Central Prostate Pathology Review: Should It Be Mandatory? Eur Urol. 2013 Aug; **64**(2): 199–201; discussion 202–03. doi: 10.1016/j.eururo.2013.04.002. Epub 2013 Apr 16. No abstract available.

Mazzucchelli R, Scarpelli M, Barbisan F, Santinelli A, Lopez-Beltran A, Cheng L, Montironi R.

Table 3.2 Factors Resulting in the Diagnosis of Atypical Small Acinar Proliferations Suspicious for Malignancy

Small Size of Focus
- Small number of acini in the focus of concern (invariably fewer than two dozen acini)
- Small focus size, average 0.4 mm in diameter
- Focus at core tip or biopsy edge, indicating that the focus is incompletely sampled
- Loss of focus of concern in deeper levels

Conflicting Morphologic Findings
- Distortion of acini raising concern for atrophy
- Lack of convincing features of cancer (insufficient nucleomegaly or nucleolomegaly)
- Clustered growth pattern mimicking a benign process such as atypical adenomatous hyperplasia
- Foamy cytoplasm raising concern for foamy gland carcinoma

Conflicting Immunohistochemical Findings
- Focally positive high molecular weight cytokeratin
- Focally positive p63 staining
- Negative racemase immunostain

Confounding Findings
- Histologic artifacts such as thick sections or overstained nuclei
- Tangential cutting of adjacent high grade PIN
- Architectural or cytologic changes (nucleomegaly and nucleolomegaly) owing to inflammation or other lesions

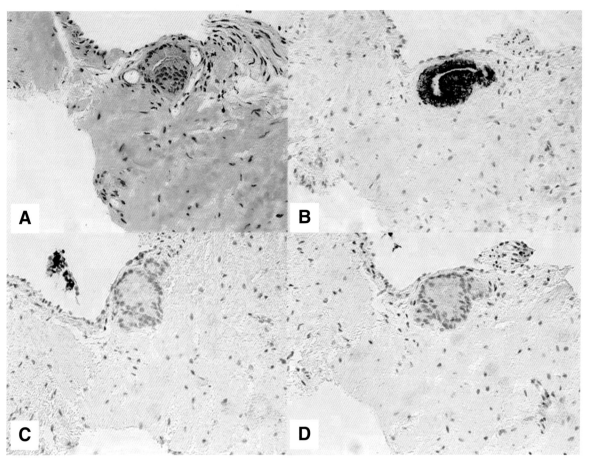

Fig 3.33 Rarely, as depicted in this case, we see single atypical acini with positive racemase expression (b) and negative p63 and 34βE12 (c and d) therefore supporting malignancy. In these cases, a re-biopsy should be performed.

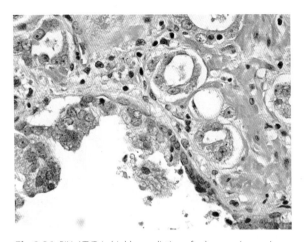

Fig 3.34 PIN ATYP is highly predictive of adenocarcinoma in re-biopsy.

Immunohistochemical Expression of Prostate Tumour Overexpressed 1 (PTOV1) in Atypical Adenomatous Hyperplasia (AAH) of the Prostate: Additional Evidence Linking (AAH) to Adenocarcinoma. Cell Oncol (Dordr). 2013 Feb; **36**(1): 37–42. doi: 10.1007/s13402-012-0111-7.

Varma M, Berney DM, Algaba F, Camparo P, Compérat E, Griffiths DF, Kristiansen G, Lopez-Beltran A, Montironi R, Fgevad L. Prostate Needle Biopsy Processing: A Survey of Laboratory Practice across Europe. J Clin Pathol. 2013 Feb; **66**(2): 120–23. doi: 10.1136/jclinpath-2012-200993.

Lee S, Han JS, Chang A, Ross HM, Montironi R, Yorukoglu K, Lane Z, Epstein JI. Small Cell-like Change in Prostatic Intraepithelial Neoplasia, Intraductal Carcinoma, and Invasive Prostatic Carcinoma: A Study of 7 Cases. Hum Pathol. 2013 Mar; **44**(3): 427–31. doi: 10.1016/j.humpath.2012.06.008.

Ukimura O, Coleman JA, de la Taille A, Emberton M, Epstein JI, Freedland SJ, Giannarini G, Kibel AS, Montironi R, Ploussard G, Roobol MJ, Scattoni V, Jones JS. Contemporary Role of Systematic Prostate

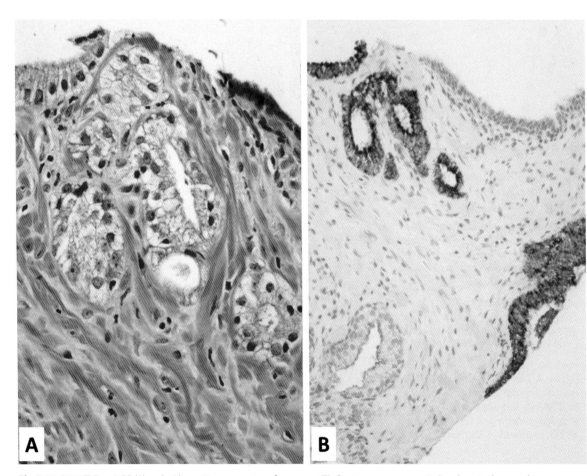

Fig 3.35 PIN ATYP on H&E (A) and with positive expression of racemase (B). Carcinoma was present elsewhere in the sample.

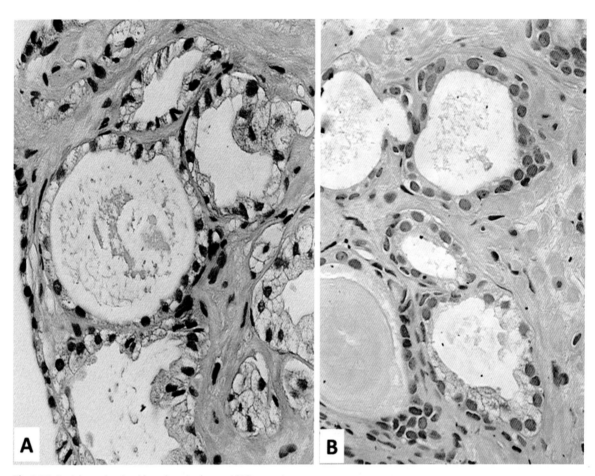

Fig 3.36 Partial atrophy should not be mistaken as ASAP or carcinoma.

Biopsies: Indications, Techniques, and Implications for Patient Care. Eur Urol. 2013 Feb; **63**(2): 214–30. doi: 10.1016/j.eururo.2012.09.033.

Montironi R, Scarpelli M, Cheng L, Lopez-Beltran A, Zhou M, Montorsi F. Do Not Misinterpret Intraductal Carcinoma of the Prostate as High-grade Prostatic Intraepithelial Neoplasia! Eur Urol. 2012 Sep; **62**(3): 518–22. Epub 2012 Jun 5.

Lopez-Beltran A, Cheng L, Blanca A, Montironi R. Cell Proliferation and Apoptosis in Prostate Needle Biopsies with Adenocarcinoma Gleason Score 6 or 7. Anal Quant Cytol Histol. 2012 Apr; **34**(2): 61–65.

Scarpelli M, Mazzucchelli R, Barbisan F, Santinelli A, Lopez-Beltran A, Cheng L, Montironi R. Is There a Role for Prostate Tumour Overexpressed-1 in the Diagnosis of HGPIN and of Prostatic Adenocarcinoma? A Comparison with Alpha-Methylacyl CoA Racemase. Int J Immunopathol Pharmacol. 2012 Jan–Mar; **25**(1): 67–74.

Camparo P, Egevad L, Algaba F, Berney DM, Boccon-Gibod L, Compérat E, Evans AJ, Grobholz R, Kristiansen G, Langner C, Lopez-Beltran A, Montironi R, Oliveira P, Vainer B, Varma M. Utility of Whole Slide Imaging and Virtual Microscopy in Prostate Pathology. APMIS. 2012 Apr; **120**(4): 298–304. doi: 10.1111/j.1600-0463.2011.02872.x. Review.

Montironi R, Mazzucchelli R, Lopez-Beltran A, Scarpelli M, Cheng L. Prostatic Intraepithelial Neoplasia: Its Morphological and Molecular Diagnosis and Clinical Significance. BJU Int. 2011 Nov; **108**(9): 1394–401. doi: 10.1111/j.1464-410X.2011.010413.x. Epub 2011 Aug 26. Review.

Lopez-Beltran A, Qian Junqi, Montironi Rodolfo, Luque Rafael J., Bostwick David G. Atypical Adenomatous Hyperplasia (Adenosis) of the Prostate: DNA Ploidy Analysis and Immunophenotype. Int J Surgical Pathology 2005, **13**: 167–173.

Montironi R, Scattoni V, Mazzucchelli R, Lopez-Beltran A, Bostwick DG, Montorsi F. Atypical Foci Suspicious but Not Diagnostic of Malignancy in Prostate Needle Biopsies (Also Referred to as "Atypical Small Acinar Proliferation Suspicious for but Not Diagnostic of Malignancy"). Eur Urol. 2006 Oct; **50**(4): 666–74.

De Marzo AM, Platz EA, Epstein JI, Ali T, Billis A, Chan TY, Cheng L, Datta M, Egevad L, Ertoy-Baydar D, Farre X, Fine SW, Iczkowski KA, Ittmann M, Knudsen BS, Loda M, Lopez-Beltran A, Magi-Galluzzi C, Mikuz G, Montironi R, Pikarsky E, Pizov G, Rubin MA, Samaratunga H, Sebo T, Sesterhenn IA, Shah RB, Signoretti S, Simko J, Thomas G, Troncoso P, Tsuzuki TT, van Leenders GJ, Yang XJ, Zhou M, Figg WD, IIoque A, Lucia MS. A Working Group Classification of Focal Prostate Atrophy Lesions. Am J Surg Pathol. 2006 Oct; 30(10): 1281–91.

Montironi R, Mazzucchelli R, Lopez-Beltran A, Cheng L, Scarpelli M. Mechanisms of Disease: High-grade Prostatic Intraepithelial Neoplasia and Other Proposed Preneoplastic Lesions in the Prostate. Nat Clin Pract Urol. 2007 Jun; 4(6): 321–32.

Mazzucchelli R, Lopez-Beltran A, Cheng L, Scarpelli M, Kirkali Z, Montironi R. Rare and Unusual Histological Variants of Prostatic Carcinoma: Clinical Significance. BJU Int. 2008 Nov; 102(10): 1369–74.

Montironi R, Lopez-Beltran A, Cheng L, Scarpelli M. Cervical-type Squamous Metaplasia and Myoepithelial Cell Differentiation in Stromal Tumor of the Prostate. Am J Surg Pathol. 2011 Nov; 35(11): 1752–54. No abstract available.

Varma M, Egevad L, Delahunt B, Kristiansen G. Reporting Intraductal Carcinoma of the Prostate: A Plea for Greater Standardization. Histopathology. 2016 Sep 10. doi: 10.1111/his.13081

Chen S, Patil PA, Lepe M, Lombardo KA, Amin A, Matoso A. Retrospective Analysis of Atypical Glands Suspicious for Carcinoma in Transurethral Resection of Prostate. Appl Immunohistochem Mol Morphol. 2016 Jun 13. [Epub ahead of print]

Morais CL, Guedes LB, Hicks J, Baras AS, De Marzo AM, Lotan TL. ERG and PTEN Status of Isolated High-grade PIN Occurring in Cystoprostatectomy Specimens without Invasive Prostatic Adenocarcinoma. Hum Pathol. 2016 Sep; 55: 117–25.

Packer JR, Maitland NJ. The Molecular and Cellular Origin of Human Prostate Cancer. Biochim Biophys Acta. 2016 Jun; 1863(6 Pt A): 1238–60.

Torabi-Nezhad S, Malekmakan L, Mashayekhi M, Daneshian A. Histopathological Features of Intra-ductal Carcinoma of Prostatic and High Grade Prostatic Intraepithelialneoplasia and Correlation with PTEN and P63. Prostate. 2016 Mar; 76(4): 394–401.

De Marzo AM, Haffner MC, Lotan TL, Yegnasubramanian S, Nelson WG. Premalignancy in Prostate Cancer: Rethinking What We Know. Cancer Prev Res (Phila). 2016 Aug; 9(8): 648–56.

Kowalewski A, Szylberg Ł, Skórczewska A, Marszałek A. Diagnostic Difficulties with Atrophy, Atypical Adenomatous Hyperplasia, and Atypical Small Acinar Proliferation: A Systematic Review of Current Literature. Clin Genitourin Cancer. 2016 Oct; 14(5): 361–65.

Leone A, Gershman B, Rotker K, Butler C, Fantasia J, Miller A, Afiadata A, Amin A, Zhou A, Jiang Z, Sebo T, Mega A, Schiff S, Pareek G, Golijanin D, Yates J, Karnes RJ, Renzulli J. Atypical Small Acinar Proliferation (ASAP): Is a Repeat Biopsy Necessary ASAP? A Multi-institutional Review. Prostate Cancer Prostatic Dis. 2016 Mar; 19(1): 68–71.

De Luca S, Passera R, Cappia S, Bollito E, Randone DF, Porpiglia F. Pathological Patterns of Prostate Biopsy in Men with Fluctuations of Prostate Cancer Gene 3 Score: A Preliminary Report. Anticancer Res. 2015 Apr; 35(4): 2417–22.

Adenocarcinoma of the Prostate

4.1 Diagnostic Criteria for Prostate Adenocarcinoma

- Most clinically palpable prostate cancers diagnosed on needle biopsy are predominantly located posterolateral. Large transition zone tumors may extend into the peripheral zone and become palpable.
- Cancers detected on TURP are predominantly within the transition zone. Non-palpable cancers detected on needle biopsy are predominantly located peripherally, although 20% have tumors predominantly within the transition zone. Large tumors may extend into the central zone, yet cancers uncommonly arise in this zone. Multifocal adenocarcinoma of the prostate is seen in about 85% of prostates.
- Grossly evident cancers are firm, solid and range in color from white-grey to yellow-orange, the latter having increased cytoplasmic lipids; the tumors contrast with the adjacent benign parenchyma, which is typically tan and spongy. Tumors usually extend microscopically beyond their macroscopic border. Fig 4.1

Fig 4.1 Grossly yellow prostate carcinoma.

- Gross hemorrhage and necrosis are rare. Subtle tumors may be grossly recognized by structural asymmetry; for example, peripheral zone tumors may deform the periurethral fibromuscular concentric band demarcating the periurethral and peripheral prostate centrally, and peripherally may expand or obscure the outer boundaries of the prostate. Anterior and apical tumors are difficult to grossly identify because of admixed stromal and nodular hyperplasia.
- Grossly recognizable tumors tend to be larger, of higher grade and stage and are frequently palpable, compared with grossly unapparent tumors (usually < 5 mm) which are often non-palpable, small, low grade and low stage. Some large tumors are diffusely infiltrative, and may not be evident grossly.
- In countries with widespread PSA testing, grossly evident prostate cancer has become relatively uncommon.

4.2 Histologic Features of Prostate Cancer

- The diagnosis of carcinoma relies on a combination of architectural and cytological findings. More than 95% of all carcinomas of the prostate seen in needle biopsy specimens are referred to as acinar or conventional type. Table 4.1; Figs 4.2–4.5

4.3 Architectural Features

- Prostate adenocarcinoma is a prototypic example of heterogeneous neoplasm, which is reflected by its variable morphology.
- Architectural features are usually assessed at low to medium power magnification, with emphasis on spacing, size and shape of acini.

Table 4.1 Differential Diagnoses of Prostate Adenocarcinoma

Common:

- Atrophy
- Post-atrophic hyperplasia
- Partial atrophy
- Basal cell hyperplasia
- Atypical adenomatous hyperplasia (adenosis)
- Inflammatory-associated atypia
- High grade PIN

Less common:

- Cowper's gland
- Nephrogenic metaplasia
- Clear cell cribriform hyperplasia
- Seminal vesicle/ejaculatory ducts
- Paraganglia
- Xanthoma

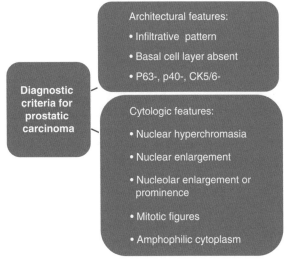

Diagnostic criteria for prostatic carcinoma

Architectural features:
- Infiltrative pattern
- Basal cell layer absent
- P63-, p40-, CK5/6-

Cytologic features:
- Nuclear hyperchromasia
- Nuclear enlargement
- Nucleolar enlargement or prominence
- Mitotic figures
- Amphophilic cytoplasm

Fig 4.2 Diagnostic criteria for prostate cancer.

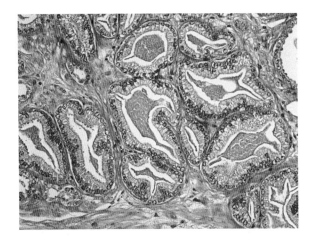

Fig 4.3 Microscopic appearance of acinar (conventional) prostate cancer showing infiltrating acini, amphophilic cytoplasm, eosinophilic luminal material and minimal nuclear atypia.

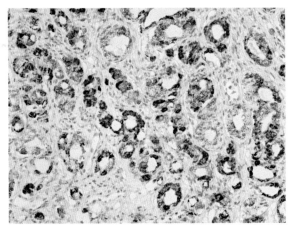

Fig 4.4 Racemase intense expression in prostate carcinoma. Anti-racemase immunohistochemistry.

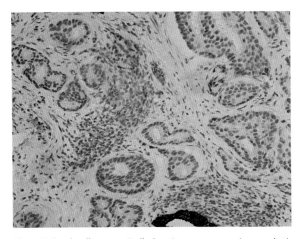

Fig 4.5 Basal cells are typically lost in prostate carcinoma. Anti-34βE12 immunohistochemistry.

The arrangement of the acini is diagnostically useful and is the basis of the Gleason grade.

- Malignant acini usually have an irregular, haphazard arrangement, randomly scattered in the stroma in clusters or singly. The spacing between malignant acini often varies widely. Variation in acinar size is a useful criterion for cancer, particularly when small, irregular, abortive acini with primitive lumens are seen at the periphery of a focus of well-differentiated carcinoma.
- The acini in suspicious foci are usually small or medium sized, with irregular contours that contrast with the typical smooth, round to

elongated contours of benign and hyperplastic acini. Comparison with the adjacent benign prostatic acini is always of value in the diagnosis of cancer.

- Well-differentiated carcinoma and the large acinar variant of Gleason 3 carcinoma are particularly difficult to separate from benign acini in needle biopsies because of the uniform size and spacing of acini; in such cases, greater emphasis is placed on cytologic features, immunohistochemical findings and the presence of smaller diagnostic acini at the edge of the focus. Figs 4.6–4.16
- The basal cell layer is absent in prostate cancer, whereas an intact basal cell layer is present with benign acini. This is an important diagnostic

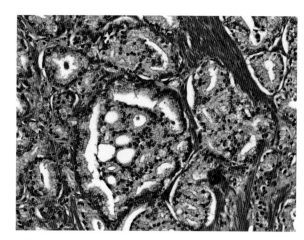

Fig 4.6 Glomeruloid pattern of prostate adenocarcinoma.

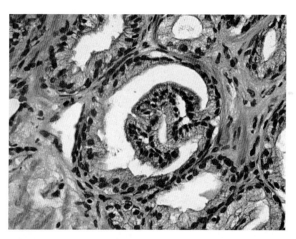

Fig 4.7 Glomeruloid-like structures (so-called telescoping) may be seen in normal prostate glands and should not be mistaken as prostatic adenocarcinoma.

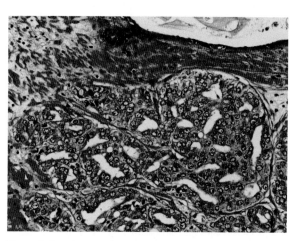

Fig 4.8 Fused acini forming cribriform pattern of prostate adenocarcinoma.

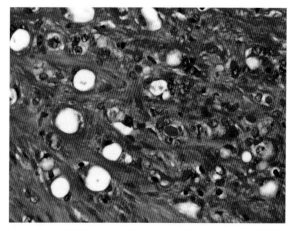

Fig 4.9 Atrophic pattern of prostate adenocarcinoma should not be mistaken as atrophy.

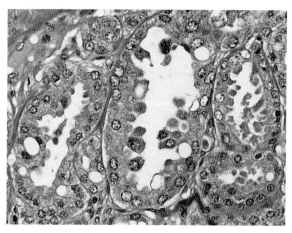

Fig 4.10 Occasionally, prostate adenocarcinoma may show apocrine differentiation.

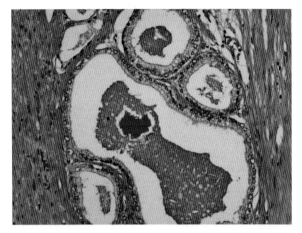

Fig 4.11 Variable sized acini are frequently seen in prostate adenocarcinoma.

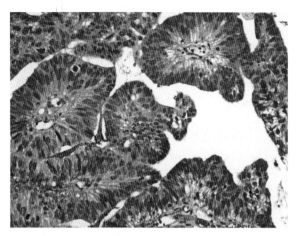

Fig 4.12 Papillary formations with pseudostratified epithelium may be seen in some prostate adenocarcinoma.

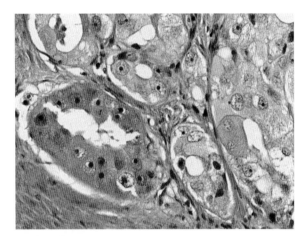

Fig 4.13 Occasionally, prostate adenocarcinoma may show onco-cyte-type differentiation.

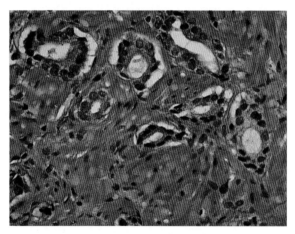

Fig 4.14 Retraction artifact is one frequent hallmark of prostate adenocarcinoma.

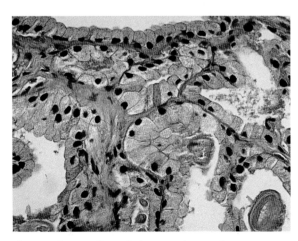

Fig 4.15 Foamy cell morphology may be seen in some prostate adenocarcinoma.

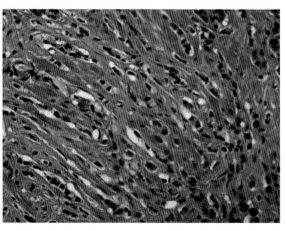

Fig 4.16 Some prostate adenocarcinoma may show these com-pressed poorly formed acini.

feature that is not always easy to evaluate in routine tissue sections, owing to false negative findings with atrophy and other mimics of cancer. Compressed stromal fibroblasts may mimic basal cells, but are usually seen only focally at the periphery of acini. Figs 4.17–4.18

4.4 Cytological and Nuclear Features

- The cytological features of adenocarcinoma include nuclear and nucleolar enlargement, which occurs in most malignant cells. Every cell has a nucleolus at least 1.50 μm in diameter or larger.
- Artifacts such as overstaining and differences in fixation often obscure the nuclei and nucleoli, so comparison with non-neoplastic cells (internal control) from the same specimen is a useful diagnostic clue.
- Intracytoplasmic vacuoles (signet-ring-like) can also be seen frequently. Figs 4.19–4.26

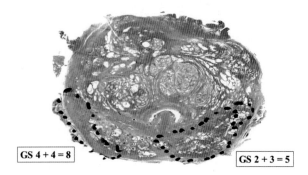

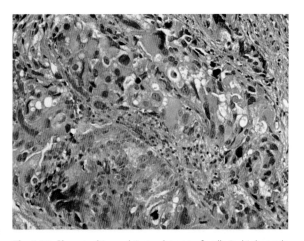

GS 4 + 4 = 8

GS 2 + 3 = 5

Fig 4.18 Prostate adenocarcinoma is typically multicentric.

4.5 Luminal Findings

- Crystalloids are sharp, needle-like eosinophilic structures that are often present in the lumens of well-differentiated and moderately differentiated

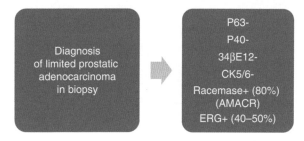

| Diagnosis of limited prostatic adenocarcinoma in biopsy | ⇨ | P63-
P40-
34βE12-
CK5/6-
Racemase+ (80%) (AMACR)
ERG+ (40–50%) |

Fig 4.17 Diagnostic criteria of prostate adenocarcinoma in limited biopsy samples.

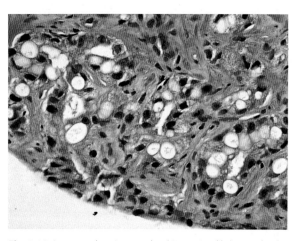

Fig 4.19 Intracytoplasmic vacuoles (signet-ring-like) can also be seen in prostate adenocarcinoma.

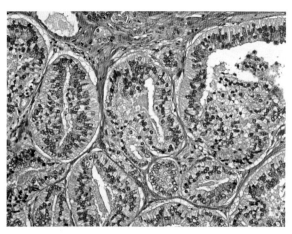

Fig 4.20 Pleomorphic nuclei may be seen focally in high grade prostate adenocarcinoma.

Fig 4.21 Occasionally, prostate adenocarcinoma may show subnuclear vacuoles simulating secretory endometrial carcinoma.

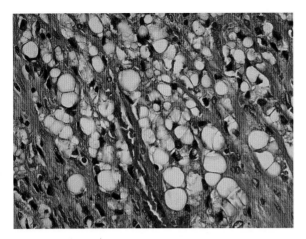

Fig 4.22 Intracytoplasmic vacuoles (signet-ring-like) seen in prostate adenocarcinoma may rarely present lipoblast-like morphology.

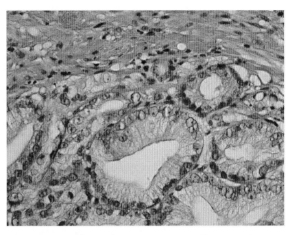

Fig 4.23 Vesicular nuclei are a common feature in prostate adenocarcinoma.

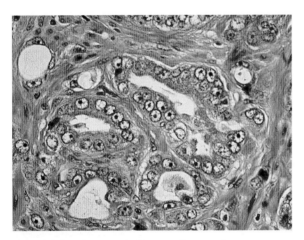

Fig 4.24 Prominent nucleoli are a feature of most prostate adenocarcinomas.

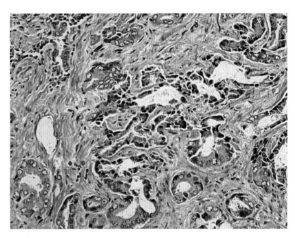

Fig 4.25 Apoptotic prostate adenocarcinoma may produce compelling morphological features in prostate adenocarcinoma.

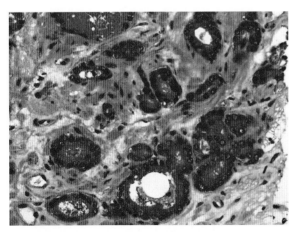

Fig 4.26 Basophilic cytoplasm may be seen rarely in some prostate adenocarcinoma.

carcinoma. They are not specific for carcinoma and can be found in other conditions. The presence of crystalloids in metastatic adenocarcinoma of unknown site of origin is strong presumptive evidence of prostatic origin, although it is an uncommon finding.

- Luminal acidic sulfated and nonsulfated mucin is often seen in acini of adenocarcinoma, appearing as amorphous, faintly basophilic secretions in routine sections. This mucin stains with Alcian blue at pH 2.5, whereas normal prostatic epithelium contain periodic acid Schiff-reactive mucin that is neutral.
- Acidic mucin is not specific for carcinoma. It may be found in prostatic intraepithelial

51

neoplasia (PIN), atypical adenomatous hyperplasia, sclerosing adenosis and, rarely, nodular hyperplasia.

- Intraluminal corpora amylacea may be seen occasionally in prostate cancer. Figs 4.27–4.32

4.6 Stromal Findings

- The stroma in cancer frequently contains young collagen, which appears lightly eosinophilic, although desmoplasia may be prominent. Muscle fibers in the stroma are sometimes split or distorted, but most frequently resemble the stroma associated with benign prostate.
- Collagenous micronodules (mucinous fibroplasia) are a specific but infrequent and incidental finding

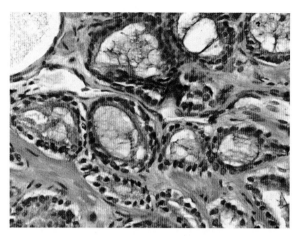

Fig 4.27 Prostate adenocarcinoma with luminal mucin.

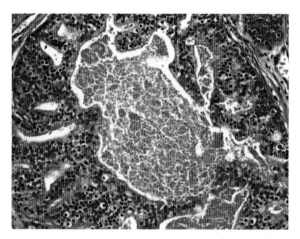

Fig 4.28 Prostate adenocarcinoma with proteinaceous material that should not be mistaken as necrosis.

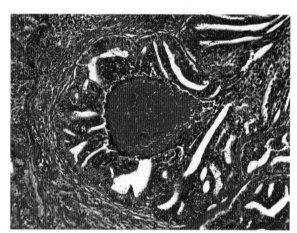

Fig 4.29 Prostate adenocarcinoma with luminal necrosis.

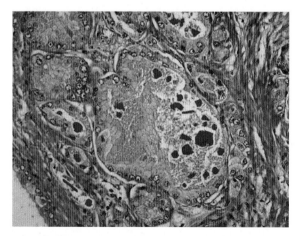

Fig 4.30 Prostate adenocarcinoma with luminal crystalloids.

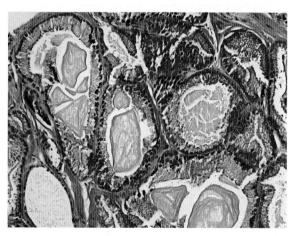

Fig 4.31 Prostate adenocarcinoma with luminal corpora amylacea.

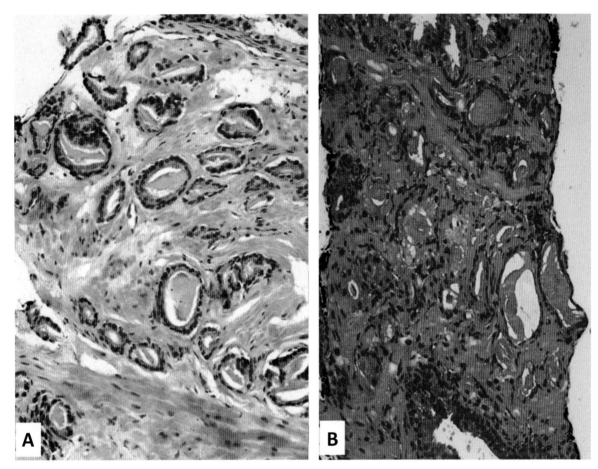

Fig 4.32 Prostate adenocarcinoma with luminal proteinaceous material (A and B).

in prostatic adenocarcinoma. They consist of microscopic nodular masses of paucicellular eosinophilic fibrilar stroma that impinge on acinar lumens. They are usually present in mucin-producing adenocarcinoma and result from extravasation of acidic mucin into the stroma.

- Collagenous micronodules are present in about 14% of cases of adenocarcinoma. Collagenous micronodules may be particularly valuable in challenging needle biopsy specimens. They are not observed in PIN, nodular hyperplasia or benign epithelium. (Table 4.2; Figs 4.33–4.40)

4.7 Immunohistochemical Findings

- Important immunohistochemical markers in prostate pathology are PSA, PAP, PSMA,

high-molecular-weight keratin clone 34ßE12, CK 5/6, p63 and AMACR.

- Immunohistochemical expression of Prostate-Specific Antigen (PSA) is useful for distinguishing high grade prostate cancer from urothelial carcinoma, colonic carcinoma, granulomatous prostatitis and lymphoma. PSA also facilitates identification of the site of tumor origin in metastatic adenocarcinoma. PSA can be detected in frozen and paraffin-embedded sections and is preserved in decalcified specimens. Staining is invariably heterogeneous.
- The use of PSMA adds specificity over PSA, according to some authors. Prostatic Acid Phosphatase (PAP) is a valuable immunohistochemical marker for identifying

prostate cancer when used in combination with PSA.

- High-molecular-weight cytokeratin (clone 34ßE12) and CK5/6 may be useful for evaluation of the basal cell layer. It is most useful in confirming the benignancy of a suggestive focus by showing an immunoreactive basal cell layer. Anti-keratin 34ßE12 stains nearly all of the

normal basal cells of the prostate; no staining occurs in the secretory and stromal cells.

- Uniform absence of a basal cell layer is one important diagnostic feature of invasive carcinoma and basal cells may be inapparent by Hematoxilin-Eosin (H&E) stain. Basal cell-specific immunostains may help to distinguish invasive prostatic adenocarcinoma from benign small acinar cancer mimics which retain their basal cell layer, e.g. glandular atrophy, post-atrophic hyperplasia, atypical adenomatous hyperplasia, sclerosing adenosis and radiation induced atypia.
- Because the basal cell layer may be interrupted or not demonstrable in small numbers of benign

Table 4.2 Diagnostic Criteria for Prostatic Carcinoma

- Architectural features
  - infiltrative pattern of malignant acini, e.g.:
    - arrangement: irregular and haphazard
    - spacing between acini varies widely
    - variation in size
    - irregular contour
  - basal cell layer
    - absent
- Cytological features (secretory cells in single layer)
  - Nuclear hyperchromasia
  - Nuclear enlargement
  - Nucleolar enlargement or prominence
  - Mitotic figures
  - Amphophilic cytoplasm
- Luminal findings
  - Crystalloids
  - Intraluminal blue mucin and/or pink amorphous secretions
- Stromal findings
  - Collagenous micronodules
- Immunohistochemical findings
  - Prostate-specific antigen
  - Prostatic acid phosphatase
  - 34βE12
  - p63/p40
  - Racemase
- Additional feature
  - Adjacent prostatic intraepithelial neoplasia frequent

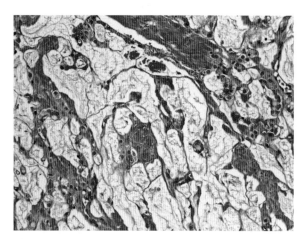

Fig 4.33 Mucinous adenocarcinoma of the prostate with extensive mucinous stroma.

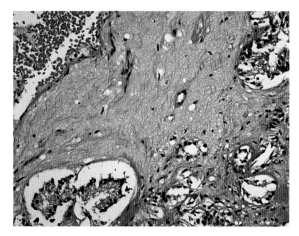

Fig 4.34 Prostate adenocarcinoma with proteinaceous stroma.

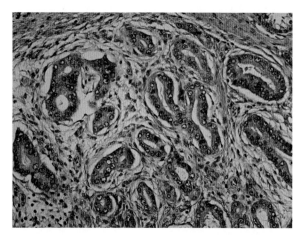

Fig 4.35 Prostate adenocarcinoma with fibrous/myxoid stroma.

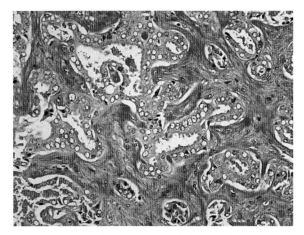

Fig 4.36 Prostate adenocarcinoma with fibrous-collagenic stroma (so-called stromogenic carcinoma).

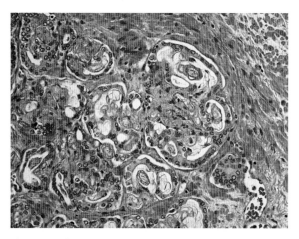

Fig 4.37 Collagenous micronodules (mucinous fibroplasia) seen in prostate adenocarcinoma.

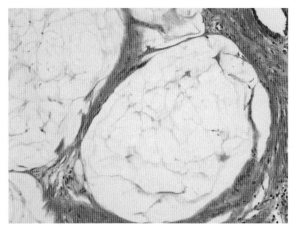

Fig 4.38 Acellular mucin lakes can also be seen in prostate adenocarcinoma.

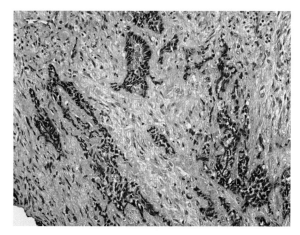

Fig 4.39 Pseudosarcomatous stroma may be seen in some high grade prostate adenocarcinoma.

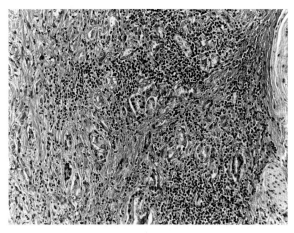

Fig 4.40 Prostate adenocarcinoma with heavy inflammatory stroma.

glands, the complete absence of a basal cell layer in a small focus of acini cannot be used alone as a definitive criterion for malignancy; rather, absence of a basal cell layer is supportive of invasive carcinoma only in acinar proliferations which exhibit suspicious cytological and/or architectural features on H&E stain.

- Conversely, some early invasive prostatic carcinomas, e.g. microinvasive carcinomas arising in association with or independent of high grade prostatic intraepithelial neoplasia, may have residual basal cells (transitive glands). Intraductal spread of invasive carcinoma and entrapped benign glands are other proposed explanations for residual basal cells. Rare prostatic adenocarcinomas contain sparse neoplastic glandular cells which are immunoreactive for 34βE12, yet these are not in a basal cell distribution. The use of antibodies for 34βE12 is especially helpful for the diagnosis of deceptively benign-appearing variants of prostate cancer.

- Immunohistochemistry for cytokeratins 7 and 20 have a limited diagnostic use in prostate pathology, with the exception that negative staining for both markers, which can occur in prostate adenocarcinoma, would be unusual for transitional cell carcinoma.

- p63 is a nuclear protein encoded by a gene on chromosome 3q27-29 with homology to p53 (a tumor suppressor gene), and has been shown to regulate growth and development in epithelium of the skin, cervix, breast and urogenital tract.

- Specific isotypes are expressed in basal cells of stratified and pseudostratified epithelia (prostate, bronchial), reserve cells of simple columnar epithelium (endocervical, pancreatic ductal), myoepithelial cells (breast, salivary glands, cutaneous apocrine/eccrine glands), urothelium and squamous epithelium. High molecular weight cytokeratins and p63 have similar applications in the diagnosis of prostatic adenocarcinoma, but with the advantages that p63 is less susceptible to the staining variability of 34βE12 (particularly in TURP specimens with cautery artifact), stains a subset of 34βE12 negative basal cells and is easier to interpret because of its strong nuclear staining intensity.

- Interpretative limitations related to presence or absence of basal cells in small numbers of glands for 34βE12 apply to p63, requiring correlation with morphology. Prostatic adenocarcinomas have occasional p63 immunoreactive cells, most representing entrapped benign glands or intraductal spread of carcinoma with residual basal cells, but some true p63 positive carcinomas have been reported. Fig 4.41

- An immunohistochemical cocktail containing monoclonal antibodies to cytokeratin 34betaE12 and p63 is in use by some authorities.

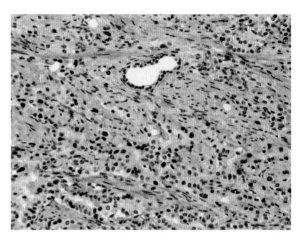

Fig 4.41 Prostate adenocarcinoma with positive expression of p63 (anti-p63 immunohistochemistry).

- AMACR (α-Methyl-CoA racemase, P504S) is a racemase protein for which polyclonal and monoclonal antibodies have been produced which are active in formalin-fixed, paraffin-embedded tissue. Over 80% of prostatic adenocarcinomas are labeled with racemase.

- Certain subtypes of prostate cancer, such as foamy gland carcinoma, atrophic carcinoma, pseudohyperplastic and treated carcinoma show lower AMACR expression. However, AMACR is not specific for prostate cancer and is present in nodular hyperplasia (12%), atrophic glands (35%), HGPIN (90%) and atypical adenomatous hyperplasia (18%).

- AMACR may be used as a confirmatory stain for prostatic adenocarcinoma, in conjunction with histology and basal cell specific markers. AMACR is expressed in other non-prostatic neoplasms, including urothelial, renal and colon cancer.

- A cocktail containing 34betaE12, p63 and racemase is used by some authorities.

4.8 Focal Neuroendocrine Differentiation

- About 10% of prostatic carcinomas have zones with a large number of single or clustered neuroendocrine cells detected by chromogranin A immunohistochemistry; some cells may also be serotonin positive. Immunostaining for neuron-specific enolase, synaptophysin, bombesin/gastrin-releasing peptide and a variety of other neuroendocrine peptides may also occur in individual neoplastic neuroendocrine cells, or in a more diffuse pattern, and receptors for serotonin may also be present.

- There are conflicting studies as to whether advanced androgen independent and androgen deprived carcinomas show increased neuroendocrine differentiation. The prognostic significance of focal neuroendocrine differentiation in primary untreated prostatic carcinoma is controversial.

- In advanced prostate cancer, especially androgen independent cancer, focal neuroendocrine differentiation portends a poor prognosis. Fig 4.42

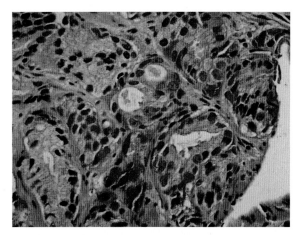

Fig 4.42 Neuroendocrine cells in acinar prostate adenocarcinoma.

Suggested Reading

Kim MJ, Divatia MK, Lee JH, Shen S, Miles BJ, Hwang JH, Ayala AG, Ro JY. Collagenous Micronodules in Prostate Cancer Revisited: Are They Solely Associated with Gleason Pattern 3 Adenocarcinomas? Int J Clin Exp Pathol. 2015 Apr 1; **8**(4): 3469–76.

Santoni M, Scarpelli M, Mazzucchelli R, Lopez-Beltran A, Cheng L, Epstein JI, Cascinu S, Briganti A, Catto JW, Montorsi F, Montironi R. Current Histopathologic and Molecular Characterisations of Prostate Cancer: Towards Individualised Prognosis and Therapies. Eur Urol. 2016 Feb; **69**(2): 186–90.

Mazzucchelli R, Galosi AB, Santoni M, Lopez-Beltran A, Scarpelli M, Cheng L, Montironi R. Role of the Pathologist in Active Surveillance for Prostate Cancer. Anal Quant Cytopathol Histpathol. 2015 Feb; **37**(1): 65–68.

Epstein JI, Egevad L, Amin MB, Delahunt B, Srigley JR, Humphrey PA. Grading Committee. The 2014 International Society of Urological Pathology (ISUP) Consensus Conference on Gleason Grading of Prostatic Carcinoma: Definition of Grading Patterns and Proposal for a New Grading System. Am J Surg Pathol. 2016 Feb; **40**(2): 244–52. doi: 10.1097/PAS.0000000000000530.

Gasparrini S, Mazzucchelli R, Scarpelli M, Massari F, Raspollini MR, Lopez-Beltran A, Cheng L, Montironi R. Prostate Cancer Grading in 2016. *Minerva Urol Nefrol.* 2016 Nov 4; [Epub ahead of print].

Berney DM, Algaba F, Camparo P, Compérat E, Griffiths D, Kristiansen G, Lopez-Beltran A, Montironi R, Varma M, Egevad L. Variation in Reporting of Cancer Extent and Benign Histology in Prostate Biopsies among European Pathologists. Virchows Arch. 2014 Mar 4; [Epub ahead of print].

Montironi R, Cheng L, Lopez-Beltran A, Montironi MA, Galosi AB, Scarpelli M. A Low Grade PIN-like Neoplasm of the Transition Zone Immunohistochemically Negative for Basal Cell Markers: A Possible Example of Low Grade Adenocarcinoma with Stratified Epithelium. Pathology. 2014 Jan; **46**(1): 88–91.

Berney DM, Algaba F, Camparo P, Compérat E, Griffiths D, Kristiansen G, Lopez-Beltran A, Montironi R, Varma M, Egevad L. The Reasons behind Variation in Gleason Grading of Prostatic Biopsies: Areas of Agreement and Misconception among 266 European Pathologists. Histopathology. 2014 Feb; **64**(3): 405–11. doi: 10.1111/his.12284. Epub 2013 Nov 6.

Yossepowitch O, Briganti A, Eastham JA, Epstein J, Graefen M, Montironi R, Touijer K. Positive Surgical Margins after Radical Prostatectomy: A Systematic Review and Contemporary Update. Eur Urol. 2014 Feb; **65**(2): 303–13. doi: 10.1016/j.eururo.2013.07.039. Epub 2013 Aug 3.

Schelling LA, Williamson SR, Zhang S, Yao JL, Wang M, Huang J, Montironi R, Lopez-Beltran A, Emerson RE, Idrees MT, Osunkoya AO, Man YG, Maclennan GT, Baldridge LA, Compérat E, Cheng L. Frequent TMPRSS2-ERG Rearrangement in Prostatic Small Cell Carcinoma Detected by Fluorescence in Situ Hybridization: The Superiority of Fluorescence in Situ Hybridization over ERG Immunohistochemistry. Hum Pathol. 2013 Oct; **44**(10): 2227–33. doi: 10.1016/j.humpath.2013.05.005. Epub 2013 Jul 12.

Montironi R, Cheng L, Lopez-Beltran A, Mazzucchelli R, Scarpelli M. Combined Handling of Prostate Base/Bladder Neck and Seminal Vesicles in Radical Prostatectomy Specimens: Our Approach with the Whole Mount Technique. Histopathology. 2013 Sep; **63**(3): 431–35. doi: 10.1111/his.12158. Epub 2013 Jun 24. No abstract available.

Montironi R, Lopez-Beltran A, Cheng L, Montorsi F, Scarpelli M. Central Prostate Pathology Review: Should It Be Mandatory? Eur Urol. 2013 Aug; **64**(2): 199–201.

57

Discussion 202–03. doi: 10.1016/j.eururo.2013.04.002. Epub 2013 Apr 16. No abstract available.

Montironi R, Scarpelli M, Cheng L, Lopez-Beltran A, Montorsi F, Kirkali Z. Somatostatin Receptor Expression in Prostate Carcinoma: The Urological Pathologist's Role in the Era of Personalised Medicine. Pathology. 2013 Jan; 45(1): 93–96. doi: 10.1097/PAT.0b013e32835bae76. No abstract available.

Cheng L, MacLennan GT, Lopez-Beltran A, Montironi R. Anatomic, Morphologic and Genetic Heterogeneity of Prostate Cancer: Implications for Clinical Practice. Expert Rev Anticancer Ther. 2012 Nov; 12(11): 1371–74. doi: 10.1586/era.12.127.

Egevad L, Ahmad AS, Algaba F, Berney DM, Boccon-Gibod L, Compérat E, Evans AJ, Griffiths D, Grobholz R, Kristiansen G, Langner C, Lopez-Beltran A, Montironi R, Moss S, Oliveira P, Vainer B, Varma M, Camparo P. Standardization of Gleason Grading among 337 European Pathologists. Histopathology. 2013 Jan; 62(2): 247–56. doi: 10.1111/his.12008.

Varma M, Berney DM, Algaba F, Camparo P, Compérat E, Griffiths DF, Kristiansen G, Lopez-Beltran A, Montironi R, Egevad L. Prostate Needle Biopsy Processing: A Survey of Laboratory Practice across Europe. J Clin Pathol. 2013 Feb; 66(2): 120–23. doi: 10.1136/jclinpath-2012-200993.

Brimo F, Montironi R, Egevad L, Erbersdobler A, Lin DW, Nelson JB, Rubin MA, van der Kwast T, Amin M, Epstein JI. Contemporary Grading for Prostate Cancer: Implications for Patient Care. Eur Urol. 2013 May; 63(5): 892–901. doi: 10.1016/j.eururo.2012.10.015.

Ukimura O, Coleman JA, de la Taille A, Emberton M, Epstein JI, Freedland SJ, Giannarini G, Kibel AS, Montironi R, Ploussard G, Roobol MJ, Scattoni V, Jones JS. Contemporary Role of Systematic Prostate Biopsies: Indications, Techniques, and Implications for Patient Care. Eur Urol. 2013 Feb; 63(2): 214–30. doi: 10.1016/j.eururo.2012.09.033.

Quick Charles M. MDa, Gokden N., Sangoi Ankur R. MDb, Brooks James D. MDc, McKenney Jesse K. MDa. The distribution of PAX-2 Immunoreactivity in the Prostate Gland, Seminal Vesicle, and Ejaculatory Duct: Comparison with Prostatic Adenocarcinoma and Discussion of Prostatic Zonal Embryogenesis. Human Pathology. 2010; 41: 1145–49.

Harvey Aaron M. MD, Grice Beverly HTL, Hamilton Candice HTL, Truong Luan D. MD, Ro Jae Y. MD, Ayala Alberto G. MD, Zhai Qihui "Jim" MD. Diagnostic Utility of P504S/p63 Cocktail Prostate-specific Antigen, and Prostatic Acid Phosphatase in Verifying Prostatic Carcinoma Involvement in Seminal Vesicles: A Study of 57 Cases of Radical Prostatectomy Specimens of Pathologic Stage pT3b. Arch Pathol Lab Med. 2010; 134: 983–88.

Lopez-Beltran A, Cheng L, Blanca A, Montironi R. Cell Proliferation and Apoptosis in Prostate Needle Biopsies with Adenocarcinoma Gleason Score 6 or 7. Anal Quant Cytol Histol. 2012 Apr; 34(2): 61–65.

Scarpelli M, Mazzucchelli R, Barbisan F, Santinelli A, Lopez-Beltran A, Cheng L, Montironi R. Is There a Role for Prostate Tumour Overexpressed-1 in the Diagnosis of HGPIN and of Prostatic Adenocarcinoma? A Comparison with Alpha-Methylacyl CoA Racemase. Int J Immunopathol Pharmacol. 2012 Jan–Mar; 25(1): 67–74.

Camparo P, Egevad L, Algaba F, Berney DM, Boccon-Gibod L, Compérat E, Evans AJ, Grobholz R, Kristiansen G, Langner C, Lopez-Beltran A, Montironi R, Oliveira P, Vainer B, Varma M. Utility of Whole Slide Imaging and Virtual Microscopy in Prostate Pathology. APMIS. 2012 Apr; 120(4): 298–304. doi: 10.1111/j.1600-0463.2011.02872.x. Review.

Montironi R, Scarpelli M, Mazzucchelli R, Cheng L, Lopez-Beltran A, Montorsi F. Extent of Cancer of Less Than 50% in Any Prostate Needle Biopsy Core: How Many Millimeters Are There? Eur Urol. 2012 Apr; 61(4): 751–56. Epub 2012 Jan 5. No abstract available.

Cheng L, Montironi R, Bostwick DG, Lopez-Beltran A, Berney DM. Staging of Prostate Cancer. Histopathology. 2012 Jan; 60(1): 87–117. doi: 10.1111/j.1365-2559.2011.04025.x.

Montironi R, Lopez-Beltran A, Cheng L, Scarpelli M. Cervical-type Squamous Metaplasia and Myoepithelial Cell Differentiation in Stromal Tumor of the Prostate. Am J Surg Pathol. 2011 Nov; 35(11): 1752–54. No abstract available.

Mazzucchelli R, Barbisan F, Santinelli A, Lopez-Beltran A, Cheng L, Scarpelli M, Montironi R. Immunohistochemical Expression of Prostate Tumor Overexpressed 1 in Cystoprostatectomies with Incidental and Insignificant Prostate Cancer. Further Evidence for Field Effect in Prostatic Carcinogenesis. Hum Pathol. 2011 Dec; 42(12): 1931–36. Epub 2011 Jun 14.

Williamson SR, Zhang S, Yao JL, Huang J, Lopez-Beltran A, Shen S, Osunkoya AO, MacLennan GT, Montironi R, Cheng L. ERG-TMPRSS2 Rearrangement Is Shared by Concurrent Prostatic Adenocarcinoma and Prostatic Small Cell Carcinoma and Absent in Small Cell Carcinoma of the Urinary Bladder: Evidence Supporting Monoclonal Origin. Mod Pathol. 2011 Aug; 24(8): 1120–27. doi: 10.1038/modpathol.2011.56.

Capitanio U, Cheng L, Lopez-Beltran A, Scarpelli M, Freschi M, Montorsi F, Montironi R. The Importance of Interaction between Urologists and Pathologists in Incidental Prostate Cancer Management. Eur Urol. 2011 Jul; 60(1): 75–77.

Montironi R, Cheng L, Lopez-Beltran A, Mazzucchelli R, Scarpelli M. Editorial Comment to When Should We Expect No Residual Tumor (pT0) Once We Submit

Incidental T1a-b Prostate Cancers to Radical Prostatectomy? Int J Urol. 2011 Feb; **18**(2): 153–54. doi: 10.1111/j.1442-2042.2010.02717.x.

Mazzucchelli R, Nesseris I, Cheng L, Lopez-Beltran A, Montironi R, Scarpelli M. Active Surveillance for Low-risk Prostate cancer. Anticancer Res. 2010 Sep; **30**(9): 3683–92.

Montironi R, Mazzucchelli R, Lopez-Beltran A, Cheng L. Words of Wisdom. Re: Peripheral Zone Prostate Cancers: Location and Intraprostatic Patterns of Spread at Histopathology. Eur Urol. 2010 Jul; **58**(1): 180–82.

Montironi R, Cheng L, Lopez-Beltran A, Scarpelli M, Mazzucchelli R, Mikuz G, Kirkali Z, Montorsi F. Original Gleason System Versus 2005 ISUP Modified Gleason System: The Importance of Indicating Which System Is Used in the Patient's Pathology and Clinical Reports. Eur Urol. 2010 Sep; **58**(3): 369–73.

Montironi R, Vela Navarrete R, Lopez-Beltran A, Mazzucchelli R, Mikuz G, Bono AV. Histopathology Reporting of Prostate Needle Biopsies. 2005 Update. Virchows Arch. 2006; **449**(1): 1–13.

Lopez-Beltran A, Mikuz G, Luque RJ, Mazzucchelli R, Montironi R. Current Practice of Gleason Grading of Prostate Carcinoma. Virchows Arch. 2006 Feb; **448**(2): 111–18.

Epstein JI, Allsbrook WC, Amin MB, Egevad LL, Bastacky S, Lopez-Beltran A, et al. The 2005 International Society of Urological Pathology (ISUP) Consensus Conference on Gleason Grading of Prostatic Carcinoma. Am J Surg Pathol. 2005; **29**: 1228–42.

Lopez-Beltran A, Qian Junqi, Montironi Rodolfo, Luque Rafael J, Bostwick David G. Atypical Adenomatous Hyperplasia (Adenosis) of the Prostate: DNA Ploidy Analysis and Immunophenotype. Int J Surgical Pathology. 2005; **13**: 167–73.

Lopez-Beltran A, Eble John N, Bostwick David G. Pleomorphic Giant Cell Carcinoma of the Prostate. Archives of Pathology and Laboratory Medicine. 2005; **129**: 683–85.

Montironi R, Scattoni V, Mazzucchelli R, Lopez-Beltran A, Bostwick DG, Montorsi F. Atypical Foci Suspicious but Not Diagnostic of Malignancy in Prostate Needle Biopsies (Also Referred to as "Atypical Small Acinar Proliferation Suspicious for but Not Diagnostic of Malignancy"). Eur Urol. 2006 Oct; **50**(4): 666–74.

De Marzo AM, Platz EA, Epstein JI, Ali T, Billis A, Chan TY, Cheng L, Datta M, Egevad L, Ertoy-Baydar D, Farre X, Fine SW, Iczkowski KA, Ittmann M, Knudsen BS,

Loda M, Lopez-Beltran A, Magi-Galluzzi C, Mikuz G, Montironi R, Pikarsky E, Pizov G, Rubin MA, Samaratunga H, Sebo T, Sesterhenn IA, Shah RB, Signoretti S, Simko J, Thomas G, Troncoso P, Tsuzuki TT, van Leenders GJ, Yang XJ, Zhou M, Figg WD, Hoque A, Lucia MS. A Working Group Classification of Focal Prostate Atrophy Lesions. Am J Surg Pathol. 2006 Oct; **30**(10): 1281–91.

Marks RA, Koch MO, Lopez-Beltran A, Montironi R, Juliar BE, Cheng L. The Relationship between the Extent of Surgical Margin Positivity and Prostate Specific Antigen Recurrence in Radical Prostatectomy Specimens. Hum Pathol. 2007 Aug; **38**(8): 1207–11.

Cheng L, Bishop E, Zhou H, Maclennan GT, Lopez-Beltran A, Zhang S, Badve S, Baldridge LA, Montironi R. Lymphatic Vessel Density in Radical Prostatectomy Specimens. Hum Pathol. 2008 Apr; **39**(4): 610–15.

Cheng L, MacLennan GT, Abdul-Karim FW, Lopez-Beltran A, Montironi R. Eosinophilic Metaplasia of the Prostate: A Newly Described Lesion Distinct from Other Eosinophilic Changes in Prostatic Epithelium. Anal Quant Cytol Histol. 2008 Aug; **30**(4): 226–30.

Mazzucchelli R, Lopez-Beltran A, Cheng L, Scarpelli M, Kirkali Z, Montironi R. Rare and Unusual Histological Variants of Prostatic Carcinoma: Clinical Significance. BJU Int. 2008 Nov; **102**(10): 1369–74.

Mazzucchelli R, Morichetti D, Lopez-Beltran A, Cheng L, Scarpelli M, Kirkali Z, Montironi R. Neuroendocrine Tumours of the Urinary System and Male Genital Organs: Clinical Significance. BJU Int. 2009 Jun; **103**(11): 1464–70. Epub 2009 Feb 27. Review.

Montironi R, Cheng L, Mazzucchelli R, Lopez-Beltran A. Pathological Definition and Difficulties in Assessing Positive Margins in Radical Prostatectomy Specimens. BJU Int. 2009 Feb; **103**(3): 286–88.

Lopez-Beltran A, Cheng L, Prieto R, Blanca A, Montironi R. Lymphoepithelioma-like Carcinoma of the Prostate. Hum Pathol. 2009 Jul; **40**(7): 982–87.

Montironi R, Cheng L, Lopez-Beltran A, Mazzucchelli R, Scarpelli M, Kirkali Z, Montorsi F. Joint Appraisal of the Radical Prostatectomy Specimen by the Urologist and the Uropathologist: Together, We Can Do It Better. Eur Urol. 2009 Dec; **56**(6): 951–55.

Morichetti D, Mazzucchelli R, Lopez-Beltran A, Cheng L, Scarpelli M, Kirkali Z, Montorsi F, Montironi R. Secondary Neoplasms of the Urinary System and Male Genital Organs. BJU Int. 2009 Sep; **104**(6): 770–76.

Gleason Grading of Prostate Cancer

5.1 Gleason Grading of Prostate Cancer

- The Gleason grading system for prostate cancer is the predominant grading system for prostate cancer around the world. The Gleason grading system is based on glandular architecture, which can be divided into five patterns of growth (also known as grades) with decreasing differentiation. Table 5.1; Fig 5.1

- The primary and secondary pattern or grade, i.e. the most prevalent and the second most prevalent pattern or grade, are added to obtain a Gleason score or sum that is to be reported. Nuclear atypia or cytoplasmic features are not evaluated. An important issue is that the initial grading of prostate carcinoma should be

Table 5.1 Diagnostic Reporting of Gleason Score: General Features

- Perform Gleason grading at low magnification using a 4x or 10x lens
- Report primary pattern and secondary pattern and assign Gleason score
- If only one pattern is present, double it to yield Gleason score. A Gleason score is usually assignable even if the cancer is extremely small
- In a needle biopsy with more than two patterns (tertiary pattern), the worst pattern must be reflected in the Gleason score even if it is not the predominant or secondary pattern; use the rule "the most and the worst"
- In a radical prostatectomy with more than two patterns, the primary and secondary patterns must be reflected in the Gleason score. Add tertiary pattern as a note in the report as an option
- Provide Gleason score for each separately involved core when identified and give overall Gleason score when mixed in one container
- In general, a diagnosis of Gleason score 2–4 should not be made
- Do not report Gleason score after hormonal or radiation therapy except if cancer shows no treatment effect
- Provide percent of tumor with Gleason pattern 4 in Gleason score 7
- Provide percent of tumor with Gleason patterns 4 and 5 in tumors with Gleason scores 8–10

performed at low magnification. Then one may proceed with high power objectives to look for rare fused glands or a few individual cells.

- Gleason grading remains as one of the most significant factors in the clinical decision-making activity both in needle biopsy specimens and after radical prostatectomy is performed; i.e., it predicts pathologic stage, margin status, biochemical failure, local recurrences, lymph node, disease progression or distant metastasis after prostatectomy. Radiation therapy, radical prostatectomy and other therapies are initially based on the Gleason score.

- In practice, Gleason score of 7 is considered on intermediate risk, Gleason score 8 is a high risk and Gleason scores 9–10 are associated with worse prognosis; meanwhile Gleason scores 5–6 are associated with lower progression rates after therapy. Gleason score has been included in clinical nomograms, which are used with increasing frequency to predict disease progression.

5.2 Gleason Patterns

- Pattern 1: Very well-circumscribed nodule of separate, closely packed glands which do not infiltrate into adjacent benign prostatic tissue. The glands are of intermediate size and approximately equal in size and shape. The nucleus is typically small and cytoplasm frequently is abundant and pale-staining. Nuclear and cytoplasm appearance are not taken into account in diagnosis. This pattern is exceedingly rare and usually seen in transition zone cancers. It is suggested to not report this pattern since more of the cases might be considered adenosis if properly investigated. Figs 5.2–5.3

- Pattern 2: Round to oval glands with smooth ends. The glands are more loosely arranged and not quite as uniform in size and shape as those of

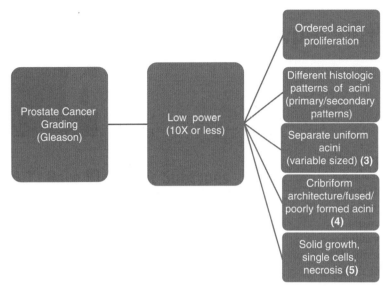

Fig 5.1 Basic Criteria to Apply Gleason Grading.

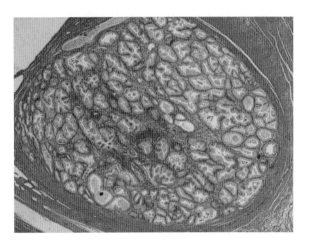

Fig 5.2 Low power view of Gleason pattern 1.

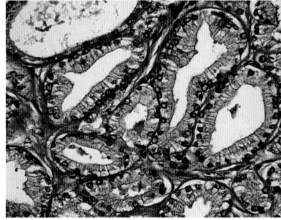

Fig 5.3 Cellular details of Gleason pattern 1.

Gleason pattern 1. There may be minimal invasion by neoplastic glands into the surrounding non-neoplastic prostatic tissue. The glands are of intermediate size and larger than in Gleason pattern 1. The variation in glandular size and separation between glands is less than that seen in pattern 3. Although not evaluated in Gleason grading, the cytoplasm of Gleason pattern 2 cancers is abundant and pale-staining. Gleason pattern 2 is usually seen in transition zone cancers, but may occasionally be found in the peripheral zone. It is not recommended to report Gleason pattern 2 in needle prostate biopsies and only rarely in TURP specimens. Figs 5.4–5.5

- Pattern 3: The most common pattern, but is morphologically heterogeneous. The glands are infiltrative and the distance between them is more variable than in patterns 1 and 2. Malignant glands often infiltrate between adjacent non-neoplastic glands. The glands of pattern 3 vary in size and shape and are often angular. Small glands are typical for pattern 3, but they may also be large and irregular. Each gland has an open lumen and is circumscribed by stroma. This heterogeneous expression of Gleason grade 3 raised an initial subdivision in patterns known as A, B and C, respectively. Figs 5.6–5.16 show the variability of Gleason pattern 3.

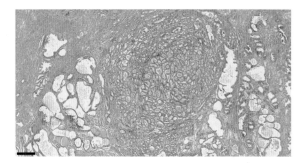

Fig 5.4 Low power view of Gleason pattern 2.

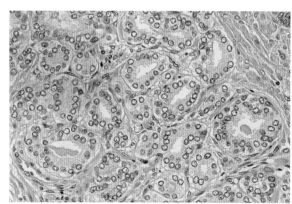

Fig 5.5 Cellular details of Gleason pattern 2.

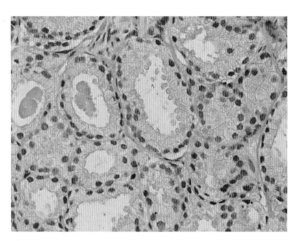

Fig 5.6 Close packed acini in Gleason pattern 3.

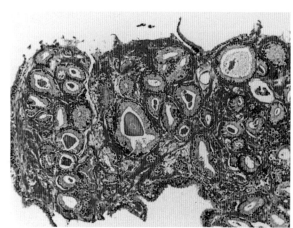

Fig 5.7 Variable sized acini in Gleason pattern 3.

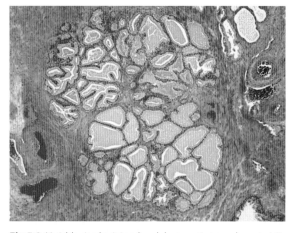

Fig 5.8 Variable sized acini and nodular grouping are characteristic of some Gleason pattern 3.

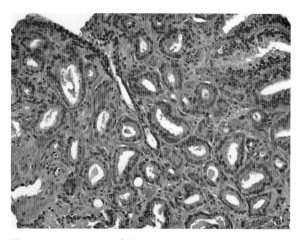

Fig 5.9 Close up view of Gleason pattern 3 showing small acini pattern.

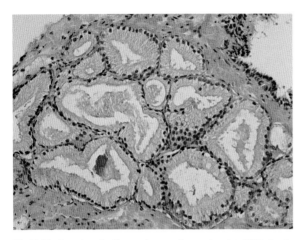

Fig 5.10 Occasionally Gleason pattern 3 may simulate BPH glands.

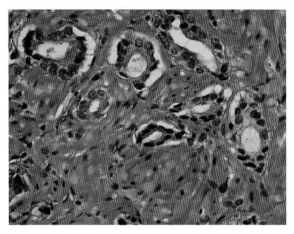

Fig 5.11 Slightly distorted acini with asymmetric lumens of Gleason pattern 3. Some authors might include this morphology as pattern 4 poorly formed glands.

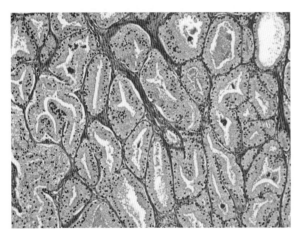

Fig 5.12 Large acini Gleason pattern 3.

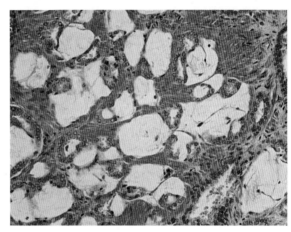

Fig 5.13 Most mucinous adenocarcinoma fall into Gleason pattern 3.

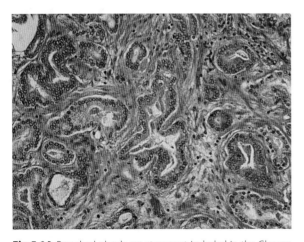

Fig 5.14 Branched glands are at present included in the Gleason pattern 3.

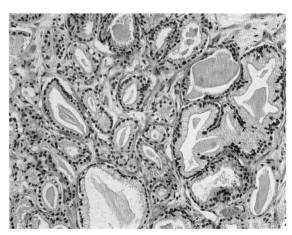

Fig 5.15 Size variability of acini with corpora amylacea in Gleason pattern 3.

- Pattern 4: Glands appear fused, cribriform or they may be poorly defined and small. Fused glands are composed of a group of glands that are no longer completely separated by stroma. The edge of a group of fused glands is scalloped and there are occasionally thin strands of connective tissue within this group. The hypernephroid pattern described by Gleason is a rare variant of fused glands with clear or very pale-staining cytoplasm that is now included within the spectrum of foamy cell carcinoma. Cribriform pattern 4 glands (currently all cribriform patterns are Gleason 4 except those with necrosis) are large or they may be irregular with jagged edges. As opposed to fused glands, there are no strands of stroma within a cribriform gland. Poorly defined glands do not have a lumen that is completely encircled by epithelium. Figs 5.17–5.30

- Pattern 5: Almost complete loss of glandular lumina, which are only occasionally present. The epithelium forms solid sheets, solid strands or single cells invading the stroma; comedonecrosis may be present. Care must be applied when assigning a Gleason pattern 4 or 5 to limited cancer on needle biopsy to exclude an artifact of tangential sectioning of lower grade cancer. Figs 5.31–5.39

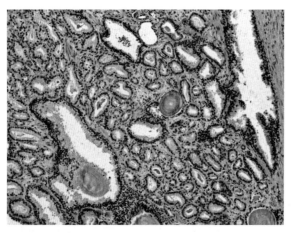

Fig 5.16 Acini proliferating between non-neoplastic glands is seen in this Gleason pattern 3.

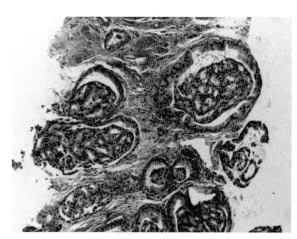

Fig 5.17 Glomeruloid pattern of Gleason 4.

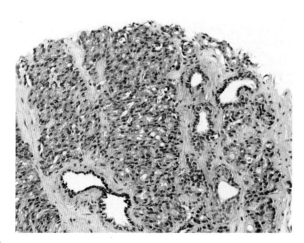

Fig 5.18 Fused acini pattern of Gleason 4.

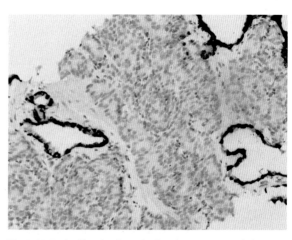

Fig 5.19 Lack of basal cells in this fused acini pattern of Gleason 4 (anti-34βE12 immunohistochemistry).

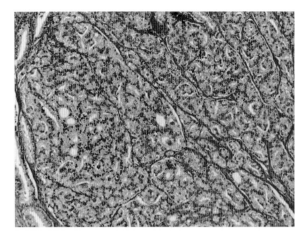

Fig 5.20 Fused acini pattern of Gleason 4 with some cribriform morphology.

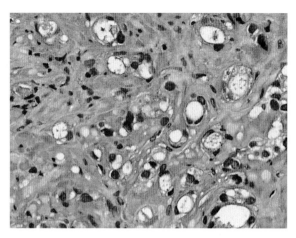

Fig 5.21 Poorly formed glands pattern of Gleason 4.

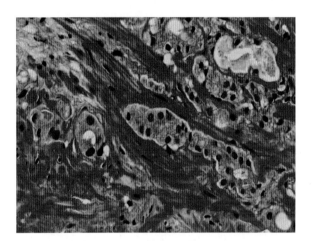

Fig 5.22 Poorly formed glands pattern of Gleason 4.

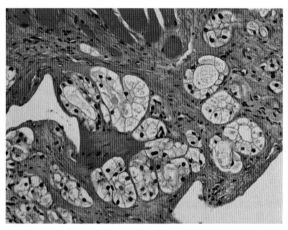

Fig 5.23 Poorly formed glands pattern of Gleason 4.

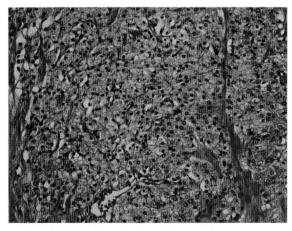

Fig 5.24 Hypernephroid pattern of Gleason 4 now considered with the spectrum of foamy cell carcinoma Gleason 4.

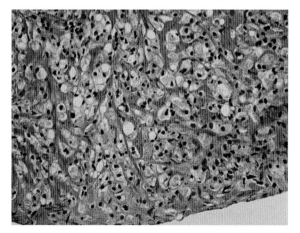

Fig 5.25 Poorly formed glands pattern of Gleason 4 with some individual looking cells most probably as result of tangential sectioning.

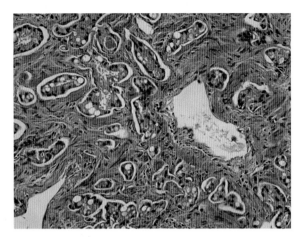

Fig 5.26 Poorly formed glands pattern of Gleason 4.

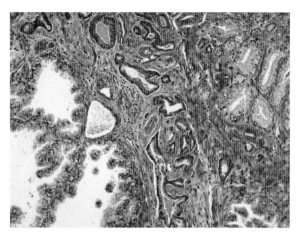

Fig 5.27 Poorly formed glands pattern of Gleason 4. Some authors might consider this as Gleason pattern 3, but the level of architectural atypia supports its inclusion as Gleason 4.

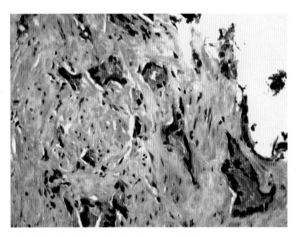

Fig 5.28 Poorly formed glands pattern of Gleason 4.

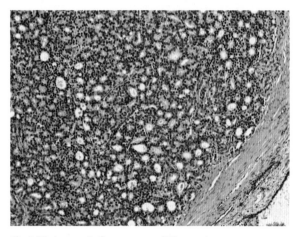

Fig 5.29 Large cribriform pattern of Gleason 4.

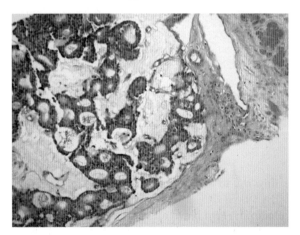

Fig 5.30 Mucinous adenocarcinoma of the prostate. In this case, a cribriform morphology is recognized, which support inclusion as Gleason 4.

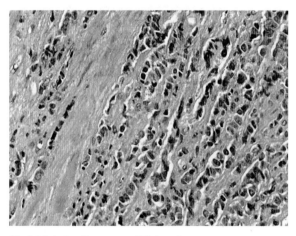

Fig 5.31 Indian file pattern of Gleason 5.

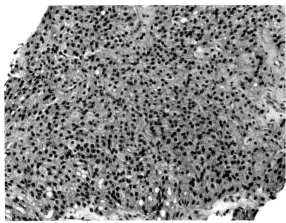

Fig 5.32 Solid growth pattern of Gleason 5.

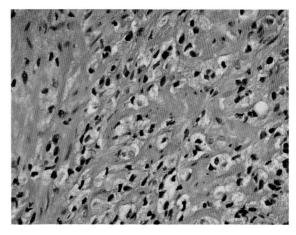

Fig 5.33 Individual clear cells of Gleason 5.

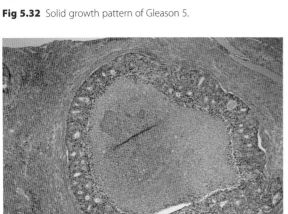

Fig 5.34 Comedo-type necrosis of Gleason 5.

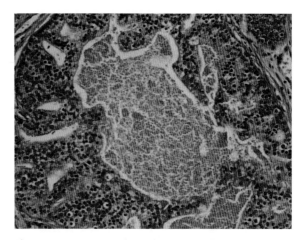

Fig 5.35 Proteinaceous luminal material in Gleason pattern 4 should not be misdiagnosed as comedo-type necrosis.

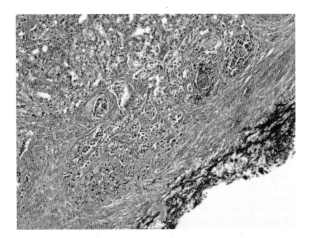

Fig 5.36 Apoptotic cells should not be mistaken as Gleason 5.

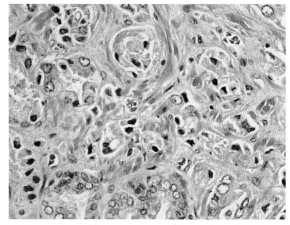

Fig 5.37 Individual-looking cells as depicted in this case should not be misdiagnosed as Gleason 5, since most of these cells represent tangential sectioning. Deeper levels may be useful to arrive to correct diagnoses.

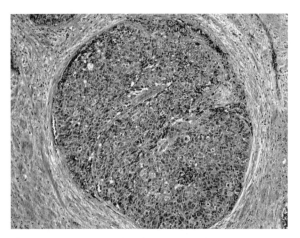

Fig 5.38 Solid growth with early necrosis in Gleason 5.

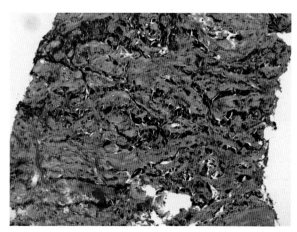

Fig 5.39 These distorted-looking cells represent typically Gleason 5.

5.3 Reporting Gleason Scores in Prostate Needle Biopsies

5.3.1 Gleason Score 2–4

- The diagnosis of Gleason score 2–4 on needle biopsies should be made "rarely, if ever," as agreed by the International Society of Urological Pathology, and the reasons are compelling: 1) Gleason score 2–4 cancer is extraordinarily rare in needle biopsies as compared to transurethral resection specimens; 2) poor reproducibility among experts; 3) the correlation with the prostatectomy score is poor and 4) a "low" score of Gleason 2–4 may misguide clinicians into believing that there is an indolent tumor.
- Gleason score of 1+1=2 is a grade that should not be diagnosed regardless of the type of specimen, since most of these cases in the era of Gleason would today be referred to as atypical adenomatous hyperplasia (adenosis). Cribriform morphology is not allowed within Gleason pattern 2.

5.3.2 Gleason Pattern 3

- Cribriform morphology is not allowed within Gleason pattern 3. Therefore, the majority of cribriform patterns should be diagnosed as Gleason pattern 4. As agreed by the International Society of Urological Pathology, "Individual cells" would not be allowed within Gleason pattern 3.

5.3.3 Gleason Pattern 4

- The importance of the percentage of Gleason 4 pattern in Gleason score 7 tumors accumulates rapidly. In recently generated nomograms, patients with Gleason score 4+3 vs. 3+4 are stratified differently. Whether or not the percentage of pattern 4 tumors should be included in the report remains optional at present time. Small, ill-defined glands with poorly formed glandular lumina also warrant the diagnosis of Gleason pattern 4.

5.3.4 Gleason Pattern 5

- Comedonecrosis when seen in solid nests or cribriform masses should be regarded as Gleason pattern 5. However, the definition of comedonecrosis requires intraluminal necrotic cells and/or nuclear debris (karyorrhexis).

5.3.5 Tertiary Pattern

- Another important issue in current practice is the recognition and reporting of the tertiary pattern in needle biopsies.
- This includes tumors with patterns 3, 4 and 5 in various proportions on a biopsy. Tertiary patterns are uncommon, but when the worst Gleason grade is the tertiary pattern, it should influence the final

Gleason score, and therefore the primary pattern and the highest grade should be recorded following the rule of "the most and the worst." A case with primary Gleason pattern 3, secondary pattern 4 and tertiary pattern 5 should be assigned a Gleason score of 8.

5.3.6 Needle Biopsy with Different Cores Showing Different Grades

- This is related to when one or more of the cores show pure high grade cancer (i.e., Gleason score 4+4=8) and the other cores show pattern 3 (3+3, 3+4 or 4+3) cancer. If one reports the grades of each core separately, the highest grade tumor (Gleason score 8) would typically be the one selected by the clinician as the grade of the entire case.
- Others give instead an overall score for the entire case. For example, in a case with Gleason score 4+4=8 on one core with pattern 3 (3+3=6, 3+4=7, 4+3=7) on other cores, the overall score for the entire case would be Gleason score 4+3=7 or 3+4=7, depending on whether pattern 4 or 3 predominated.
- Likewise, it was demonstrated that when one core is Gleason score 4+4=8 with other cores having pattern 3, the pathological stage at radical prostatectomy is comparable to cases with all needle cores having Gleason score 4+4=8. The use of the highest core grade of the given case in cases where there are multiple cores of different grades advocated in current tables and nomograms gives additional support for giving cores a separate grade rather than an overall score for the entire case.
- Consequently, it has been recommended to assign individual Gleason scores to separate cores as long as the cores were submitted in separate containers or the cores were in the same container, yet specified by the urologist as to their location (i.e. by different color inks). In addition, one has the option to also give an overall score at the end of the case.
- In cases where a container contains multiple pieces of tissue and one cannot be sure if one is looking at an intact core, it is recommended that one should only give an overall score for that container.

5.4 Reporting Gleason Scores in Radical Prostatectomies

- In these specimens, one should assign the Gleason score based on the primary and secondary patterns with a comment if present on the tertiary pattern.

5.4.1 Gleason Scores 2–4

- Gleason scores 2–4 are rarely seen as the grade of the main tumor in radical prostatectomies performed for stages T1c or T2 disease. These tumors are typically seen in multifocal incidental adenocarcinoma of the prostate found within the transition zone in transurethral resection (TURP) specimens.
- The situation where Gleason scores 2–4 tumor represents the major tumor at radical prostatectomy performed for tumor incidentally found on TURP (stages T1a and T1b) is uncommon. In one study, Gleason score 2–4 was the grade of the main tumor in 2% of the radical prostatectomy specimens; this represents a disproportionate number of T1a and T1b tumors as compared to what would be currently seen in today's practice. All men with only Gleason scores 2–4 tumor at radical prostatectomy are cured.

5.4.2 Gleason Scores 5–6

- It is important to recognize that the majority of tumors with Gleason scores 5–6 are cured after radical prostatectomy.

5.4.3 Gleason Score 7

- Tumors with a Gleason score of 7 have a significantly worse prognosis than those with a Gleason score of 6. Given the adverse prognosis associated with Gleason pattern 4, one would expect that whether a tumor is Gleason score 3+4 versus 4+3 would influence prognosis. There have been several studies addressing Gleason score 3+4 as compared to Gleason score 4+3 at radical prostatectomy with somewhat conflicting results. In one study, they reported no significant survival advantage for Gleason pattern 3+4 over 4+3, but other studies showed Gleason score 3+4 versus 4+3 correlated with both stage and progression in men with serum PSA values <10 ng/ml and organ confined disease.

- Several other investigations have shown that Gleason score 4+3 have a worse prognosis. This is an issue in which much work needs to be done.

5.4.4 Gleason Scores 8–10

- Gleason scores 8–10 may account for only 7% of the grades seen at radical prostatectomy, but these patients have highly aggressive tumors with advanced stage such that they are not amenable to surgical therapy alone. Overall, patients with Gleason scores 8–10 at radical prostatectomy have a 15% chance of having no evidence of disease at 15 years following surgery.

5.4.5 Percent Gleason Pattern 4/5

- The proportion of high grade tumor as the preferred method for grading prostate cancer has been proposed as it is predictive for progression at the extremes (greater than 70% or less than 20% pattern 4/5). It has been recently demonstrated that classifying tumors based on the combined percent of pattern 4/5 is more predictive than stratifying patients into Gleason score alone. Therefore, it has been recommended being included in the report.

5.4.6 Tertiary Gleason Pattern

- In radical prostatectomies, a higher proportion of cases are found to contain more than two grades and over 50% of them contain at least three different grades. The progression rate of Gleason scores 5–6 tumors with a tertiary component of Gleason pattern 4 is almost the same as those of pure Gleason score 7 tumors. Gleason score 7 tumors with tertiary pattern 5 experience progression rates following radical prostatectomy approximating pure Gleason 8 tumors. On the other hand, no such significance could be seen in cases of Gleason (4+4) score 8 with tertiary pattern 5; since Gleason score 8 tumors are already aggressive, the existence of pattern 5 elements adds no difference. These tumors should be graded routinely (primary and secondary patterns) with a comment in the report noting the presence of the tertiary element. In the setting of high grade cancer (score 8–10), one should ignore

lower grade patterns if they occupy less than 5% of the area of the tumor.

5.4.6.1 Tumors with One Predominant Pattern and a Small Percentage of Higher Grade Tumor

- Some controversy still exists on how to grade tumors, which are over 95% of one pattern, where there is only a very small percentage of higher grade tumor. For example, if a tumor composed of >95% Gleason pattern 3 and <5% pattern 4, some experts would assign a Gleason score 3+3=6, as it has been proposed that one needs over 5% of a pattern to be present for it to be incorporated within the Gleason score. Others might grade the tumor as Gleason score 3+4=7. It seems like the existence of a high grade component, even if it constitutes less than 5% of the whole tumor, has a significant adverse influence.

5.4.6.1 Radical Prostatectomy Specimens with Separate Tumor Nodules

- It was recommended that radical prostatectomy specimens should be processed in an organized fashion where one can make some assessment as to whether one is dealing with a dominant nodule or separate tumor nodules. One should assign a separate grade to each dominant tumor nodule(s). With only a couple of exceptions, pathologists within the consensus conference who were authors of large radical prostatectomy series had already adopted this method of grading, and the prognostic impact of the Gleason score within these series already reflects this approach. Most often, the dominant nodule is the largest tumor, which is also the tumor associated with the highest stage and highest grade.

5.5 Grading Variants and Variations of Adenocarcinoma of the Prostate

- Ductal adenocarcinoma should be graded as Gleason score 4+4=8, while retaining the diagnostic term of ductal adenocarcinoma to denote their unique clinical and pathological features.
- There is no consensus on how mucinous (colloid) carcinoma should be scored. Some authors suggest that a Gleason score of 8 is to be assigned, while others recommend ignoring mucin and grading

Table 5.2 Gleason Grades in Histological Variants and Variations of Prostate Cancer

Variations of Acinar Adenocarcinoma
- Atrophic carcinoma (underlying glandular pattern most pattern 3 or 4)
- Pseudohyperplastic and microcystic (pattern 3)
- Glomeruloid (pattern 4)
- Cribriform carcinoma (pattern 4)
- Collagenous micronodules (mucinous fibroplasia) (underlying glandular pattern [most pattern 3])
- Foamy gland carcinoma (underlying glandular pattern [most pattern 3])
- Non-mucinous signet-ring cell features (cytoplasmic vacuoles) (underlying glandular pattern [pattern 3, 4 or 5])
- Hypernephroid (now recognize as pattern 4 foamy carcinoma)
- Other variations (underlying glandular pattern)

Variants of Prostate Adenocarcinoma
- Ductal carcinoma (pattern 4)
- Small cell carcinoma (no grade applies)
- Mucinous (colloid) carcinoma (grade according to underlying pattern 3 or 4)
- Mucinous signet-ring cell carcinoma (no grade applies)
- Sarcomatoid carcinoma (no grade applies)
- Pleomorphic giant cell (pattern 5)
- Adenosquamous carcinoma (no grade applies)
- Lymphoepithelioma-like (no grade applies)
- Basal cell/adenoid cystic carcinoma (no grade applies)
- Urothelial carcinoma (involving prostatic ducts and acini with or without stromal invasion) (no grade applies)
- Squamous cell carcinoma (no grade applies)

the tumor based on the underlying architectural pattern. Small cell, sarcomatoid and mucinous signet-ring cell carcinomas should not be assigned a Gleason grade. It has been suggested that the rare pleomorphic giant cell carcinoma of the prostate should be assigned a pattern 5. Table 5.2

5.6 Correlation between Needle Biopsy and RP Gleason Scores

- There have been several studies addressing the correlation between Gleason scores in needle biopsies and corresponding radical prostatectomy specimens. Although earlier studies used the thicker (14-gauge) needle biopsies, more recent series are based on thin-core (18-gauge) needles used in conjunction with biopsy guns attached to trans-rectal ultrasound. Sextant or other modes of systematic sampling are typically performed in the more current series. In a recent compilation of data on 3,789 patients from 18 studies, exact correlation of Gleason scores was found in 43% of cases and correlation plus or minus one Gleason core unit in 77% of cases.

- Under-grading of carcinoma in needle biopsy is the most common problem, occurring in 42% of all reviewed cases. Importantly, over-grading of carcinoma in needle biopsies may also occur, but this was only found in 15% of cases. In general, adverse findings on needle biopsy accurately predict adverse findings in the radical prostatectomy specimen, whereas favorable findings on the needle biopsy do not necessarily predict favorable findings in the radical prostatectomy specimens, in large part due to sampling error.

5.6.1 Sources of Discrepancies between Needle Biopsy and RP Gleason Scores

5.6.1.1 Sampling Error

- Perhaps the most important factor is sampling error, which relates to the small amount of tissue removed by thin-core needle biopsies. The average 20-mm, 18-gauge core samples approximately 0.04% of the average gland volume (40 cc). The most common type of sampling error occurs when there is a higher grade component present within the radical prostatectomy specimen which is not sampled on needle biopsy. This typically occurs when a needle biopsy tumor is graded as Gleason score 3 + 3 = 6. In the radical prostatectomy, there exists a Gleason pattern 4 which was not sampled on the biopsy, resulting in a prostatectomy Gleason 3 + 4 = 7.

- In some instances, under-grading results from an attempt to grade very tiny areas of carcinoma, so-called minimal or limited adenocarcinoma. Scores of minimal adenocarcinoma in needle biopsies show a reasonably strong correlation with radical prostatectomy scores, but the Gleason scores do not have the same power to predict extra-prostatic extension and positive margin status as they do in non-minimal carcinomas.

- Over-grading can result from sampling error in cases where the high grade pattern is selectively represented in needle biopsy. It may only represent a very minor element in the radical prostatectomy specimen. Even the same cancer focus may have different grades depending on the area sampled.

5.6.1.2 Borderline Cases

- The other source of discrepancy between biopsy and radical prostatectomy is borderline cases. In the description of the Gleason grading system, there are some cases that are right at the interface between two different patterns where there will be inter-observer variability and possible even intra-observer variability.

5.6.1.3 Pathology Error

- Pathology error is most frequently seen when pathologists assign a Gleason score of ≤4 on a needle biopsy which in fact was Gleason score 5–6. Many pathologists under-grade needle biopsies by confusing quantitative changes with qualitative changes. When there is a limited focus of small glands of cancer on needle biopsy, by definition, this is a Gleason pattern 3. Gleason pattern 3 consists of small glands with an infiltrative pattern. Biopsying truly low grade adenocarcinoma of the prostate could not result in just a few neoplastic glands, but rather would be more extensive, as low grade adenocarcinoma grows as nodules of closely packed glands rather than infiltrating in and among normal glands.
- Under-grading may result from difficulty in recognizing an infiltrative growth pattern or failing to recognize the presence of small areas of gland fusion.

5.6.1.4 Pathologists' Education and Experience

- The pathologists' experience in grading thin-core needle biopsies can also influence overall correlation with radical prostatectomy results. With experience, pathologists recognize grading pitfalls; in particular, the fact that Gleason scores of 4 and lower are almost non-existent in needle biopsy situations. Furthermore, small areas of fusion in the presence of a predominantly grade 3 background are recognized and will yield a Gleason score of 7, which often correlates well with radical prostatectomy results.

5.6.1.5 Intra-observer and Inter-observer Variability

- Reproducibility studies can be categorized as intra-observer and inter-observer. For investigations of intra-observer agreement of Gleason grades, exact agreement was reported in 43% to 78% of cases, and agreement within plus or minus one Gleason score unit was reported in 72% to 87% of cases. Gleason wrote that he duplicated exactly his previous histological scores approximately 50% of the time.

- Highly variable levels of inter-observer agreement on Gleason scores have also been reported, with range of 36% to 81% for exact agreement and 69% to 86% observers within plus or minus one Gleason score unit. Improvements in Gleason grading reproducibility can be achieved by recognizing problematic areas and educating physicians via meetings, courses, website tutorials and publications that specifically focus on the Gleason grading system.

5.7 2014 ISUP Modified Gleason System

- The major changes, compared with the previous 2005 ISUP revision, are a better definition of the Gleason pattern 4, resulting in shrinkage of the pattern 3 and expansion of the pattern 4. Gleason pattern 4 now includes cribriform, glomeruloid, fused and poorly formed glands. Cribriform glands are all considered as a Gleason pattern 4, regardless of their morphology.
- Glands with glomeruloid features are considered as pattern 4. In cases with borderline histology between Gleason pattern 3 and pattern 4, the lower grade is favored. All this means that only discrete well-formed glands, including branched glands, are at present included in the 2014 modified Gleason pattern 3.
- Such modifications have resulted in a grading shift, with an increase in the percentage of Gleason score 7 compared to Gleason score 6 Pca. In addition, since certain patterns previously included in the pattern 3 are now pattern 4, Pcas graded as Gleason score 3+3=6 by the 2014 ISUP modified Gleason system have a far better prognosis compared to Gleason score 6 Pcas based on the 2005 revision. The concordance between biopsy and subsequent radical prostatectomy (RP) grades has improved.
- Another important change is that in the setting of high grade Pca on needle biopsy, the lower pattern is included in the Gleason score if it is less than 5% of the tumor. With three distinct patterns (such as pattern 3, 4 and 5) on needle biopsy, the most prevalent pattern is added to the highest one, instead of to the second most common pattern. The presence of a tertiary pattern 5 on RP

Table 5.3 ISUP 2014 Modified Gleason and Grade Groups

ISUP 2014 Modified Gleason	Grade Group
GS ≤ 6 (3 + 3)	1
GS 7 (3 + 4)	2
GS 7 (4 + 3)	3
GS 8 (4 + 4) / GS 8 (3 + 5) (5+3)	4
GS 9 – 10	5

specimens has been a controversial item; the recommendation in the 2005 ISUP modified system was to report it as a tertiary pattern if it occupied less than 5% of the tumor and to include pattern 5 in the final Gleason score if it represented more than 5% of the tumor. In the 2014 ISUP modified Gleason system, the tertiary is only recorded for RPs with either 3+4=7 or 4+3=7 with tertiary pattern 5.

- The 2014 ISUP modified Gleason system requires that the percentage of pattern 4 in Gleason score 7 tumors, particularly in Gleason score 3+4=7 cancers, has to be reported, due to the fact that patients with a minor component (<5%) of pattern 4 may be considered still eligible for active surveillance (AS), although others may accept up to 20% of pattern 4.

5.7 Five-tiered Grading Prognostic System (Grade Groups 1–5)

- In 2016, the WHO classification of urologic tumors included a different scheme to report grading of prostate adenocarcinoma to avoid the fact that patients diagnosed with Gleason score 6 prostate tumors erroneously think that their cancer is of intermediate risk, despite the fact that Gleason score 6 is the lowest grade used on needle biopsies of the prostate. Table 5.3; Figs 5.40–5.41
- The intermediate grade category includes Gleason score 3+4=7 and 4+3=7 Pcas, despite the fact that several studies have shown worse prognosis for patients with Gleason score 7 with primary pattern 4 versus 3. In addition, Gleason score 9–10 cancers have a worse prognosis than Gleason score 4+4=8 Pcas.
- In 2013, a new grading system for Pca was proposed by Pierorazio et al. to address some of the limitations of the modified Gleason system. The new system, based on data collected at the Johns Hopkins Hospital, suggested five distinct Grade Groups (GGs).

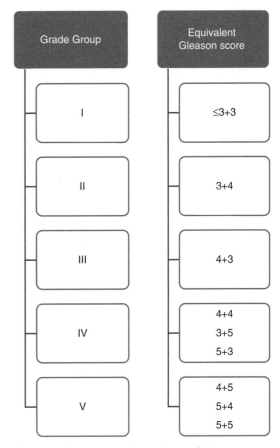

Fig 5.40 Gleason score and equivalent grade group.

- Grade Group 1 includes tumors composed only of individual discrete well-formed glands (Gleason score ≤6); Grade Group 2 includes tumors composed predominantly of well-formed glands with a lesser component of poorly formed/fused/cribriform glands (Gleason score 3+4=7); Grade Group 3 includes tumors with predominantly poorly formed/fused/cribriform glands with a lesser component of well-formed glands (Gleason score 4+3=7); Grade Group 4 includes tumors composed only of poorly formed/fused/cribriform glands or tumors with well-formed glands and lesser component lacking glands, or tumors predominantly lacking glands with a lesser component of well-formed glands (Gleason score 4+4=8; 3+5=8; 5+3=8); and Grade Group 5 includes tumors lacking gland formation (or with necrosis) with or without poorly formed/fused/cribriform glands (Gleason score 9/10).

Grade group I (GS ≤ 6): Only individual discrete well-formed glands

Grade group II (GS 3+4=7):Predominantly well-formed glands with lesser component of poorly-formed/fused/cribriform glands

Grade group III (GS 3+4=7): Predominantly poorly formed/fused/cribriform glands with lesser component of well-formed glands

Grade group IV (GS 4+4=8; 3+5=8; 5+3=8): Only poorly-formed/fused/cribriform glands or

Predominantly well-formed glands and lesser component lacking glands or

Predominantly lacking glands and lesser component of well-formed glands

Grade group V (GS 9–10): Lacks gland formation (or with necrosis) with or w/o poorly formed/fused/cribriform glands

Fig 5.41 Basic criteria to apply to grade groups.

- Tertiary pattern 5 on 3+4=7 and 4+3=7 tumors at RP would be recorded as Grade Group 2 and 3, respectively, with a minor higher grade pattern; likewise, other possible recording is to the grade group with a plus at the end – for example, Groups 2+ or 3+.
- The five-tiered grading prognostic system has been validated in a large multi-institutional study and in a nationwide population-based cohort of men with prostate cancer treated by RP or radiation therapy, and in a series of patients with long-term follow-up treated conservatively.
- This new prostate grading system has been accepted by the World Health Organization (WHO) for the 2016 edition of WHO classification of Tumors of the Urinary System and Male Genital Organs.
- The editors of the major uro-oncology journals are recommending authors to use the new system in the reporting of Pca in their papers. The updated protocols from the College of American Pathologists and the 8th edition of the American Joint Committee on Cancer staging manual incorporate the five-tiered grading prognostic system. For the time being, it is suggested to report the five-tiered grading prognostic system with the 2014 ISUP modified Gleason system
- Genomic analysis identified distinct genomic profiles between the 5 GGs, supporting GG 1

through GG 3 as distinct classes, but with genomic similarity for GG 4 and GG 5. Such observations have given support for increasing genomic changes with increasing GGs.

Suggested Reading

Minardi D, Mazzucchelli R, Scarpelli M, Massari F, Ciccarese C, Lopez-Beltran A, Cheng L, Montironi R. Prostate Cancer Glands with Cribriform Architecture and with Glomeruloid Features Should Be Considered as Gleason Pattern 4 and Not Pattern 3. Future Oncol. 2016 Jun; **12**(12): 1431–33.

McKenney Jesse K. MD, Wei Wei MS, Hawley Sarah MS, Auman Heidi PhD, Newcomb Lisa F. PhD, Boyer Hilary D. BSc, Fazli Ladan MD, Simko Jeff MD PhD, Hurtado-Coll Antonio MD, Troyer Dean A. MD PhD, Tretiakova Maria S. MD PhD, Vakar-Lopez Funda MD, Carroll Peter R. MD MPH, Cooperberg Matthew R. MD MPH, Gleave Martin E. MD, Lance Raymond S. MD, Lin Dan W. MD, Nelson Peter S. MD, Thompson Ian M. MD, True Lawrence D. MD, Feng Ziding PhD, Brooks James D. MD. Histologic Grading of Prostatic Adenocarcinoma Can Be Further Optimized: Analysis of the Relative Prognostic Strength of Individual Architectural Patterns in 1275 Patients from the Canary Retrospective Cohort. Am J Surg Pathol. 2016; **40**(11): 1439–56.

Lopez-Beltran A, Mikuz G, Luque RJ, Mazzucchelli R, Montironi R. Current Practice of Gleason Grading of Prostate Carcinoma. Virchows Arch. 2006 Feb; **448**(2): 111–18.

Montironi R, Santoni M, Mazzucchelli R, Burattini L, Berardi R, Galosi AB, Cheng L, Lopez-Beltran A, Briganti A, Montorsi F, Scarpelli M. Prostate Cancer: From Gleason Scoring to Prognostic Grade Grouping. Expert Rev Anticancer Ther. 2016; 16(4): 433–40.

Montironi R, Cheng L, Scarpelli M, Lopez-Beltran A. Pathology and Genetics: Tumours of the Urinary System and Male Genital System: Clinical Implications of the 4th Edition of the WHO Classification and Beyond. Eur Urol. 2016 Jul; 70(1): 120–23.

Brimo F, Montironi R, Egevad L, Erbersdobler A, Lin DW, Nelson JB, Rubin MA, van der Kwast T, Amin M, Epstein JI. Contemporary Grading for Prostate Cancer: Implications for Patient Care. Eur Urol. 2013; 63: 892–901.

Partin AW, Yoo J, Carter HB, Pearson JD, Chan DW, Epstein JI, Walsh PC. The Use of Prostate Specific Antigen, Clinical Stage and Gleason Score to Predict Pathological Stage in Men with Localized Prostate Cancer. J Urol. 1993; 150: 110–14.

Ohori M, Kattan MW, Koh H, Maru N, Slawin KM, Shariat S, Muramoto M, Reuter VE, Wheeler TM, Scardino PT. Predicting the Presence and Side of Extracapsular Extension: A Nomogram for Staging Prostate Cancer. J Urol. 2004; 171: 1844–49.

Cooperberg, MR, Pasta DJ, Elkin EP, Litwin MS, Latini DM, Du Chane J, Carroll PR. The University of California, San Francisco Cancer of the Prostate Risk Assessment Score: A Straightforward and Reliable Preoperative Predictor of Disease Recurrence after Radical Prostatectomy. J Urol. 2005; 173: 1938–42.

Egevad L, Mazzucchelli R, Montironi R. Implications of the International Society of Urological Pathology Modified Gleason Grading System. Arch Pathol Lab Med. 2012; 136: 426–34.

Montironi R, Cheng L, Lopez-Beltran A, Scarpelli M, Mazzucchelli R, Mikuz G, Kirkali Z, Montorsi F. Original Gleason System versus 2005 ISUP Modified Gleason System: The Importance of Indicating Which System Is Used in the Patient's Pathology and Clinical Reports. Eur Urol. 2010; 58: 369–73.

Magi-Galluzzi C, Montironi R, Epstein JI. Contemporary Gleason Grading and Novel Grade Groups in Clinical Practice. Curr Opin Urol. 2016 Sep; 26(5): 488–92.

Samaratunga H, Delahunt B, Yaxley J, Srigley JR, Egevad L. From Gleason to International Society of Urological Pathology (ISUP) Grading of Prostate Cancer. Scand J Urol. 2016 Oct; 50(5): 325–29.

Epstein JI, Allsbrook WC, Jr., Amin MB, Egevad LL, Committee IG. The 2005 International Society of Urological Pathology (ISUP) Consensus Conference on Gleason Grading of Prostatic Carcinoma. Am J Surg Pathol. 2005 Sep; 29(9): 1228–42. PubMed PMID: 16096414.

Epstein JI, Egevad L, Amin MB, Delahunt B, Srigley JR, Humphrey PA, et al. The 2014 International Society of Urological Pathology (ISUP) Consensus Conference on Gleason Grading of Prostatic Carcinoma: Definition of Grading Patterns and Proposal for a New Grading System. Am J Surg Pathol. 2016 Feb; 40(2): 244–52.

Pierorazio PM, Walsh PC, Partin AW, Epstein JI. Prognostic Gleason Grade Grouping: Data Based on the Modified Gleason Scoring System. BJU international. 2013 May; 111(5): 753–60. PubMed PMID: 23464824. Pubmed Central PMCID: 3978145.

Epstein JI, Zelefsky MJ, Sjoberg DD, Nelson JB, Egevad L, Magi-Galluzzi C, et al. A Contemporary Prostate Cancer Grading System: A Validated Alternative to the Gleason Score. European Urology. 2016 Mar; 69(3): 428–35. PubMed PMID: 26166626.

Loeb S, Folkvaljon Y, Robinson D, Lissbrant IF, Egevad L, Stattin P. Evaluation of the 2015 Gleason Grade Groups in a Nationwide Population-based Cohort. European Urology. 2015 Dec 17; (Epub ahead of print). PubMed PMID: 26707871.

Rubin MA, Girelli G, Demichelis F. Genomic Correlates to the Newly Proposed Grading Prognostic Groups for Prostate Cancer. European Urology. 2016 Nov 9; 69: 557–60.

Epstein JI. Gleason Score 2–4 Adenocarcinoma of the Prostate on Needle Biopsy: A Diagnosis that Should Not Be Made. Am J Surg Pathol. 2000 Apr; 24(4): 477–78.

Berg KD, Thomsen FB, Nerstrom C, Roder MA, Iversen P, Toft BG, et al. The Impact of the 2005 International Society of Urological Pathology Consensus Guidelines on Gleason Grading – A Matched Pair Analysis. BJU international. 2016 Jan 28; PubMed PMID: 26823232.

Billis A, Guimaraes MS, Freitas LL, Meirelles L, Magna LA, Ferreira U. The Impact of the 2005 International Society of Urological Pathology Consensus Conference on Standard Gleason Grading of Prostatic Carcinoma in Needle Biopsies. The Journal of Urology. 2008 Aug; 180 (2): 548–52. Discussion 52–53. PubMed PMID: 18550106.

Epstein JI. An Update of the Gleason Grading System. The Journal of Urology. 2010 Feb; 183(2): 433–40. PubMed PMID: 20006878.

Amin MB, Lin DW, Gore JL, Srigley JR, Samaratunga H, Egevad L, et al. The Critical Role of the Pathologist in Determining Eligibility for Active Surveillance as a Management Option in Patients with Prostate Cancer: Consensus Statement with Recommendations Supported by the College of American Pathologists, International Society of Urological Pathology, Association of Directors of Anatomic and Surgical Pathology, the New Zealand Society of Pathologists, and the Prostate Cancer Foundation. Archives of Pathology & Laboratory Medicine. 2014 Oct; 138(10): 1387–405.

Humphrey PA. Prostate Pathology. Chicago, IL: ASCP Press; 2003.

D'Amico AV, Whittington R, Malkowicz SB, Fondurulia J, Chen MH, Tomaszewski JE, et al. The Combination of

Preoperative Prostate Specific Antigen and Postoperative Pathological Findings to Predict Prostate Specific Antigen Outcome in Clinically Localized Prostate Cancer. The Journal of Urology. 1998 Dec; 160(**6** Pt 1): 2096–101. PubMed PMID: 9817331.

Chan TY, Partin AW, Walsh PC, Epstein JI. Prognostic Significance of Gleason Score 3+4 versus Gleason Score 4+3 Tumor at Radical Prostatectomy. Urology. 2000 Nov 1; **56**(5): 823–27. PubMed PMID: 11068310.

Makarov DV, Sanderson H, Partin AW, Epstein JI. Gleason Score 7 Prostate Cancer on Needle Biopsy: Is the Prognostic Difference in Gleason Scores 4 + 3 and 3 + 4 Independent of the Number of Involved Cores? The Journal of Urology. 2002 Jun; **167**(6): 2440–42. PubMed PMID: 11992053.

Amin A, Partin A, Epstein JI. Gleason Score 7 Prostate Cancer on Needle Biopsy: Relation of Primary Pattern 3 or 4 to Pathological Stage and Progression after Radical Prostatectomy. The Journal of Urology. 2011 Oct; **186**(4): 1286–90. PubMed PMID: 21862072.

Matoso A, Epstein JI. Grading of Prostate Cancer: Past, Present, and Future. Current Urology Reports. 2016 Mar; **17**(3): 25. PubMed PMID: 26874537.

Humphrey PA, Amin MB, Berney DM, Billis A, Cao D, Cheng L, et al. *Acinar Adenocarcinoma: WHO Classification of Tumours of the Urinary System and Male Genital Organs.* Moch H, Humphrey PA, Ulbright TM, Reuter VE, editors. Lyon: IARC; 2016.

Zietman A, Smith J, Klein E, Droller M, Dasgupta P, Catto J. Consensus Guidelines for Reporting Prostate Cancer Gleason Grade. Urology. 2016 Mar 22; PubMed PMID: 27015942.

Smith JA, Jr., Zietman A, Klein E, Droller MJ, Dasgupta P, Catto J, et al. Stage Grouping. The Journal of Urology. 2016 Mar 17; PubMed PMID: 26995538.

Zietman A, Smith J, Klein E, Droller M, Dasgupta P, Catto J. Describing the Grade of Prostate Cancer: Consistent Use of Contemporary Terminology Is Now Required. European Urology. 2016 Mar 21; PubMed PMID: 27012550.

Ross HM, Kryvenko ON, Cowan JE, Simko JP, Wheeler TM, Epstein JI. Do Adenocarcinomas of the Prostate with Gleason Score (GS) </=6 Have the Potential to Metastasize to Lymph Nodes? Am J of Surg Pathol. 2012 Sep; **36**(9): 1346–52. PubMed PMID: 22531173. Pubmed Central PMCID: 3421030.

Sauter G, Steurer S, Clauditz TS, Krech T, Wittmer C, Lutz F, et al. Clinical Utility of Quantitative Gleason Grading in Prostate Biopsies and Prostatectomy Specimens. European Urology. 2016 Apr; **69**(4): 592–98. PubMed PMID: 26542947.

Tsao CK, Gray KP, Nakabayashi M, Evan C, Kantoff PW, Huang J, et al. Patients with Biopsy Gleason 9 and 10 Prostate Cancer Have Significantly Worse Outcomes Compared to Patients with Gleason 8 Disease.

The Journal of Urology. 2015 Jul; **194**(1): 91–97. PubMed PMID: 25623747.

Berney DM, Beltran L, Fisher G, North BV, Greenberg D, Moller H, et al. Validation of a Contemporary Prostate Cancer Grading System Using Prostate Cancer Death as Outcome. Br Jnl Cancer. 2016 (in press).

Ploussard G, Isbarn H, Briganti A, Sooriakumaran P, Surcel CI, Salomon L, et al. Can We Expand Active Surveillance Criteria to Include Biopsy Gleason 3+4 Prostate Cancer? A Multi-institutional Study of 2,323 Patients. Urologic Oncology. 2015 Feb; **33**(2): 71e1–9. PubMed PMID: 25131660.

Chen RC, Rumble RB, Jain S. Active Surveillance for the Management of Localized Prostate Cancer (Cancer Care Ontario guideline): American Society of Clinical Oncology Clinical Practice Guideline Endorsement Summary. Journal of Oncology Practice / American Society of Clinical Oncology. 2016 Mar;**12**(3): 267–9. PubMed PMID: 26883405.

Montironi R, Scarpelli M, Mazzucchelli R, Lopez-Beltran A, Santoni M, Briganti A, Montorsi F, Cheng L. Does Prostate Acinar Adenocarcinoma with Gleason Score 3+3=6 Have the Potential to Metastasize? Diagn Pathol. 2014 Oct 18; **9**: 190. doi: 10.1186/s13000-014-0190-z.

Siadat F, Sykes J, Zlotta AR, Aldaoud N, Egawa S, Pushkar D, Kuk C, Bristow RG, Montironi R, van der Kwast T. Not All Gleason Pattern 4 Prostate Cancers Are Created Equal: A Study of Latent Prostatic Carcinomas in a Cystoprostatectomy and Autopsy Series. Prostate. 2015 Sep; **75**(12): 1277–84.

Epstein JI, Egevad L, Humphrey PA, Montironi R. Members of the ISUP Immunohistochemistry in Diagnostic Urologic Pathology Group. Best Practices Recommendations in the Application of Immunohistochemistry in the Prostate: Report from the International Society of Urologic Pathology Consensus Conference. Am J Surg Pathol. 2014 Aug; **38**(8): e6–e19. doi: 10.1097/PAS.0000000000000238.

Amin MB, Epstein JI, Ulbright TM, Humphrey PA, Egevad L, Montironi R, Grignon D, Trpkov K, Lopez-Beltran A, Zhou M, Argani P, Delahunt B, Berney DM, Srigley JR, Tickoo SK, Reuter VE. Members of the ISUP Immunohistochemistry in Diagnostic Urologic Pathology Group. Best Practices Recommendations in the Application of Immunohistochemistry in Urologic Pathology: Report from the International Society of Urological Pathology Consensus Conference. Am J Surg Pathol. 2014 Aug; **38**(8): 1017–22. doi: 10.1097/PAS.0000000000000254.

Montironi R, Lopez-Beltran A, Mazzucchelli R, Scarpelli M, Galosi AB, Cheng L. Contemporary Update on Pathology-related Issues on Routine Workup of Prostate Biopsy: Sectioning, Tumor Extent Measurement, Specimen Orientation, and Immunohistochemistry. Anal Quant Cytopathol Histpathol. 2014 Apr; **36**(2): 61–70. Review.

Histologic Subtypes of Prostatic Carcinoma

6.1 Rare Histologic Subtypes of Prostatic Carcinoma

- A wide variety of histologic subtypes and variants of acinar adenocarcinoma may be seen in the prostate. Table 6.1

6.2 Pseudohyperplastic Adenocarcinoma

- Pseudohyperplastic prostate cancer resembles benign prostate glands in that the neoplastic glands are large with branching and papillary infolding. Most occur in the transition zone, which is the usual site for benign prostatic hyperplasia.
- The recognition of cancer with this pattern is based on the architectural pattern of numerous closely packed glands as well as nuclear features more typical of carcinoma. Pseudohyperplastic cancer is considered Gleason score 3+3=6.

Table 6.1 Histological Classification of Carcinoma of the Prostate

| 1 | Adenocarcinoma (acinar, conventional, usual type) |
| 2 | Variants and variations of adenocarcinoma and other carcinomas |

- Pseudohyperplastic adenocarcinoma and microcystic adenocarcinoma
- Foamy gland adenocarcinoma
- Atrophic adenocarcinoma
- Adenocarcinoma with glomeruloid features
- Mucinous (colloid) adenocarcinoma
- Signet-ring cell mucinous carcinoma
- Oncocytic adenocarcinoma
- Lymphoepithelioma-like carcinoma
- Pleomorphic giant cell carcinoma
- Prostatic duct adenocarcinoma and PIN-like ductal adenocarcinoma
- Small cell carcinoma and other neuroendocrine tumors
- Sarcomatoid carcinoma
- Basaloid carcinoma
- Urothelial carcinoma
- Adenosquamous carcinoma
- Squamous cell carcinoma

- One pattern of pseudohyperplastic adenocarcinoma consists of numerous large glands that are almost back-to-back with straight, even luminal borders and abundant cytoplasm. Comparably sized benign glands either have papillary infolding or are atrophic.
- The presence of cytological atypia in some of these glands further distinguishes them from benign glands. It is helpful to verify the absence of basal cells by immunohistochemistry.
- HOXB13 G84E variant-related prostate cancers show frequent pseudohyperplastic-type features and markedly low prevalence of ERG.
- A cystic variant of pseudohyperplastic carcinoma (microcystic carcinoma) has been recognized. Table 6.2; Figs 6.1–6.4

6.3 Foamy Gland Adenocarcinoma

- Foamy gland (also known as xanthomatous) cancer is a variant of acinar adenocarcinoma of the prostate that is characterized by having abundant foamy appearing cytoplasm. Although the cytoplasm has a xanthomatous appearance, it does not contain lipids, but rather empty microvacuoles.
- Typical features of adenocarcinoma such as nuclear enlargement and prominent nucleoli are frequently rare-to-absent, which makes this lesion difficult to recognize as carcinoma, especially on biopsy material. Some cases may show cystic appearance.
- Whereas most cases of foamy gland carcinoma would be graded as Gleason 3+3, higher grade foamy gland carcinoma exists and should be graded accordingly based on the pattern, most frequently, Gleason pattern 4.
- Characteristically, the nuclei in foamy gland carcinoma are small and densely hyperchromatic. Nuclei in foamy gland cancer are round, more so than those of benign prostatic secretory cells. It is recognized as carcinoma by its architectural

Table 6.2 Main Clinico-Pathological Findings in Unusual Variants of Prostate Cancer

	Clinical features	PSA	IHC	Age at	Incidence	Treatment
* Small cell carcinoma	Bladder outlet obstruction; disseminated disease; paraneoplastic syndrome	Usually elevated	Cells are positive for at least one of the neuroendocrine marker, i.e. chromogranin A, synaptophysin, neuron specific enolase, CD56 or TTF-1	65–72 years (range 24 to 89)	0.3% to 1%	Chemotherapy
Ductal adenocarcinoma	Obstruction and hematuria are common; some with metastases and advanced clinical stage at diagnosis	Most above 4 ng/ml	PSA and PSAP are almost always positive; Alpha-methylacyl CoA racemase can be detected at a reduced level	63–72 years (range of 41–89 years)	1.3% **	Androgen deprivation therapy may provide palliative relief, even though this cancer is less hormonally responsive than acinar adenocarcinoma
Sarcomatoid carcinoma (carcinosarcoma)	Urinary tract obstruction and symptoms of frequency, urgency and nocturia	Variable normal or elevated	Epithelial markers (cytokeratins, PSA, PSAP) and muscle markers can be detected vimentin; immunostains are uniformly positive, and S-100 protein is consistently found in chondrosarcomatous regions, others +	70 years of age (range 50–89)	Rare	Surgery followed by chemotherapy
Basal cell carcinoma	Urinary obstruction	Variable	stained with 34betaE12 and p63 and negative for PSA, PSAP and alpha-methylacyl-coenzyme racemase; others+	Elderly	Rare	Surgery
Squamous cell carcinoma	Some arise in prostate cancer patients following endocrine therapy or radiotherapy or schistosomiasis.	Most with normal serum PSA and PSAP.	Negative for PSA and PSAP immunostains	Average age of 68	Less than 0.6%	Surgery
Adenosquamous carcinoma	50% may arise in prostate cancer patients following endocrine therapy or radiotherapy	Most with normal serum PSA and PSAP.	Negative for PSA and PSAP immunostains	Average age of 68	Rare	Surgery
Primary urothelial carcinoma	Urinary obstruction and hematuria	Variable (limited information)	They are PSA and PSAP negative, and are frequently positive for the cytokeratins CK20, CK7, high molecular weight cytokeratins bound by antibody 34betaE12, p63, thrombomodulin and uroplakins.	Range 45 to 90 years	0.7 to 2.8%	Surgery
Pleomorphic giant cell carcinoma	Urinary obstruction; metastases	Variable (limited information)	PSA, PSAP, Cytokeratins	45–77 years	Very rare	Surgery, androgen blockade, radiation therapy
LELC	Urinary obstruction	5.5 ng/ml	Cytokeratins, PSA and PSAP	66 years	Vary rare	Surgery

* In about one-half of cases, it is pure small cell carcinoma, while in the other half, there is a mixture with prostatic acinar adenocarcinoma.
** The incidence of mixed ductal-acinar adenocarcinoma is 4.8%.

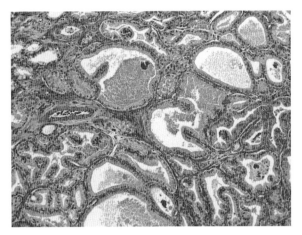

Fig 6.1 Pseudohyperplastic carcinoma may simulate benign hyperplasia of the prostate.

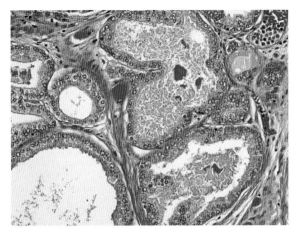

Fig 6.2 High power view of pseudohyperplastic carcinoma.

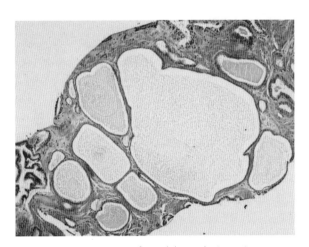

Fig 6.3 Microcystic variant of pseudohyperplastic carcinoma.

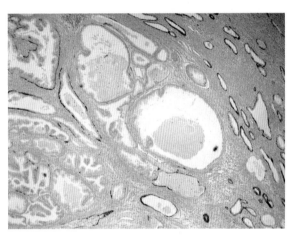

Fig 6.4 Pseudohyperplastic carcinoma lacks basal cell layer (anti-34βE12 immunohistochemistry).

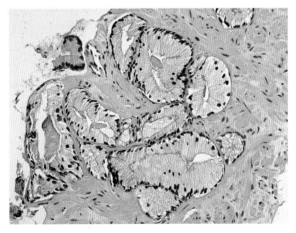

Fig 6.5 Foamy gland adenocarcinoma showing xanthomatous cytoplasm of the cells.

pattern of crowded and/or infiltrative glands, and frequently present dense pink acellular secretions.

- In most cases, foamy gland cancer is seen in association with ordinary adenocarcinoma of the prostate. Figs 6.5–6.8

6.4 Atrophic Adenocarcinoma

- An unusual variant of prostate cancer resembles benign atrophy owing to its scant cytoplasm. Atrophic prostate cancers are unrelated with a prior history of treatment.
- The diagnosis is based on several features. First, atrophic prostate cancer may demonstrate a truly infiltrative process with individual small atrophic glands situated between larger benign glands.

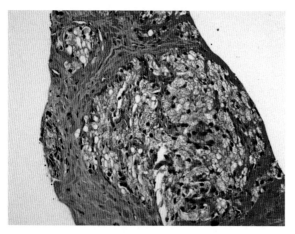

Fig 6.6 Foamy gland adenocarcinoma showing xanthomatous cytoplasm of the cells with poorly formed glands Gleason 4.

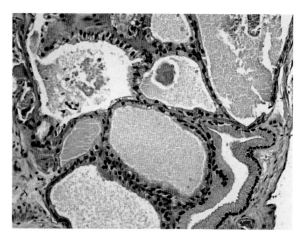

Fig 6.7 Cystic form of foamy gland adenocarcinoma.

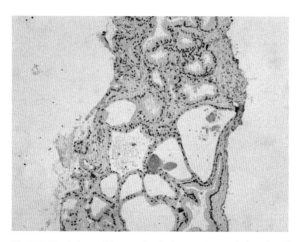

Fig 6.8 Cystic form of foamy gland adenocarcinoma lacking basal cells (anti-34βE12 immunohistochemistry).

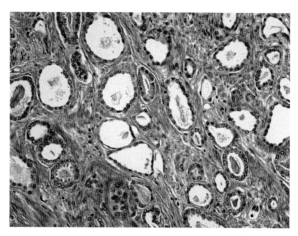

Fig 6.9 Microscopic appearance of atrophic prostate carcinoma.

In contrast, benign atrophy has a lobular configuration with a centrally dilated atrophic gland surrounded by clustered smaller glands that are not truly infiltrative.

- Whereas some forms of atrophy are associated with fibrosis, atrophic prostate cancer lacks fibrotic stroma. Atrophic prostate cancer may also be differentiated from benign atrophy by the presence of marked cytological atypia. Atrophy may show enlarged nuclei and prominent nucleoli, although not the huge eosinophilic nucleoli seen in some atrophic prostate cancers.
- Ordinary type carcinoma is usually present. The absence of basal cell layer at immunohistochemistry is of help. AMACR is expressed in 70% of atrophic carcinomas, which is lower compared to acinar adenocarcinoma.

- Most glands are well-formed with lumina (Gleason 3), and less often exhibit fusion (Gleason 4).
- Main differential diagnosis is simple atrophy which shows a lobular growth and does not exhibit gland infiltration. Benign atrophic glands retain basal cell layer that may be discontinuous and atrophic cancer has a complete loss of basal cell layer. Figs 6.9–6.11

6.5 Adenocarcinoma with Glomeruloid Features

- Prostatic adenocarcinoma with glomeruloid features is characterized by intraluminal ball-like clusters of cancer cells reminiscent of renal glomeruli. Glomeruloid structures in the prostate

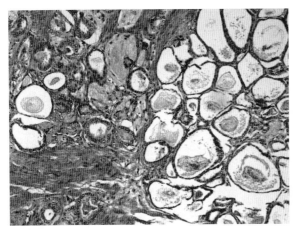

Fig 6.10 Atrophic prostate carcinoma may be occasionally cystic.

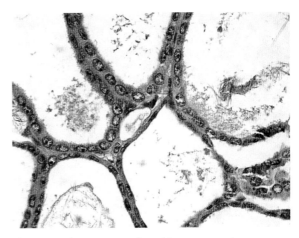

Fig 6.11 High power view of atrophic prostate carcinoma.

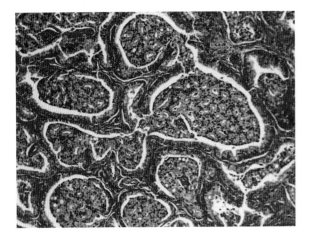

Fig 6.12 Microscopic appearance of glomeruloid prostate cancer.

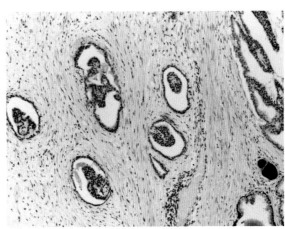

Fig 6.13 Glomeruloid prostate cancer lacks basal cells (anti-p63 immunohistochemistry).

represent an uncommon but distinctive pattern of growth that is specific for malignancy (glomeruloid-like structures in non-malignant glands are extremely rare).

- Glomeruloid features may be a useful diagnostic clue for malignancy, particularly in some challenging needle biopsy specimens. This pattern of growth is usually seen in high grade adenocarcinoma, often with extraprostatic extension. A Gleason score of 4 is assigned to this variant of prostate cancer. Figs 6.12–6.13

6.6 Mucinous and Signet-ring Cell Adenocarcinoma

- Mucinous adenocarcinoma is one of the least common morphologic variants of prostatic carcinoma. The diagnosis of mucinous (colloid) adenocarcinoma of the prostate gland should be made when at least 25% of the tumor resected contains lakes of extracellular mucin.

- Mucinous prostate adenocarcinomas behave aggressively, with most patients dead or remaining with active disease five years after therapy. Mucinous prostate adenocarcinomas have a propensity to develop bone metastases. These cases should be graded as Gleason pattern 3 or 4 (less frequent).

- Mucinous adenocarcinoma shows higher (83%) incidence of TMPRSS2-ERG fusion than usual acinar carcinoma (about 50%).

- Some carcinomas of the prostate may have a signet-ring cell appearance, yet the vacuoles do not contain mucin (prostatic carcinoma with cytoplasmic vacuoles). These vacuolated cells may

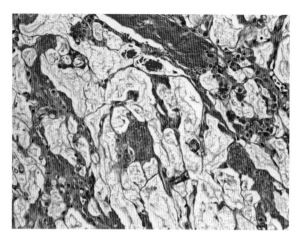

Fig 6.14 Microscopic appearance of mucinous (colloid) adenocarcinoma.

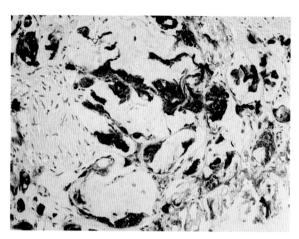

Fig 6.15 Mucinous (colloid) adenocarcinoma with PSA expression.

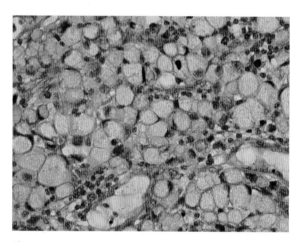

Fig 6.16 Mucinous signet-ring cell adenocarcinoma.

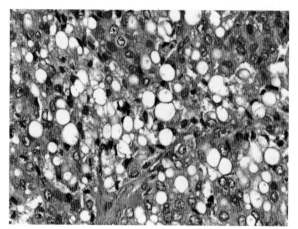

Fig 6.17 Microscopic appearance of prostate carcinoma with cytoplasmic vacuoles (signet-ring-like). This should not be misdiagnosed as mucinous signet-ring carcinoma.

be present as singly invasive cells, in single glands and in sheets of cells. These tumors should be graded as if the vacuoles were not present.

- Only a few cases of prostate cancer have been reported with mucin positive signet cells (signet-ring mucinous adenocarcinoma). These tumors seem to be very aggressive, and should be distinguished from adenocarcinoma with cytoplasmic vacuoles. Figs 6.14–6.17

6.7 Oncocytic Adenocarcinoma

- This is an exceptionally rare variant of Pca with unclear clinical significance.
- Tumor cells have round to ovoid hyperchromatic nuclei, and have granular cytoplasm with numerous mitochondria on ultrastructural or immunohistochemical examination and are

strongly positive for PSA. A high Gleason grade, elevated serum PSA and metastasis of similar morphology have been documented. Fig 6.18

6.8 Lymphoepithelioma-like Carcinoma of the Prostate

- This undifferentiated carcinoma is characterized by indistinct cytoplasmic borders with syncytial arrangement of malignant cells associated with a heavy lymphocytic infiltrate, including some plasma cells and neutrophils; one case had a prominent infiltration of eosinophils. Associated ordinary adenocarcinoma is always present and may be of acinar, adenosquamous or ductal type.

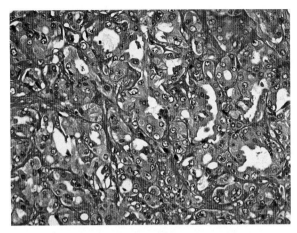

Fig 6.18 Microscopic appearance of oncocytic prostate carcinoma.

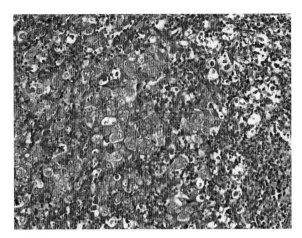

Fig 6.19 Microscopic appearance of lymphoepithelioma-like carcinoma of the prostate.

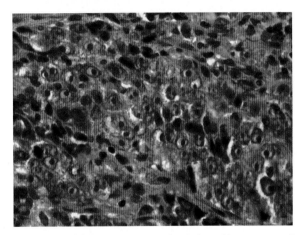

Fig 6.20 High power view of lymphoepithelioma-like carcinoma of the prostate with syncytial arrangement.

- Immunohistochemical staining demonstrated that lymphoepithelioma-like carcinoma was positive for prostate-specific antigen, prostate acid phosphatase, alpha-methylacyl coenzyme A racemase and epithelial membrane antigen; several cytokeratins (AE1/AE3, 7, 8 and 20 [rare cells]) were also immunoreactive. The mean Ki-67 labeling index was 53% (range, 40%–70%), and the p53 expression in all cases was low (10%–20%).
- The lymphoid component was mainly composed of T with a minor subset of B cells, admixed with some dendritic cells and histiocytes as seen by S100 and CD68 immunoreactivity. Latent membrane protein 1 immunostaining and in situ hybridization for Epstein-Barr virus were negative in all five lymphoepithelioma-like carcinoma cases.

- The largest series included five patients at a mean age of 76 years with obstructive symptoms and high PSA. Most presented at advanced clinical stage. Four patients died of disease from 8 to 26 months. Figs 6.19–6.20

6.9 Prostatic Ductal Adenocarcinoma

- Subtype of adenocarcinoma (also known as endometrioid carcinoma) composed of larger glands lined by tall pseudostratified columnar cells. It was originally thought to originate from prostate utricle. In pure form, ductal adenocarcinoma accounts for 0.2% to 0.8% of prostate cancers. It is assumed that almost all cases have an acinar component.
- Ductal adenocarcinoma may be located centrally around the prostatic urethra or more frequently located peripherally admixed with typical acinar adenocarcinoma. A centrally located adenocarcinoma may also be associated with a peripherally located acinar adenocarcinoma. Peripherally occurring ductal carcinomas typically show a white-gray firm appearance similar to acinar adenocarcinoma. These tumors may lead to enlargement or induration of the prostate.
- Centrally occurring tumors appear as exophytic polypoid or papillary masses protruding into the urethra around the verumontanum and may cause hematuria, urinary urgency and eventually urinary retention. In these cases, there may be no abnormalities on rectal examination. Because of the papillary growth, some of these cases may

83

Table 6.3 Subtypes of Ductal Carcinoma of the Prostate

- Micropapillary ductal adenocarcinoma
- Mucinous ductal adenocarcinoma
- Foamy gland ductal adenocarcinoma
- Cystic prostatic ductal adenocarcinoma (cystadenocarcinoma)
- Ductal adenocarcinoma with Paneth cell-like neuroendocrine differentiation
- PIN-like ductal adenocarcinoma

be misdiagnosed as papillary urothelial carcinoma of high grade arising in the urethra.

- Of importance is that serum PSA levels may be normal, particularly in patients with only centrally located tumors. In most cases, transurethral resections performed for diagnosis or relief of the urinary obstruction will provide an accurate diagnostic. Transrectal needle core biopsies may also obtain diagnostic tissue when the tumor is more peripherally located. In addition, areas of ductal adenocarcinoma may be incidentally identified in prostatectomy specimens. And in those cases, there is a tendency to find more advanced disease.
- A Gleason score of 4+4 (or 4+5 if comedonecrosis is present) applies to ductal prostatic adenocarcinoma. The recent described PIN-like ductal carcinoma should be graded as Gleason pattern 3.
- A cystic subtype of ductal adenocarcinoma has been described (cystadenocarcinoma). Table 6.3

6.9.1 Histopathology and Clinical Significance

- Ductal adenocarcinoma is aggressive with 27–39% of cases showing metastases at the time of diagnosis. Five-year survival rate is poor, ranging from14% to 40% of patients.
- Ductal adenocarcinoma is characterized by tall columnar cells with abundant usually amphophilic cytoplasm, which form a single or pseudostratified layer. The cytoplasm is often amphophilic and may occasionally appear clear. In some cases, there are numerous mitoses and marked cytological atypia. In other cases, the cytological atypia is minimal, which makes a diagnosis difficult, particularly on needle

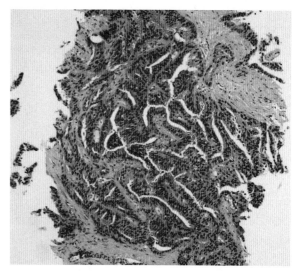

Fig 6.21 Microscopic appearance of ductal carcinoma of the prostate.

biopsy. Peripherally located tumors are often admixed with cribriform, glandular or solid patterns as seen in acinar adenocarcinoma.

- Ductal adenocarcinomas are mostly equivalent to Gleason patterns 4. In some cases, comedo-type necrosis is present and therefore considered equivalent to Gleason pattern 5.
- Ductal adenocarcinoma displays a variety of architectural patterns which are often intermingled: cribriform, papillary, individual gland or solid pattern. Immunohistochemically ductal adenocarcinoma is strongly positive for PSA and PAP and racemase. Tumor cells are typically negative for basal cell specific markers; however, a frequently incomplete basal cell layer may be present in pre-existing ducts with cancer.
- Ductal adenocarcinoma usually spreads along the urethra or into the prostatic ducts with or without stromal invasion, or may spread similar to that of acinar carcinoma with invasion to extraprostatic tissues and metastasis to pelvic lymph nodes or distal organs. Ductal adenocarcinomas appear to have a tendency to metastasize to lung and penis, but also may metastasize to bones.
- Ductal adenocarcinoma must be distinguished from urothelial carcinoma, ectopic prostatic tissue, benign prostatic polyps and papillary-polypoid urethritis. Figs 6.21–6.31

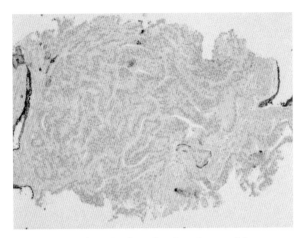

Fig 6.22 Lack of basal cells in ductal carcinoma of the prostate (anti-34βE12 immunohistochemistry).

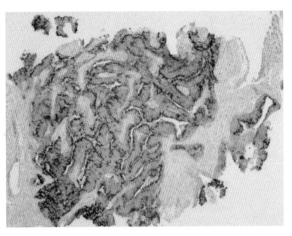

Fig 6.23 Racemase expression in ductal carcinoma of the prostate.

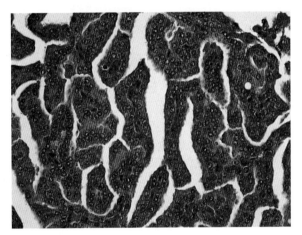

Fig 6.24 Microscopic appearance of ductal carcinoma of the prostate with papillary features.

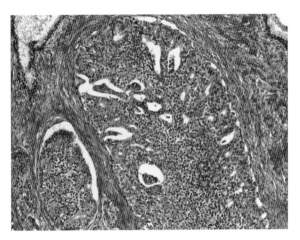

Fig 6.25 Microscopic appearance of ductal carcinoma of the prostate with cribriform features.

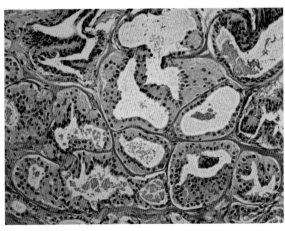

Fig 6.26 Histologic features of PIN-like ductal carcinoma of the prostate.

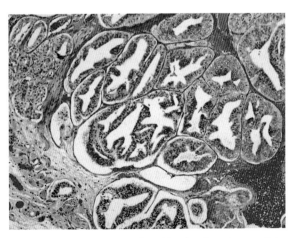

Fig 6.27 High power view of PIN-like ductal carcinoma of the prostate.

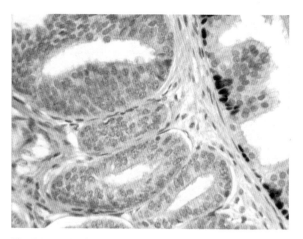

Fig 6.28 Lack of basal cells in PIN-like ductal carcinoma of the prostate (anti-p63 immunohistochemistry).

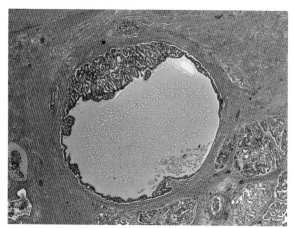

Fig 6.29 Cystadenocarcinoma of the prostate.

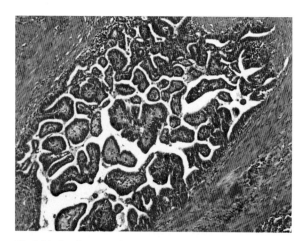

Fig 6.30 Papillary cystadenocarcinoma of the prostate.

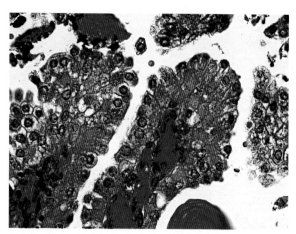

Fig 6.31 Papillary cystadenocarcinoma of the prostate with onco-cytic features.

6.10 Intraductal Carcinoma

- Intraepithelial spread of prostatic carcinoma within pre-existing non-neoplastic ducts or acini is known as intraductal carcinoma (IDC). It is characterized by the preservation of basal cells and is now regarded as tumor progression prior to cancer invasion. Others suggest that is a carcinomatous evolution of high grade PIN preceding invasion. Table 6.3; Figs 6.32–6.37

- Diagnosis of IDC in practice is limited by its problematic distinction from PIN; both lesions retain basal cells, as seen by immunohistochemistry. Most cases are seen in association with high grade Pca. IDC has been reported to occur in 18% of radical prostatectomy samples. The incidence is higher in specimens with higher stages. In needle biopsies, it might be present in about 3% of cases. Basal cell immunohistochemistry may show complete or partial basal cell layer.

- IDC as an isolated finding is rare (< 1% of biopsies) and its clinical significance remains a matter of discussion. An alternative term of atypical cribriform lesion has been suggested to report needle biopsy cases with borderline features between IDC and high grade PIN.

- Current approach to IDC is by identifying large acini and ducts containing basal cells filled with malignant epithelial cells that show solid or dense cribriform patterns. In cases with luminal pattern of loose cribriform or micropapillary, marked nuclear atypia ($\geq 6x$) or non-focal comedonecrosis is required. Other authors suggest combining a set of major and minor criteria, as follows.

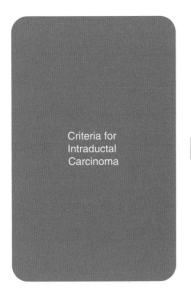

Criteria for Intraductal Carcinoma

Malignant epithelial cells filling large acini and prostatic ducts, with preservation of basal cells and:

• Solid or dense cribriform pattern

Or

Loose cribriform or micropapillary pattern with either:

• Marked nuclear atypia: nuclear size 6normal

• Necrosis

Fig 6.32 Diagnostic criteria of intraductal carcinoma of the prostate.

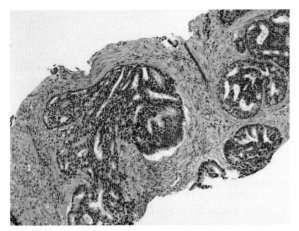

Fig 6.33 Intraductal carcinoma of the prostate as seen in needle biopsy.

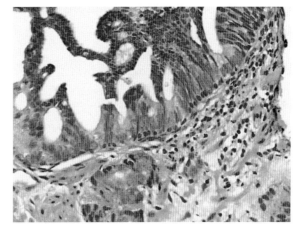

Fig 6.34 Intraductal carcinoma and associated acinar carcinoma of the prostate.

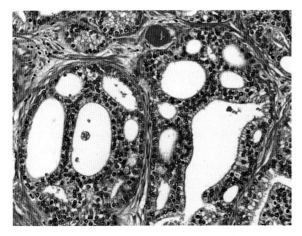

Fig 6.35 Close view of intraductal carcinoma of the prostate.

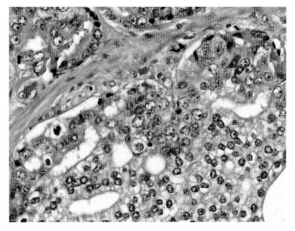

Fig 6.36 High grade nuclear features of intraductal carcinoma of the prostate.

87

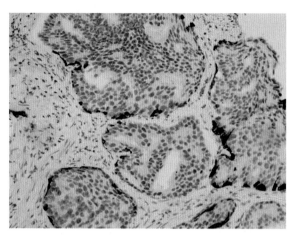

Fig 6.37 Persistence of basal cells is characteristic of intraductal carcinoma of the prostate (anti-34βE12 immunohistochemistry).

Sarcomatoid carcinoma	• Necrosis and atypical mitosis present • ALK1-, CK+, Desmin+/-, EMA+, SMA+/-, Vim+/-, S100-, p63+/-, 34βE12+/-, CK5/6+/-
Inflammatory myofibroblastic tumor	• Non-atypical mitosis. No to focal necrosis • ALK1+, CK+/-, Desmin+/-, EMA+/-, SMA+/-, Vim+, S100-, caponin+/-, h-caldesmon+/-, p63-, 34βE12-, CK5/6-

Fig 6.38 Differential diagnosis of sarcomatoid carcinoma and myofibroblastic tumor.

6.10.1 Major Criteria for Diagnosis of IDC

1 Large glands (>2x normal)
2 Presence of basal cells (confirmed by immunohistochemistry)
3 Cytologically malignant cells with frequent mitosis
4 Cells spanning gland lumen
5 Comedonecrosis

6.10.2 Minor Criteria for Diagnosis of IDC

1 Right-angle branching
2 Round, smooth gland contour
3 Frequently two populations of cells

6.11 Small Cell Carcinoma

• Small cell carcinomas of the prostate histologically are identical to small cell carcinomas of the lung and similar diagnostic criteria apply. About 50% of the patients have mixed small cell carcinoma and adenocarcinoma of the prostate. For further pathologic features, see also Chapter 7.

6.12 Sarcomatoid Carcinoma (Carcinosarcoma)

• In some series, carcinosarcoma and sarcomatoid carcinoma are considered as separate entities based on the presence of specific mesenchymal elements in the former. However, given their otherwise similar clinico-pathologic features and identically poor prognosis, these two lesions are best considered as one entity.
• Sarcomatoid carcinoma of the prostate is a rare neoplasm composed of both malignant epithelial and malignant spindle-cell and/or mesenchymal elements. Sarcomatoid carcinoma may be present in the initial pathologic material (synchronous presentation), or there may be a previous history of adenocarcinoma treated by radiation and/or hormonal therapy (metachronous). The gross appearance may resemble sarcoma. Figs 6.38–6.41
• Serum PSA is within normal limits in most cases. Nodal and distant organ metastases at diagnosis are common with less than a 35% five-year survival.

6.12.1 Histology

• Microscopically, sarcomatoid carcinoma is composed of a glandular component showing a variable Gleason score. The sarcomatoid component often consists of a non-specific malignant spindle-cell proliferation.
• Amongst the specific mesenchymal elements are osteosarcoma, chondrosarcoma, rhabdomyosarcoma, leiomyosarcoma, liposarcoma, angiosarcoma or multiple types of heterologous differentiation. Sarcomatoid

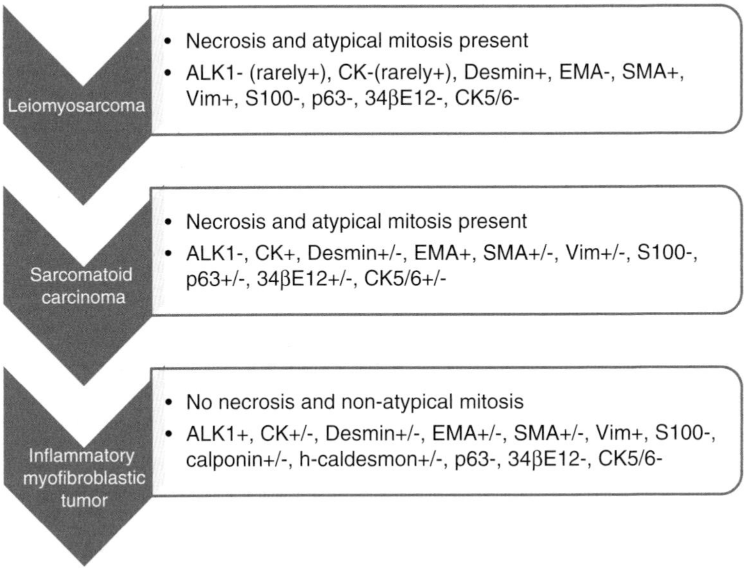

Leiomyosarcoma
- Necrosis and atypical mitosis present
- ALK1- (rarely+), CK-(rarely+), Desmin+, EMA-, SMA+, Vim+, S100-, p63-, 34βE12-, CK5/6-

Sarcomatoid carcinoma
- Necrosis and atypical mitosis present
- ALK1-, CK+, Desmin+/-, EMA+, SMA+/-, Vim+/-, S100-, p63+/-, 34βE12+/-, CK5/6+/-

Inflammatory myofibroblastic tumor
- No necrosis and non-atypical mitosis
- ALK1+, CK+/-, Desmin+/-, EMA+/-, SMA+/-, Vim+, S100-, calponin+/-, h-caldesmon+/-, p63-, 34βE12-, CK5/6-

Fig 6.39 Differential diagnosis of sarcomatoid carcinoma and leiomyosarcoma.

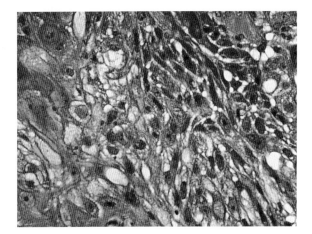

Fig 6.40 Sarcomatoid carcinoma (spindle cell carcinoma) of the prostate.

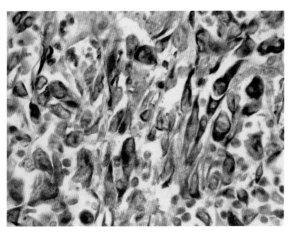

Fig 6.41 Cytokeratin expression in sarcomatoid carcinoma (spindle cell carcinoma) of the prostate.

carcinoma should be distinguished from the rare carcinoma with metaplastic, benign-appearing bone or cartilage in the stroma.
- Epithelial elements react with antibodies against PSA and/or pan-cytokeratins, whereas spindle-cell elements react with markers of soft tissue tumors and variably express cytokeratins or CD10.

6.13 PIN-like Ductal Carcinoma
- The malignant glands exhibit cellular stratification and thus morphologically resemble PIN. Patients' mean age is 68 years. The malignant glands have lumina that may be tufted, micropapillary, flat or a mixture of patterns.

- Predominance of stratified tall columnar cells is similar to ductal carcinoma and therefore it is referred to as PIN-like ductal carcinoma. It is suggested that they may behave similar to Gleason score 3+3=6 cancers.
- This unusual form of prostatic carcinoma needs to be distinguished from high grade PIN. Lack of staining for basal cell markers is a diagnostic clue.

6.14 Pleomorphic Giant Cell Carcinoma
- Extremely rare and aggressive variant of prostate cancer with large, bizarre, anaplastic giant cells.

Mean age at diagnosis is 66 years. Occurs admixed with high grade prostate carcinoma Gleason score 9. Pleomorphic giant cells are DNA aneuploidy and immunoreactive for epithelial markers and focally with PSA and PAP. Figs 6.42–6.44

Table 6.4 Gleason Grades in Histological Variants and Variations of Prostate Cancer

Variations of acinar adenocarcinoma

- Atrophic carcinoma (underlying glandular pattern [most 3 or 4])
- Pseudohyperplastic and microcystic (pattern 3)
- Glomeruloid (pattern 4)
- Cribriform carcinoma (pattern 4)
- Collagenous micronodules (mucinous fibroplasia) (underlying glandular pattern [most pattern 3])
- Foamy gland carcinoma (underlying glandular pattern [most pattern 3])
- Non-mucinous signet-ring cell features (cytoplasmic vacuoles) (underlying glandular pattern [pattern 3, 4 or 5])
- Hypernephroid (now recognized as pattern 4 foamy carcinoma)
- Other variations (underlying glandular pattern)

Variants of prostate adenocarcinoma

- Ductal carcinoma (pattern 4)
- Small cell carcinoma (no grade applies)
- Mucinous (colloid) carcinoma (grade according to underlying pattern 3 or 4)
- Mucinous signet-ring cell carcinoma (no grade applies)
- Sarcomatoid carcinoma (no grade applies)
- Pleomorphic giant cell (pattern 5)
- Adenosquamous carcinoma (no grade applies)
- Lymphoepithelioma-like (no grade applies)
- Basal cell/adenoid cystic carcinoma (no grade applies)
- Urothelial carcinoma (involving prostatic ducts and acini with or without stromal invasion) (no grade applies)
- Squamous cell carcinoma (no grade applies)

6.15 Grading Variants and Variations of Adenocarcinoma of the Prostate

- Ductal adenocarcinoma should be graded as Gleason score 4+4=8, while retaining the diagnostic term of ductal adenocarcinoma to denote their unique clinical and pathological features.
- Mucinous (colloid) carcinoma should be scored as Gleason 3 or 4 pattern. Small cell, sarcomatoid and mucinous signet-ring cell carcinomas should not be assigned a Gleason grade. It has been suggested that the rare pleomorphic giant cell carcinoma of the prostate should be assigned a pattern 5. Table 6.4

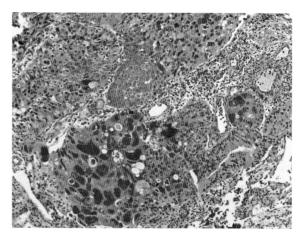

Fig 6.42 Pleomorphic giant cell carcinoma of the prostate.

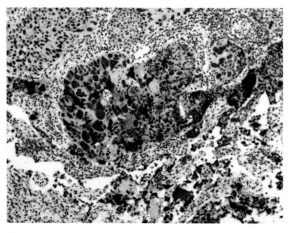

Fig 6.43 PSA expression in pleomorphic giant cell carcinoma of the prostate.

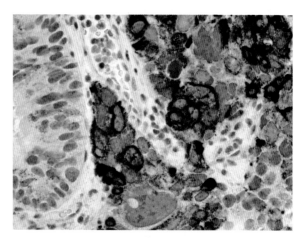

Fig 6.44 Racemase expression in pleomorphic giant cell carcinoma of the prostate.

Suggested Reading

Pacelli A, Lopez-Beltran A, Egan AJ, Bostwick DG. Prostatic Adenocarcinoma with Glomeruloid Features. Hum Pathol. 1998 May; **29**(5): 543–46.

Kato M, Tsuzuki T, Kimura K, Hirakawa A, Kinoshita F, Sassa N, Ishida R, Fukatsu A, Kimura T, Funahashi Y, Matsukawa Y, Hattori R, Gotoh M. The Presence of Intraductal Carcinoma of the Prostate in Needle Biopsy Is a Significant Prognostic Factor for Prostate Cancer Patients with Distant Metastasis at Initial Presentation. Mod Pathol. 2016 Feb; **29**(2): 166–73.

Iczkowski KA, Egevad L, Ma J, Harding-Jackson N, Algaba F, Billis A, Camparo P, Cheng L, Clouston D, Comperat EM, Datta MW, Evans AG, Griffiths DF, Guo CC, Hailemariam S, Huang W, Humphrey PA, Jiang Z, Kahane H, Kristiansen G, La Rosa FG, Lopez-Beltran A, MacLennan GT, Magi-Galluzzi C, Merrimen J, Montironi R, Osunkoya AO, Picken M M, Rao N, Shah RB, Shanks JH, Shen SS, Tawfik OW, True LD, Van der Kwast T, Varma M, Wheeler TM, Zynger DL, Sahr N, Bostwick DG. Intraductal Carcinoma of the Prostate: Interobserver Reproducibility Survey of 39 Urologic Pathologists. Ann Diagn Pathol. 2014 Dec; **18**(6): 333–42.

Montironi R, Cheng L, Lopez-Beltran A, Scarpelli M, Montorsi F. A Better Understating of the Morphological Features and Molecular Characteristics of Intraductal Carcinoma Helps Clinicians Further Explain Prostate Cancer Aggressiveness. Eur Urol. 2015 Mar; **67**(3): 504–07.

Lotan TL, Epstein JI. Gleason Grading of Prostatic Adenocarcinoma with Glomeruloid Features on Needle Biopsy. Hum Pathol. 2009 Apr; **40**(4): 471–77.

Schweizer MT, Cheng HH, Tretiakova MS, Vakar-Lopez F, Klemfuss N, Konnick EQ, Mostaghel EA, Nelson PS, Yu EY, Montgomery B, True LD, Pritchard CC. Mismatch Repair Deficiency May Be Common in Ductal Adenocarcinoma of the Prostate. Oncotarget. 2016 Oct 15; doi: 10.18632/oncotarget.12697.

Seipel AH, Delahunt B, Samaratunga H, Egevad L. Ductal Adenocarcinoma of the Prostate: Histogenesis, Biology and Clinicopathological Features. Pathology. 2016 Aug; **48**(5): 398–405.

Priemer DS, Montironi R, Wang L, Williamson SR, Lopez-Beltran A, Cheng L. Neuroendocrine Tumors of the Prostate: Emerging Insights from Molecular Data and Updates to the 2016 World Health Organization Classification. Endocr Pathol. 2016 Jun; **27**(2): 123–35.

Fisher KW, Zhang S, Wang M, Montironi R, Wang L, Baldrige LA, Wang JY, MacLennan GT, Williamson SR, Lopez-Beltran A, Cheng L. TMPRSS2-ERG Gene Fusion Is Rare Compared to PTEN Deletions in Stage T1a Prostate Cancer. Mol Carcinog. 2016 Aug 8; doi: 10.1002/mc.22535.

Wang L, Davidson DD, Montironi R, Lopez-Beltran A, Zhang S, Williamson SR, MacLennan GT, Wang C, Wang M, Emerson RE, Du X, Cheng L. Small Cell Carcinoma of the Prostate: Molecular Basis and Clinical Implications. Histol Histopathol. 2015 Apr; **30**(4): 413–24. Review.

Montironi R, Cheng L, Lopez-Beltran A, Montironi MA, Galosi AB, Scarpelli M. A Low Grade PIN-like Neoplasm of the Transition Zone Immunohistochemically Negative for Basal Cell Markers: A Possible Example of Low Grade Adenocarcinoma with Stratified Epithelium. Pathology. 2014 Jan; **46**(1): 88–91.

Berney DM, Algaba F, Camparo P, Compérat E, Griffiths D, Kristiansen G, Lopez-Beltran A, Montironi R, Varma M, Egevad L. Variation in Reporting of Cancer Extent and Benign Histology in Prostate Biopsies among European Pathologists. Virchows Arch. 2014 Mar 4; [Epub ahead of print].

Montironi R, Cheng L, Lopez-Beltran A, Montironi MA, Galosi AB, Scarpelli M. A Low Grade PIN-like Neoplasm of the Transition zone Immunohistochemically Negative for Basal Cell Markers: A Possible Example of Low Grade Adenocarcinoma with Stratified Epithelium. Pathology. 2014 Jan; **46**(1): 88–91.

Berney DM, Algaba F, Camparo P, Compérat E, Griffiths D, Kristiansen G, Lopez-Beltran A, Montironi R, Varma M, Egevad L. The Reasons Behind Variation in Gleason Grading of Prostatic Biopsies: Areas of Agreement and Misconception among 266 European Pathologists. Histopathology. 2014 Feb; **64**(3): 405–11. doi: 10.1111/his.12284. Epub 2013 Nov 6.

Schelling LA, Williamson SR, Zhang S, Yao JL, Wang M, Huang J, Montironi R, Lopez-Beltran A, Emerson RE, Idrees MT, Osunkoya AO, Man YG, Maclennan GT, Baldridge LA, Compérat E, Cheng L. Frequent TMPRSS2-ERG Rearrangement in Prostatic Small Cell Carcinoma Detected by Fluorescence in Situ Hybridization: The Superiority of Fluorescence in Situ Hybridization over ERG Immunohistochemistry. Hum Pathol. 2013 Oct; **44**(10): 2227–33. doi: 10.1016/j.humpath.2013.05.005. Epub 2013 Jul 12.

Montironi R, Cheng L, Lopez-Beltran A, Mazzucchelli R, Scarpelli M. Combined Handling of Prostate Base/Bladder Neck and Seminal Vesicles in Radical Prostatectomy Specimens: Our Approach with the Whole Mount Technique. Histopathology. 2013 Sep; **63**(3): 431–35. doi: 10.1111/his.12158. Epub 2013 Jun 24. No abstract available.

Montironi R, Lopez-Beltran A, Cheng L, Montorsi F, Scarpelli M. Central Prostate Pathology Review: Should It Be Mandatory? Eur Urol. 2013 Aug; **64**(2): 199–201. Discussion 202–03. doi: 10.1016/j.eururo.2013.04.002. Epub 2013 Apr 16. No abstract available.

Varinot J, Drouin S, Rouprêt M, Montironi R, Lopez-Beltran A, Compérat E. Prostate Cancer with Clear Cell Features and an Unusual Nested-like Pattern of Growth: A Case Report. Anal Quant Cytol Histol. 2012 Oct; **34**(5): 289–92.

Cheng L, MacLennan GT, Lopez-Beltran A, Montironi R. Anatomic, Morphologic and Genetic Heterogeneity of Prostate Cancer: Implications for Clinical Practice. Expert Rev Anticancer Ther. 2012 Nov; 12(11): 1371–74. doi: 10.1586/era.12.127.

Egevad L, Ahmad AS, Algaba F, Berney DM, Boccon-Gibod L, Compérat E, Evans AJ, Griffiths D, Grobholz R, Kristiansen G, Langner C, Lopez-Beltran A, Montironi R, Moss S, Oliveira P, Vainer B, Varma M, Camparo P. Standardization of Gleason Grading among 337 European Pathologists. Histopathology. 2013 Jan; 62(2): 247–56. doi: 10.1111/his.12008.

Mazzucchelli R, Scarpelli M, Barbisan F, Santinelli A, Lopez-Beltran A, Cheng L, Montironi R. Immunohistochemical Expression of Prostate Tumour Overexpressed 1 (PTOV1) in Atypical Adenomatous Hyperplasia (AAH) of the Prostate: Additional Evidence Linking (AAH) to Adenocarcinoma. Cell Oncol (Dordr). 2013 Feb; 36(1): 37–42. doi: 10.1007/s13402-012-0111-7.

Varma M, Berney DM, Algaba F, Camparo P, Compérat E, Griffiths DF, Kristiansen G, Lopez-Beltran A, Montironi R, Egevad L. Prostate Needle Biopsy Processing: A Survey of Laboratory Practice across Europe. J Clin Pathol. 2013 Feb; 66(2): 120–23. doi: 10.1136/jclinpath-2012-200993.

Brimo F, Montironi R, Egevad L, Erbersdobler A, Lin DW, Nelson JB, Rubin MA, van der Kwast T, Amin M, Epstein JI. Contemporary Grading for Prostate Cancer: Implications for Patient Care. Eur Urol. 2013 May; 63(5): 892–901. doi: 10.1016/j.eururo.2012.10.015.

Lee S, Han JS, Chang A, Ross HM, Montironi R, Yorukoglu K, Lane Z, Epstein JI. Small Cell-like Change in Prostatic Intraepithelial Neoplasia, Intraductal Carcinoma, and Invasive Prostatic Carcinoma: A Study of 7 Cases. Hum Pathol. 2013 Mar; 44(3): 427–31. doi: 10.1016/j.humpath.2012.06.008.

Ukimura O, Coleman JA, de la Taille A, Emberton M, Epstein JI, Freedland SJ, Giannarini G, Kibel AS, Montironi R, Ploussard G, Roobol MJ, Scattoni V, Jones JS. Contemporary Role of Systematic Prostate Biopsies: Indications, Techniques, and Implications for Patient Care. Eur Urol. 2013 Feb; 63(2): 214–30. doi: 10.1016/j.eururo.2012.09.033.

Juhasz J, Kiss P. A Hitherto Undescribed Case of 'Collision' Tumour: Liposarcoma of the Seminal Vesicle and Prostatic Carcinoma. Int Urol Nephrol. 1978; 10: 185–93.

Quick Charles M. MDa, Gokden Neriman MDa, Sangoi Ankur R. MDb, Brooks James D. MDc, McKenney Jesse K. MDa. The Distribution of PAX-2 Immunoreactivity in the Prostate Gland, Seminal Vesicle, and Ejaculatory Duct: Comparison with Prostatic Adenocarcinoma and Discussion of Prostatic Zonal Embryogenesis. Human Pathology. 2010; 41: 1145–49.

Harvey Aaron M. MD, Grice Beverly HTL, Hamilton Candice HTL, Truong Luan D. MD, Ro Jae Y.

MD, Ayala Alberto G. MD, Zhai Qihui "Jim" MD. Diagnostic Utility of P504S/p63 Cocktail Prostate-specific Antigen, and Prostatic Acid Phosphatase in Montironi R, Scarpelli M, Cheng L, Lopez-Beltran A, Zhou M, Montorsi F. Do Not Misinterpret Intraductal Carcinoma of the Prostate as High-grade Prostatic Intraepithelial Neoplasia! Eur Urol. 2012 Sep; 62(3): 518–22. Epub 2012 Jun 5.

Lopez-Beltran A, Cheng L, Blanca A, Montironi R. Cell Proliferation and Apoptosis in Prostate Needle Biopsies with Adenocarcinoma Gleason Score 6 or 7. Anal Quant Cytol Histol. 2012 Apr; 34(2): 61–65.

Scarpelli M, Mazzucchelli R, Barbisan F, Santinelli A, Lopez-Beltran A, Cheng L, Montironi R. Is There a Role for Prostate Tumour Overexpressed-1 in the Diagnosis of HGPIN and of Prostatic Adenocarcinoma? A Comparison with Alpha-Methylacyl CoA Racemase. Int J Immunopathol Pharmacol. 2012 Jan–Mar; 25(1): 67–74.

Camparo P, Egevad L, Algaba F, Berney DM, Boccon-Gibod L, Compérat E, Evans AJ, Grobholz R, Kristiansen G, Langner C, Lopez-Beltran A, Montironi R, Oliveira P, Vainer B, Varma M. Utility of Whole Slide Imaging and Virtual Microscopy in Prostate Pathology. APMIS. 2012 Apr; 120(4): 298–304. doi: 10.1111/j.1600-0463.2011.02872.x. Review.

Montironi R, Lopez-Beltran A, Cheng L, Scarpelli M. Cervical-type Squamous Metaplasia and Myoepithelial Cell Differentiation in Stromal Tumor of the Prostate. Am J Surg Pathol. 2011 Nov; 35(11): 1752–54. No abstract available.

Montironi R, Mazzucchelli R, Lopez-Beltran A, Scarpelli M, Cheng L. Prostatic Intraepithelial Neoplasia: Its Morphological and Molecular Diagnosis and Clinical Significance. BJU Int. 2011 Nov; 108(9): 1394–401. doi: 10.1111/j.1464-410X.2011.010413.x. Epub 2011 Aug 26. Review.

Egevad L, Algaba F, Berney DM, Boccon-Gibod L, Compérat E, Evans AJ, Grobholz R, Kristiansen G, Langner C, Lockwood G, Lopez-Beltran A, Montironi R, Oliveira P, Schwenkglenks M, Vainer B, Varma M, Verger V, Camparo P. Interactive Digital Slides with Heat Maps: A Novel Method to Improve the Reproducibility of Gleason Grading. Virchows Arch. 2011 Aug; 459(2): 175–82. Epub 2011 Jun 23.

Williamson SR, Zhang S, Yao JL, Huang J, Lopez-Beltran A, Shen S, Osunkoya AO, MacLennan GT, Montironi R, Cheng L. ERG-TMPRSS2 Rearrangement Is Shared by Concurrent Prostatic Adenocarcinoma and Prostatic Small Cell Carcinoma and Absent in Small Cell Carcinoma of the Urinary Bladder: Evidence Supporting Monoclonal Origin. Mod Pathol. 2011 Aug; 24(8): 1120–27. doi: 10.1038/modpathol.2011.56.

Zhang C, Montironi R, MacLennan GT, Lopez-Beltran A, Li Y, Tan PH, Wang M, Zhang S, Iczkowski KA, Cheng L.

Is Atypical Adenomatous Hyperplasia of the Prostate a Precursor Lesion? Prostate. 2011 Dec; 71(16): 1746–51. doi: 10.1002/pros.21391. Epub 2011 Apr 7.

Mazzucchelli R, Nesseris I, Cheng L, Lopez-Beltran A, Montironi R, Scarpelli M. Active Surveillance for Low-risk Prostate Cancer. Anticancer Res. 2010 Sep; 30 (9): 3683–92.

Montironi R, Mazzucchelli R, Lopez-Beltran A, Cheng L. Words of Wisdom. Re: Peripheral Zone Prostate Cancers: Location and Intraprostatic Patterns of Spread at Histopathology. Eur Urol. 2010 Jul; 58(1): 180–82.

Montironi R, Cheng L, Lopez-Beltran A, Scarpelli M, Mazzucchelli R, Mikuz G, Kirkali Z, Montorsi F. Original Gleason System Versus 2005 ISUP Modified Gleason System: The Importance of Indicating which System Is Used in the Patient's Pathology and Clinical Reports. Eur Urol. 2010 Sep; 58(3): 369–73.

Montironi R, Vela Navarrete R, Lopez-Beltran A, Mazzucchelli R, Mikuz G, Bono AV. Histopathology Reporting of Prostate Needle Biopsies. 2005 Update. Virchows Arch. 2006; 449(1): 1–13.

Lopez-Beltran A, Mikuz G, Luque RJ, Mazzucchelli R, Montironi R. Current Practice of Gleason Grading of Prostate Carcinoma. Virchows Arch. 2006 Feb; 448(2): 111–18.

Epstein JI, Allsbrook WC, Amin MB, Egevad LL, Bastacky S, Lopez-Beltran A, et al. The 2005 International Society of Urological Pathology (ISUP) Consensus Conference on Gleason Grading of Prostatic Carcinoma. Am J Surg Pathol. 2005; 29: 1228–42.

Lopez-Beltran A, Eble John N, Bostwick David G. Pleomorphic Giant Cell Carcinoma of the Prostate. Archives of Pathology and Laboratory Medicine. 2005; 129: 683–85.

De Marzo AM, Platz EA, Epstein JI, Ali T, Billis A, Chan TY, Cheng L, Datta M, Egevad L, Ertoy-Baydar D, Farre X, Fine SW, Iczkowski KA, Ittmann M, Knudsen BS, Loda M, Lopez-Beltran A, Magi-Galluzzi C, Mikuz G, Montironi R, Pikarsky E, Pizov G, Rubin MA, Samaratunga H, Sebo T, Sesterhenn IA, Shah RB, Signoretti S, Simko J, Thomas G, Troncoso P, Tsuzuki TT, van Leenders GJ, Yang XJ, Zhou M, Figg WD, Hoque A, Lucia MS. A Working Group Classification of Focal Prostate Atrophy Lesions. Am J Surg Pathol. 2006 Oct; 30(10): 1281–91.

Mazzucchelli R, Lopez-Beltran A, Cheng L, Scarpelli M, Kirkali Z, Montironi R. Rare and Unusual Histological Variants of Prostatic Carcinoma: Clinical Significance. BJU Int. 2008 Nov; 102(10): 1369–74.

Mazzucchelli R, Morichetti D, Lopez-Beltran A, Cheng L, Scarpelli M, Kirkali Z, Montironi R. Neuroendocrine Tumours of the Urinary System and Male Genital Organs: Clinical Significance. BJU Int. 2009 Jun; 103(11): 1464–70. Epub 2009 Feb 27. Review.

Lopez-Beltran A, Cheng L, Prieto R, Blanca A, Montironi R. Lymphoepithelioma-like Carcinoma of the Prostate. Hum Pathol. 2009 Jul; 40(7): 982–87.

Montironi R, Cheng L, Lopez-Beltran A, Mazzucchelli R, Scarpelli M, Kirkali Z, Montorsi F. Joint Appraisal of the Radical Prostatectomy Specimen by the Urologist and the Uropathologist: Together, We Can Do It Better. Eur Urol. 2009 Dec; 56(6): 951–55.

Morichetti D, Mazzucchelli R, Lopez-Beltran A, Cheng L, Scarpelli M, Kirkali Z, Montorsi F, Montironi R. Secondary Neoplasms of the Urinary System and Male Genital Organs. BJU Int. 2009 Sep; 104(6): 770–66.

Epstein JI, Egevad L, Amin MB, Delahunt B, Srigley JR, Humphrey PA. The 2014 International Society of Urological Pathology (ISUP) Consensus. Grading Committee. Conference on Gleason Grading of Prostatic Carcinoma: Definition of Grading Patterns and Proposal for a New Grading System. Am J Surg Pathol. 2016 Feb; 40(2): 244–52.

Varma M, Egevad L, Algaba F, Berney D, Bubendorf L, Camparo P, Comperat E, Erbersdobler A, Griffiths D, Grobholz R, Haitel A, Hulsbergen-van de Kaa C, Langner C, Loftus B, Lopez-Beltran A, Mayer N, Nesi G, Oliveira P, Oxley J, Rioux-Leclercq N, Seitz G, Shanks J, Kristiansen G. Intraductal Carcinoma of Prostate Reporting Practice: A Survey of Expert European Uropathologists. J Clin Pathol. 2016 Oct; 69(10): 852–57.

Johnson H, Zhou M, Osunkoya AO. ERG Expression in Mucinous Prostatic Adenocarcinoma and Prostatic Adenocarcinoma with Mucinous Features: Comparison with Conventional Prostatic Adenocarcinoma. Hum Pathol. 2013 Oct; 44(10): 2241–46.

Bohman KD, Osunkoya AO. Mucin-producing Tumors and Tumor-like Lesions Involving the Prostate: A Comprehensive Review. Adv Anat Pathol. 2012 Nov; 19(6): 374–87.

Mikuz G. Histologic Classification of Prostate Cancer. Anal Quant Cytopathol Histpathol. 2015 Feb; 37(1): 39–47.

Paner GP, Lopez-Beltran A, So JS, Antic T, Tsuzuki T, McKenney JK. Spectrum of Cystic Epithelial Tumors of the Prostate: Most Cystadenocarcinomas Are Ductal Type with Intracystic Papillary Pattern. Am J Surg Pathol. 2016 Jul; 40(7): 886–95.

Neuroendocrine Tumors of the Prostate

Neuroendocrine differentiation in prostatic carcinoma has five forms. Table 7.1; Fig 7.1

1 Focal neuroendocrine differentiation in acinar prostatic adenocarcinoma
2 Adenocarcinoma with Paneth cell-like neuroendocrine differentiation
3 Neuroendocrine tumor (carcinoid)
4 Small cell carcinoma
5 Large cell neuroendocrine carcinoma

7.1 Focal Neuroendocrine Differentiation in Acinar Prostatic Adenocarcinoma

- Conventional acinar prostatic adenocarcinoma may present variable neuroendocrine differentiation when evaluated with immunohistochemistry. The cells may react with antibodies to chromogranin, serotonin or many other markers in about 50% of cases, most times without clinical evidence of endocrine activity. Androgen-deprivation therapy is associated with an increased number of neuroendocrine cells. Frequently, these cells are androgen-receptor negative. It remains controversial if neuroendocrine differentiation in conventional carcinoma worsens prognosis.
- About 10% of prostatic carcinomas have zones with a large number of single or clustered neuroendocrine cells detected by chromogranin A immunohistochemistry; some cells may also be serotonin positive. Immunostaining for neuron-specific enolase, synaptophysin, bombesin/gastrin-releasing peptides and a variety of other neuroendocrine peptides may also occur in individual neoplastic neuroendocrine cells, or in a more diffuse pattern, and receptors for serotonin may also be present.
- There are conflicting studies as to whether advanced androgen independent and androgen-deprived carcinomas show increased neuroendocrine differentiation. The prognostic significance of focal neuroendocrine differentiation in primary untreated prostatic carcinoma is controversial.
- In advanced prostate cancer, especially androgen independent cancer, focal neuroendocrine differentiation portends a poor prognosis. Figs 7.2–7.6

Table 7.1 Subtypes of Neuroendocrine Tumors and Related Lesions of the Prostate

1 Focal neuroendocrine differentiation in acinar prostatic adenocarcinoma
2 Adenocarcinoma with Paneth cell-like neuroendocrine differentiation
3 Well differentiated neuroendocrine tumor (carcinoid tumor)
4 Small cell carcinoma
5 Large cell neuroendocrine carcinoma

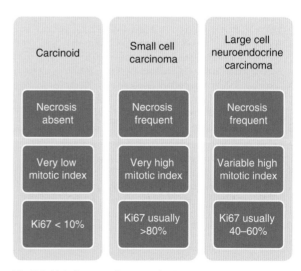

Fig 7.1 Main features of neuroendocrine tumors.

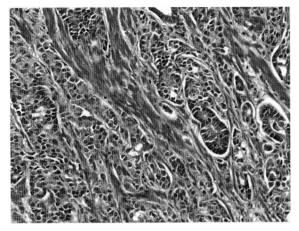

Fig 7.2 Prostate adenocarcinoma with carcinoid-like morphology.

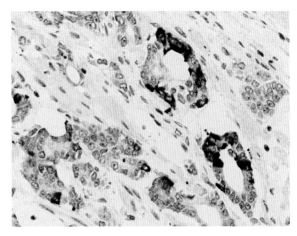

Fig 7.3 Positive synaptophysin expression in prostate adenocarcinoma with carcinoid-like morphology.

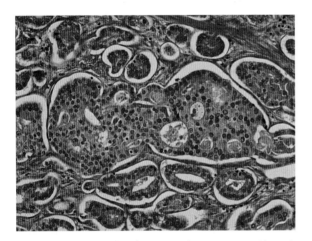

Fig 7.4 High power view of prostate adenocarcinoma with carcinoid-like morphology.

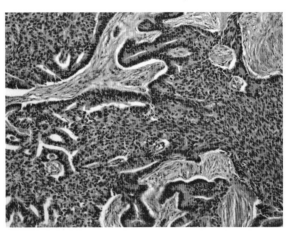

Fig 7.5 Prostate adenocarcinoma with neuroendocrine features.

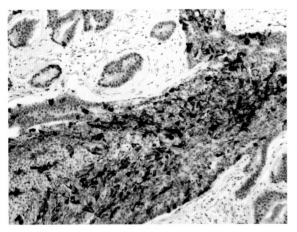

Fig 7.6 Positive synaptophysin expression in prostate adenocarcinoma with neuroendocrine features.

7.2 Adenocarcinoma with Paneth cell-like Neuroendocrine Differentiation

- The term Paneth cell-like has been used to describe chromogranin positive, eosinophilic and granular neuroendocrine cells basally located, in PIN and conventional prostatic carcinoma. Most frequently, these cells are seen isolated, patchy in small solid nests or diffusely involving glands. Gleason grading of these tumors should be assigned only to the areas of conventional adenocarcinoma. Paneth cell-like change seems not to be related to aggressiveness of the tumor. Fig 7.7

7.3 Well Differentiated Neuroendocrine Tumor (Carcinoid)

- True carcinoid tumors of the prostate are exceedingly rare, and most lesions reported as

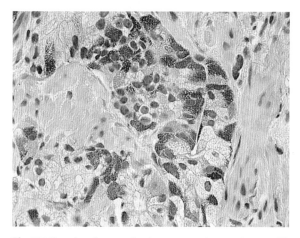

Fig 7.7 Paneth cell expression in prostate adenocarcinoma with neuroendocrine features.

carcinoid tumors represent prostatic adenocarcinoma with focal neuroendocrine differentiation. Most of them are positive for prostatic markers and behave as conventional carcinomas.

- The term "carcinoid-like tumors" has been applied by some authorities to label these carcinomas. True carcinoid tumors of the prostate show classic cytological features of carcinoid tumors seen elsewhere, are reactive for neuroendocrine markers and negative for PSA and PAP. The prognosis is uncertain due to the small number reported. Fig 7.8

7.4 Small Cell Carcinoma

- Prostate small cell carcinoma is rare and might represent less than 2% of prostatic carcinomas. It is most frequently seen in elderly patients with obstructive symptoms. Some cases may present paraneoplastic symptoms due to ACTH or ADH

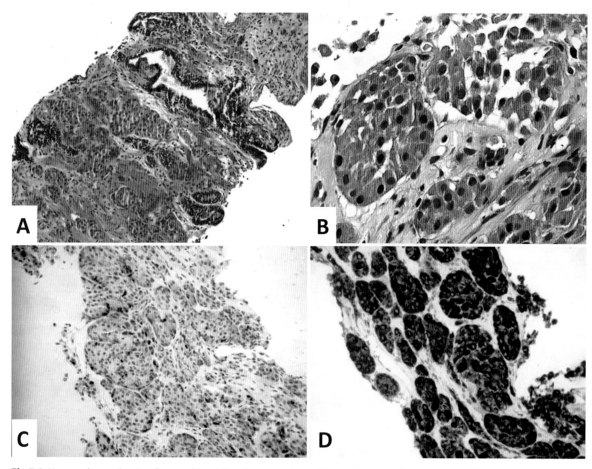

Fig 7.8 Neuroendocrine (carcinoid) tumor (A and B), with synaptophysin (C) and chromogranin A expression (D).

overproduction. Serum PSA is variable, with some cases having normal PSA even in metastatic disease. Most are of advanced stage at time of diagnosis and the prognosis is dismal, with survival of less than two year, in most cases.

- The average survival of patients with small-cell carcinoma of the prostate is less than a year. There is no difference in prognosis between patients with pure small cell carcinomas and those with mixed glandular and small cell carcinomas.
  The appearance of a small cell component within the course of adenocarcinoma of the prostate indicates a terminal phase of the disease.
- Using immunohistochemistry, small cell components are negative for PSA and PAP but positive for neuroendocrine markers and ERG. By FISH analysis, small cell carcinoma from prostate may be differentiated from small cell carcinoma of the bladder since the former retains *ERG-TMPRSS2* molecular alterations.
- There are conflicting studies as to whether small cell carcinoma of the prostate is positive for thyroid transcription factor-1 (TTF-1), in order to distinguish them from a metastasis of the lung.

- Small cell carcinoma of the prostate needs to be differentiated from Gleason pattern 5, which is negative for neuroendocrine markers. No Gleason grade applies to small cell carcinoma. Fig 7.9–7.15

7.4.1 Histology

- Histologically similar to those arising in the lung, with tumor cells showing scant cytoplasm and round, oval or spindled nuclei usually smaller than three times the size of lymphocytes. Chromatin is finely granular, and nucleoli are absent to inconspicuous. Other cases show intermediate cells with larger cytoplasm and more visible nucleoli.
- About half of small cell carcinoma cases arising in the prostate are pure, with the remaining cases admixed with prostatic adenocarcinoma, most frequently of Gleason score 8–10.

7.4.2 Immunohistochemistry

- In addition to the positivity of neuroendocrine markers (synaptophysin, chromogranin, CD56),

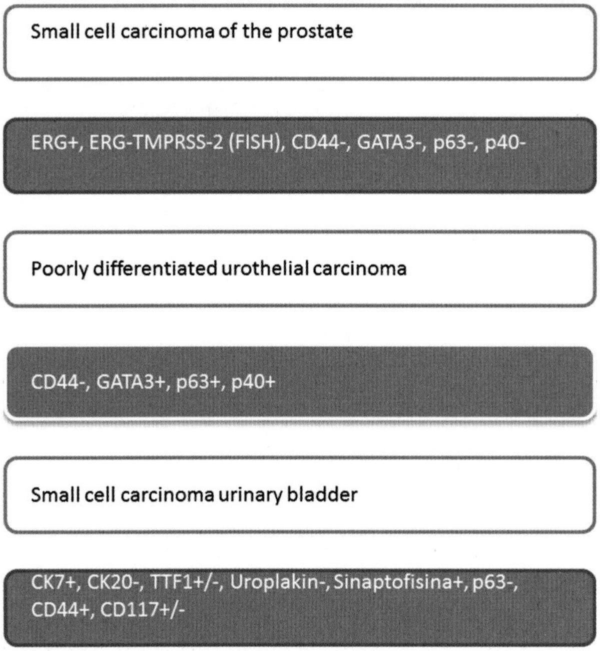

Fig 7.9 Differential diagnosis of small cell carcinoma of the prostate.

Small cell carcinoma of the prostate

ERG+, ERG-TMPRSS-2 (FISH), CD44-, GATA3-, p63-, p40-

Poorly differentiated urothelial carcinoma

CD44-, GATA3+, p63+, p40+

Small cell carcinoma urinary bladder

CK7+, CK20-, TTF1+/-, Uroplakin-, Sinaptofisina+, p63-, CD44+, CD117+/-

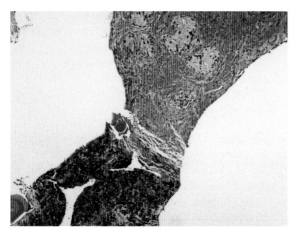

Fig 7.10 Small cell carcinoma and acinar adenocarcinoma of the prostate.

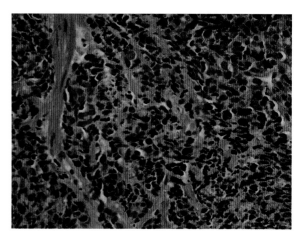

Fig 7.11 High power view of small cell carcinoma of the prostate.

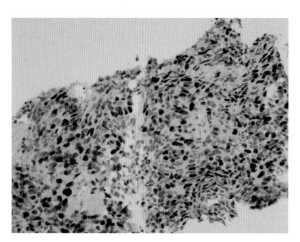

Fig 7.12 Ki67 expression in small cell carcinoma of the prostate.

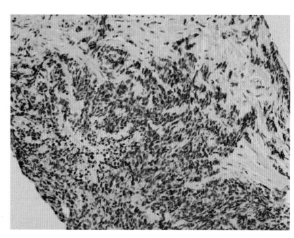

Fig 7.13 Negative PSA expression in small cell carcinoma of the prostate.

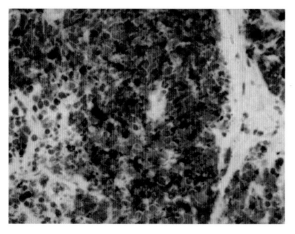

Fig 7.14 Synaptophysin expression in small cell carcinoma of the prostate.

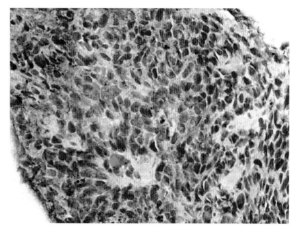

Fig 7.15 Racemase expression in small cell carcinoma of the prostate.

focal positivity for PSA or PSMA is seen in some cases. TTF1 and AMACR are frequently positive, and p63, CK7, CK20 and 34βE12 are typically negative. CKAE1/AE3 is usually positive, showing a dot-like (paranuclear) pattern. Ki67 is present in >70% of cells. Some reports suggest that CD44 is positive in small cell carcinoma of the prostate and negative in non-prostatic small cell carcinoma.

7.4.3 Differential Diagnosis

- Small cell carcinoma arising in the prostate is diagnosed based on morphologic. Immunohistochemistry is useful in equivocal cases; in particular, those with intermediate type of cells are likely to be underdiagnosed and may benefit from immunohistochemistry. Main differential diagnosis includes Gleason 5+5 conventional adenocarcinoma. Immunohistochemistry can be helpful. Synaptophysin may be focally seen in conventional adenocarcinoma; therefore, it is advisable to use a panel also including additional neuroendocrine markers. Single cell pattern of infiltrative growth, prominent nucleoli, abundant cytoplasm, negative CD44, strong positivity for prostatic markers and diffuse 34βE12 expression favors poorly differentiated adenocarcinoma.
- Small cell carcinomas of the prostate histologically are identical to small cell carcinomas of the lung, and similar diagnostic criteria apply. About 50% of the patients have mixed small cell carcinoma and adenocarcinoma of the prostate.

7.5 Large Cell Neuroendocrine Carcinoma

- There is limited experience on this type of neuroendocrine carcinoma, since it is extremely rare in the prostate. Most cases are diagnosed after long-standing hormonal therapy (mean four years). Large cell neuroendocrine carcinomas are aggressive tumors that usually present at advanced stage and metastatic disease.
- Histologically, sheets and ribbons of amphophilic cells with large nuclei, high mitotic rate and foci of tumor necrosis are characteristically present. The cells strongly react with neuroendocrine markers with focal or negative PSA and PAP expression. AMACR may be positive. Figs 7.16–7.18

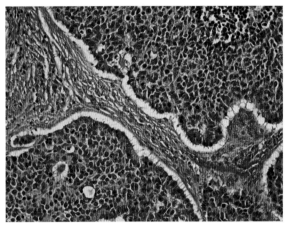

Fig 7.16 Large cell neuroendocrine carcinoma of the prostate.

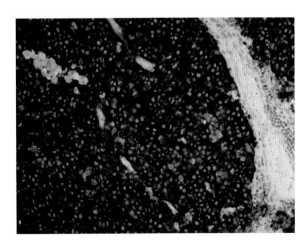

Fig 7.17 Synaptophysin expression in large cell neuroendocrine carcinoma of the prostate.

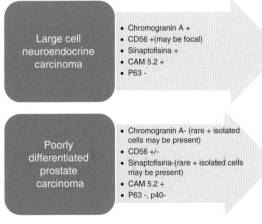

Large cell neuroendocrine carcinoma	• Chromogranin A + • CD56 +(may be focal) • Sinaptofisina + • CAM 5.2 + • P63 -
Poorly differentiated prostate carcinoma	• Chromogranin A- (rare + isolated cells may be present) • CD56 +/- • Sinaptofisina-(rare + isolated cells may be present) • CAM 5.2 + • P63 -, p40-

Fig 7.18 Differential diagnosis of large cell neuroendocrine carcinoma of the prostate.

Suggested Reading

Priemer DS, Montironi R, Wang L, Williamson SR, Lopez-Beltran A, Cheng L. Neuroendocrine Tumors of the Prostate: Emerging Insights from Molecular Data and Updates to the 2016 World Health Organization Classification. Endocr Pathol. 2016 Jun; 27(2): 123–35.

Guadagno E, De Rosa G, Del Basso De Caro M. Neuroendocrine Tumours in Rare Sites: Differences in Nomenclature and Diagnostics—A Rare and Ubiquitous Histotype. J Clin Pathol. 2016; **69**: 563–74.

Mazzucchelli R, Morichetti D, Lopez-Beltran A, Cheng L, Scarpelli M, Kirkali Z, Montironi R. Neuroendocrine Tumours of the Urinary System and Male Genital Organs: Clinical Significance. BJU Int. 2009; **103**: 1464–70.

Wang X, MacLennan GT, Lopez-Beltran A, Cheng L. Small Cell Carcinoma of the Urinary Bladder–Histogenesis, Genetics, Diagnosis, Biomarkers, Treatment, and Prognosis. Appl Immunohistochem Mol Morphol. 2007; **15**: 8–18.

Parimi V, Goyal R, Poropatich K, Yang XJ. Neuroendocrine Differentiation of Prostate Cancer: A Review. Am J Clin Exp Urol. 2014; **2**: 273–85.

Terry S, Beltran H. The Many Faces of Neuroendocrine Differentiation in Prostate Cancer Progression. Front Oncol. 2014; **4**: 60.

Epstein JI, Amin MB, Beltran H, Lotan TL, Mosquera JM, Reuter VE, Robinson BD, Troncoso P, Rubin MA. Proposed Morphologic Classification of Prostate Cancer with Neuroendocrine Differentiation. Am J Surg Pathol. 2014; **38**: 756–67.

Furtado P, Lima MV, Nogueira C, Franco M, Tavora F. Review of Small Cell Carcinomas of the Prostate. Prostate Cancer. 2011; **2011**: 543272.

Monn M. Francesca, Montironi Rodolfo, Lopez-Beltran Antonio, Cheng Liang. Emerging Molecular Pathways and Targets in Neuroendocrine Prostate Cancer. Transl Cancer Res. 2016; **5**(S2): S282–85.

Mosquera JM, Beltran H, Park K, et al. Concurrent AURKA and MYCN Gene Amplifications Are Harbingers of Lethal Treatment-related Neuroendocrine Prostate Cancer. Neoplasia. 2013; **15**: 1–10.

Chapter

8

Pathologic Prognostic Factors of Prostate Cancer

8.1 Prostate Biopsy

- The surgical pathology report should thus be comprehensive and yet succinct in providing relevant information to urologists, radiation oncologists and oncologists. Parameters to include are as follows: (Table 8.1); Figs 8.1–8.2

8.2 Histological Type

- Since acinar adenocarcinoma is the overwhelming histological type of cancer in needle biopsy specimens, it is not necessary to specify such cancers as acinar or conventional type in biopsy pathology reports.

Table 8.1 Prognostic Factors to be Reported in Prostate Biopsies with Adenocarcinoma

- Histopathologic type
- Gleason score including primary and secondary pattern
- Grade group 1–5
- Extent of involvement (percentage and or cancer extension in millimeters)
- Location and distribution of tumor
- Local invasion: extraprostatic extension and seminal vesicle involvement
- Perineural invasion: extent (focal vs. multifocal) and diameter of nerve bundles
- Lymphovascular invasion

- Morphologic variations such as atrophic, pseudohyperplastic, hypernephroid (foamy) and other patterns are descriptive terms used to help pathologists recognize potential diagnostic pitfalls, but have no known prognostic significance, and therefore do not deserve specific mention in the final diagnostic report.
- Several variants of prostate cancer have been described, including ductal, mucinous, signet-ring cell, adeno-squamous, small cell carcinoma and sarcomatoid carcinoma. The former three are diagnoses tenable only on examination of radical prostatectomy or transurethral resection specimens.
- When present in needle biopsies, the diagnostic terminology used must be: adenocarcinoma of prostate with ductal features; adenocarcinoma of prostate with signet-ring cell features; and adenocarcinoma of prostate with mucinous differentiation. Small cell carcinoma, sarcomatoid carcinoma and adeno-squamous carcinoma may be diagnosed on needle biopsies.
- Some prostate adenocarcinomas produce desmoplastic stroma (so-called stromogenic carcinoma), which is considered an aggressive feature; therefore, it can be reported as a note. Fig 8.3

Reporting prostate biopsies with cancer:

Minimal criteria

→

- Histopathologic type
- Gleason score (primary and secondary pattern)
- Extent of involvement (percentage or cancer extension in millimeters)
- Extraprostatic extension and seminal vesicle involvement if present
- Perineural invasion
- Lymphovascular invasion

Fig 8.1 Reporting prostate biopsies with cancer (minimal criteria).

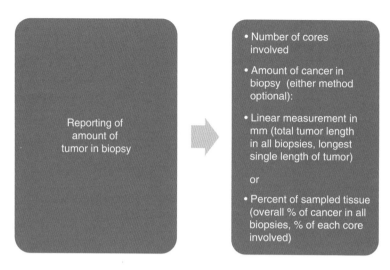

Fig 8.2 Reporting the amount of tumor in prostate biopsies.

- Number of cores involved

- Amount of cancer in biopsy (either method optional):

- Linear measurement in mm (total tumor length in all biopsies, longest single length of tumor)

or

- Percent of sampled tissue (overall % of cancer in all biopsies, % of each core involved)

Reporting of amount of tumor in biopsy

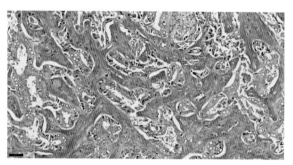

Fig 8.3 Stromogenic prostate cancer.

8.3 Gleason Grade (Score)

- The Gleason grading system is recommended as the international standard for grading prostate cancer (see Chapter 5).

8.4 Extent of Tumor Involvement of Needle Core

- The amount of tumor in prostate needle cores is an important pathologic parameter that must be reported. The extent of involvement of needle cores by prostatic adenocarcinoma has been shown to correlate with the Gleason score, tumor volume, surgical margins and pathologic stage in radical prostatectomy specimens. The extent of needle core involvement including bilateral involvement has also been shown to predict biochemical recurrence, post-prostatectomy progression and radiation therapy failure in univariate and often in multivariate analysis.

- There is lack of consensus in the literature as to the best method of reporting the extent of tumor involvement. The report should provide the number of involved cores. In addition, one or both of the following more detailed methods of tumor extent should be performed. One method is to report the linear length of cancer in mm (total tumor length in all biopsies; longest single length of tumor). The other method is to provide a percentage estimate of involvement of each of the cores derived by visual estimation (overall percent of cancer in all biopsies, percent of each core involved; reporting the percentage of cancer involvement in increments of 5 or 10% is appropriate).

- One problem encountered with this otherwise straightforward method is when there is extreme fragmentation of the needle biopsy specimen, making assessment of the number of cores and the percentage of cancer within each core difficult. In case of highly fragmented tissue, this may be overcome by providing a composite (global) percentage of involvement of cancer in all needle biopsy tissue, and this may be a slightly more accurate correlate of the amount of cancer in the prostate gland itself. Each container submitted needs to receive a separate report including Gleason score and tumor extent in positive cases.

- Bilateral cancer, which indicates multifocality, is indirectly suggestive of greater tumor volume. This parameter is easily deduced from the pathology report findings of each of the cores submitted. In patients not subsequently treated by

Table 8.2 Reporting of Amount of Adenocarcinoma in Prostate Biopsies

- Number of cores involved
- Amount of cancer in biopsy (either method optional)
  - Linear measurement in mm (total tumor length in all biopsies, longest single length of tumor)
  - Percent of sampled tissue (overall percent of cancer in all biopsies, percent of each core involved)
- Bilaterality if present

radical prostatectomy, this is a critical factor in assigning clinical stage. Table 8.2

8.5 Local Invasion

- Routine biopsy sampling may occasionally contain extraprostatic fat or seminal vesicle tissue. If cancer is noted to involve these structures, the findings would indicate pT3 disease. The presence of seminal vesicle invasion or extraprostatic fat involvement in the staging biopsy is highly correlative of similar findings at radical prostatectomies. Extraprostatic fat invasion at needle biopsy is highly predictive of biochemical recurrence (78% compared to 41% failure rate in cases with extraprostatic extension not detected by needle biopsy).
- Only exceptionally rarely is fat present within the normal prostate. Hence, tumor in adipose tissue in a needle biopsy specimen can safely be interpreted as extraprostatic extension. Fig 8.4
- Ganglion cells and skeletal muscle involvement by tumor is not equivalent to extraprostatic extension as they may both be found frequently within the prostate.
- Distinction between the seminal vesicle epithelium and ejaculatory duct epithelium may be impossible in limited samples, although occasionally the seminal vesicle can be distinguished if its smooth muscle wall is present. In contrast, ejaculatory duct epithelium have a rim of fibrous tissue that is rich in thin blood vessels.
- If the distinction between seminal vesicle tissue/ ejaculatory duct is not feasible, diagnostic terminology such as "adenocarcinoma of the prostate with invasion of seminal vesicle/ ejaculatory duct tissue" may be used.
- Using immunohistochemistry might be relevant in separating seminal vesicle/ejaculatory ducts from prostate carcinoma. SVs are typically CKAE1/AE3 +, p63+, PAX-2 +, PSA-, PAP-, P504S-.

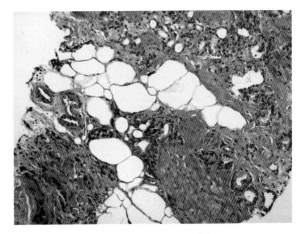

Fig 8.4 Extraprostatic extension in prostate biopsy.

8.6 Perineural Invasion

- Perineural, circumferential or intraneural invasion is defined as the presence of prostate cancer juxtaposed intimately along, around or within a nerve. Other descriptors of perineural invasion that may strengthen the prognostic significance of this parameter include extensive (multifocal) perineural invasion and greater nerve diameter. Involvement of nerves present within adipose tissue (extraprostatic nerves) by cancer indicates extraprostatic extension and deserves notation in the pathology report when present. Figs 8.5–8.6
- Although perineural invasion in needle biopsy specimens is not an independent predictor of prognosis when the Gleason score, serum PSA and extent of cancer are factored in, most studies indicate that its presence variably correlates with extraprostatic extension in some reports, with data suggesting that this finding may independently predict lymph node metastasis and post-surgical progression.
- Some of the data from the radiation oncology literature suggests that it is an independent risk factor for predicting adverse outcome after external beam radiation therapy.

8.7 Vascular/Lymphatic Invasion

- Microvascular invasion consists of tumor cells within endothelial-lined spaces. Also, we do not differentiate between vascular and lymphatic channels because of the difficulty

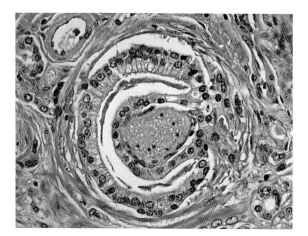

Fig 8.5 Perineural invasion by carcinoma.

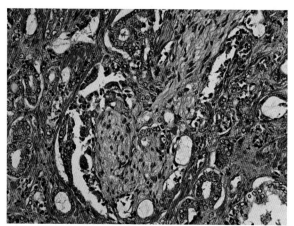

Fig 8.6 Perineural and intra-neural invasion by carcinoma.

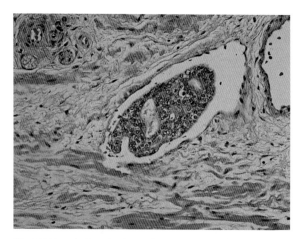

Fig 8.7 Vascular invasion by carcinoma.

8.8 Microvessel Density

- A significant increase in microvessel density (MVD) occurs in prostatic intraepithelial neoplasia and carcinoma compared with normal prostatic tissue. Mean blood vessel count is higher in tumors with metastases than in those without, and most studies, but not all, show a correlation with pathologic stage. MVD appears to be an independent predictor of cancer progression in some studies. Some studies suggest that increased MVD contributes to extraprostatic spread of adenocarcinoma. MVD reporting remains an option.

8.9 Prognostic Factors after Radical Prostatectomy (Table 8.3; Figs 8.8–8.9)

8.10 Histological Type of Prostatic Carcinoma

- Rare and other infrequent histological variants or subtypes of prostatic carcinoma have been identified. These variants represent the spectrum of changes which can occur in adenocarcinoma. The biological behavior of many of these variants may differ from typical adenocarcinoma and proper clinical management relies on accurate diagnosis and reporting. Mixtures of different histological types should be indicated.

and lack of reproducibility among different observers by routine light microscopic examination. Microvascular invasion may be confused with fixation-associated retraction artifact of acini. Immunohistochemical stains directed against endothelial cells such as CD31 or CD34 may increase the detection rate, although this is not necessary in routine work. Fig 8.7

- Lymphovascular invasion as studied in radical prostatectomy specimens correlates with lymph node metastasis, biochemical recurrence and distinct metastasis; its presence in the needle biopsy is likely to have similar correlations. This feature is very rarely seen in needle biopsy specimens.

Table 8.3 Histologic Parameters to be Reported in Radical Prostatectomy Specimens

1 Histologic type of carcinoma
2 Gleason score, including primary and secondary pattern (if three patterns are present, record the predominant and second most common patterns; the tertiary pattern should be recorded in a comment if higher than primary and secondary patterns). Add percent of Gleason 4 or 5 when present.
3 Grade group 1–5
4 Tumor location
5 Margin status

   Extent if positive
   Focal
   Non-focal
   Location of positive margins
   Specify status of following margins: bladder neck, apical, vas deferentia (optional)
   Nature of positive margins
   In area of extra-prostatic extension
   Iatrogenic (pT2+)

6 Extra-prostatic extension (EPE)

   Extent of EPE
   Focal
   Non-focal
   Location of EPE

7 Vascular invasion
8 Seminal vesicle invasion
9 Tumor volume (optional)
10 Gleason grade and grade group in tumor index
11 Pathologic Staging (pTNM 2016 revision)
12 Comments: as appropriate

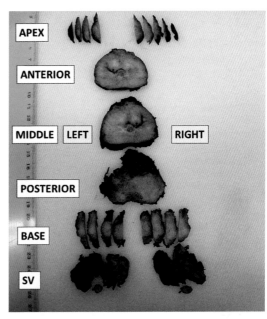

Fig 8.8 Model of handling radical prostatectomy that allows a proper partial sampling.

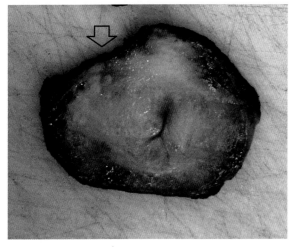

Fig 8.9 Radical prostatectomy showing a missing part of the specimen (arrow).

8.11 Histological Grade of Cancer

- The Gleason score assigned to the tumor at radical prostatectomy is a powerful predictor of progression following radical prostatectomy.

8.12 Staging

- The protocol recommends the use of the most recent revision of the TNM Staging System for carcinoma of the prostate of the American Joint Committee on Cancer (AJCC) and the International Union against Cancer (UICC).
- Clinical classification (cTNM) is usually carried out by the referring physician before treatment during initial evaluation of the patient or when pathologic classification is not possible. The prefix symbol "p" refers to the pathologic classification of the TNM (pTNM), as opposed to the clinical classification.
- Tumor remaining in a resection specimen following previous treatment of any type (radiation therapy alone, chemotherapy therapy alone or any combined modality treatment) is codified by the TNM using a prescript "y" to indicate the post-treatment status of the tumor (e.g., ypT1). The classification of residual disease may be a predictor of postoperative outcome.
- Tumor that is locally recurrent after a documented disease-free interval following surgical resection is classified according to the TNM categories, but modified with the prefix "r" (e.g., rpT1). Table 8.4

Table 8.4 Pathologic (pT) Tumor, Node, Metastasis Classification of Prostate Adenocarcinoma (2016 Revision)

Primary Tumor (T)

(There is no pathologic T1 category)

- pT2: Organ confined
- pT3: Extraprostatic extension
- pT3a: Extraprostatic extension
- pT3b: Seminal vesicle extension
- pT4: Invasion of bladder, rectum

Regional Lymph Nodes (N)

- NX: Regional lymph nodes cannot be assessed
- N0: No regional lymph node metastasis
- N1: Metastasis in regional lymph node or nodes

Distant Metastasis (M) (When more than one site of metastasis is present, the most advanced category (pM1 c) is used).

- MX: Distant metastasis cannot be assessed
- M0: No distant metastasis
- M1: Distant Metastasis
- M1a: non-regional lymph node(s)
- M1b: bone(s)
- M1 c: other site(s)

* Invasion into the prostatic apex or into (but not beyond) the prostatic capsule is not classified as T3, but as T2. Tumor extension into periprostatic soft tissue is T3. Bladder neck invasion is T3.

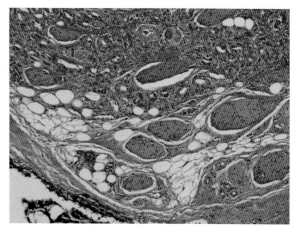

Fig 8.10 Radical prostatectomy with extraprostatic extension and negative surgical margin (pT3a).

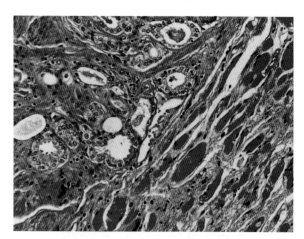

Fig 8.12 Adenocarcinoma of the anterior prostate with adenocarcinoma within muscle fibers should be staged as pT2.

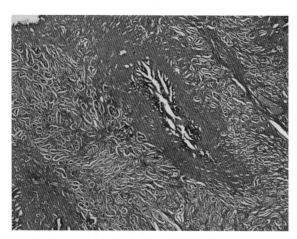

Fig 8.11 Radical prostatectomy with extension to seminal vesicle (pT3b).

8.13 Extent of Local Invasion

- This includes extraprostatic extension (pT3a) and seminal vesicle involvement (pT3b). Microscopic involvement of bladder neck muscle fibers in radical prostatectomy specimens should also be defined as pT3b. Because the prostate lacks a discrete capsule, the term "extraprostatic extension" (EPE) has replaced "capsular penetration" to describe a tumor that has extended out of the prostate into periprostatic soft tissue.
- Histologically, the prostatic capsule is not well-defined. In some areas, there may appear to be a fibrous or fibro-muscular band at the edge of the prostate, although in other areas, normal prostatic glands extend out to the edge of the prostate without any appearance that there is a capsule. Figs 8.10–8.12
- Tumor abutting on or admixed with fat constitutes extraprostatic extension. EPE may also be reported when a tumor involves perineural spaces in the neurovascular bundles, even in the absence of periprostatic fat involvement.

- Difficulty in diagnosing EPE arises when a tumor extends out of the prostatic gland and induces a dense desmoplastic response in the periprostatic adipose tissue. This is most commonly seen in prostatectomy specimens obtained after endocrine neoadjuvant therapy. Because of the desmoplastic response, it can be difficult to judge whether the tumor has extended out of the gland or is within the fibrous tissue of the prostate.

- The best way of assessing whether extraprostatic extension has occurred is to look at the adjacent edge of the prostate on scanning magnification where there is no tumor and follow the edge of the gland to the area in question to see whether the normal rounded contour of the gland has been altered by a protuberance corresponding to extension of a tumor into the periprostatic tissue.

- In certain locations, such as the anterior prostate and bladder neck regions, there is paucity of fat. In these locations, EPE is determined when the tumor extends beyond the confines of the normal glandular prostate. At the apex, tumor admixed with skeletal muscle elements does not constitute extraprostatic extension.

- The degree of extraprostatic extension varies from only a few glands outside the prostate (focal EPE) to cases with more extensive extraprostatic spread (non-focal or established). The amount of EPE carries prognostic importance.

- Different ways have been used to define the amount of EPE. If it is equal to, or less than, two high-power (40X) microscopic fields, then EPE is focal. Any amount in excess of two high-power fields is considered to be either non-focal or extensive.

- Others define focal EPE as an extraprostatic tumor occupying less than one high power field on ≤ 2 separate histologic sections.

- Cases showing focal EPE have a progression rate of 20% versus about 60% progression for cases with established (non-focal) EPE, a fact that seems to be relevant since organ-confined (pT2) disease shows about 13% progression rate.

- Seminal vesicle invasion is defined as cancer invading into the muscular coat of the seminal vesicle. It has been shown in numerous studies to be a significant prognostic indicator. While in most cases, seminal vesicle invasion occurs in glands with EPE, the latter cannot be documented in a minority of these cases.

- Some of these patients had only minimal involvement of the seminal vesicles, or involve only the portion of the seminal vesicles that is at least partially intraprostatic. Patients in this category were reported to have a favorable prognosis similar to patients without seminal vesicle invasion.

- Histologic patterns of seminal vesicle invasion are: extension up the ejaculatory duct complex; spread across the base of the prostate without other evidence of EPE or involvement from tumor invading the seminal vesicles from the periprostatic and peri-seminal vesicle adipose tissue; an isolated tumor deposit without continuity with the primary prostate cancer tumor focus.

8.14 Positive Surgical Margins

- Patients with positive margins have a significantly increased risk of progression as compared to those with negative margins. Surgical margins should be designated as "negative" if tumor is not present at the inked margin and is "positive" if tumor cells touch the ink at the margin. Figs 8.13–8.19

- There are two main causes for positive margins. In non-iatrogenic positive margins, positive margins can result from a failure to excise extraprostatic extension of tumor; in capsular incision, one cause of a positive resection margin is transection of intra-prostatic tumor.

- Positive surgical margins should not be interpreted as extra-prostatic extension. If the surgical margin is positive, the pathologist should

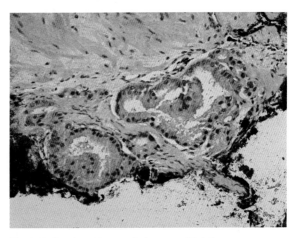

Fig 8.13 Focal positive margin (contact with ink).

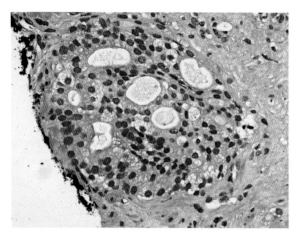

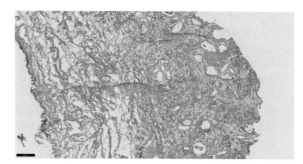

Fig 8.15 Frozen section allows proper margin status evaluation (negative in this case).

Fig 8.14 Adenocarcinoma glands close to ink, but with no contact, should be considered negative.

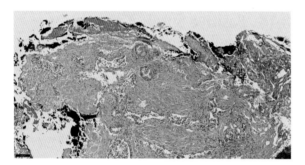

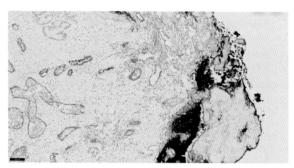

Fig 8.17 Distorted surgical margin may occasionally require immunohistochemistry (anti-CK5/6 immunohistochemistry).

Fig 8.16 Distorted surgical margin may be difficult to assess.

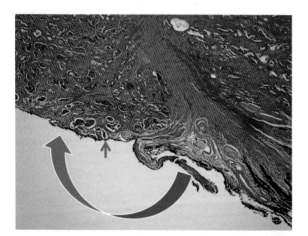

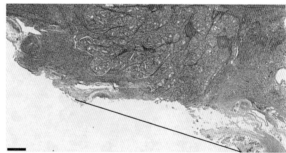

Fig 8.19 Missing part of the surgical margin, which can be present deeper in the paraffin block.

Fig 8.18 False positive (iatrogenic) surgical margin.

state this explicitly in the report. Surgical margin positivity predicts disease progression.

- The location of positive margin is also important since it is not the same as positive margin extraprostatic vs. intra-prostatic.

- The pathologist should be aware of "false positive" margins due to the penetration of ink into cracks present on the external surface.
- The main cause for discrepancy in the definition of a positive margin is seen in situations in which cancer was very close, but not clearly touching, the inked margin or when the color used to identify the margin appeared very pale. The apex should be

closely examined because of its unusual susceptibility to positive margins.

- The specific locations of the positive margins should be documented since they provide feedback to the urologist, and there should be some indication (e.g., number of positive blocks, linear extent in millimeters) of the extent of margin positivity. It is currently preferred to provide linear extent of positive margins in millimeters, with focal ≤ 3 mm vs. extensive >3 mm. It is also recommended to report when tumor cells are close (<1 mm) to the inked margin, though in this case, surgical margin is still considered negative and should be reported accordingly.
- The pathology report should also indicate the presence of normal prostate tissue at the resection margin level. This might help the urologist explain why the serum PSA in patients with such a feature remains detectable after radical prostatectomy. In fact, the serum PSA value, even though very low, is not linked to tumor recurrence and persistence, but to incomplete resection of the prostate gland.

8.15 Vascular Invasion

- It is recommended to report vessel invasion (lymphatic or venous) in prostatic samples even if its independent prognostic significance remains unclear.

8.16 Perineural Invasion

- Perineural invasion is one of the major mechanisms by which prostate cancer spreads out of the gland. Perineural invasion is almost ubiquitously present in radical prostatectomy specimens. As with all of the other parameters, the key question is whether the presence of (intra-prostatic) perineural invasion in the prostatectomy specimen is an independent prognosticator. At this time, it is not entirely clear whether there are differences in terms of prognosis between intra-prostatic and extra-prostatic perineural invasion. Fig 8.20

8.17 Volume of Cancer

- One of the most controversial aspects of the pathological assessment of radical prostatectomy

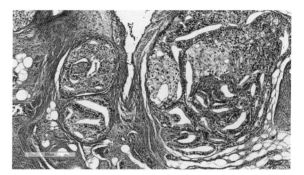

Fig 8.20 Extraprostatic and perineural invasion.

specimens is the measurement of tumor volume. The critical and controversial question concerns whether tumor volume is an independent prognostic parameters once other routinely assessed variables are accounted for.

- There is one situation where it is important to give some estimate of tumor volume at radical prostatectomy. As a consequence of screening for prostate cancer, we have seen an increase in the resection of prostates harboring cancers that are so small that they are histologically difficult to identify. These cases currently account for approximately 4% of radical prostatectomy specimens.
- The pathologist has to specify in the pathology report that these tumors are "small" or "minute" (i.e., less than 0.5 cc), since these tumors carry on low clinical significance. Most of them, if not all, are cured by surgery.

8.18 Biomarkers to Predict Progression Following Radical Prostatectomy

- The drive to identify prognostic markers in prostate cancer is based on the perceived need to develop objective markers to either supplant or supplement more subjective markers such as conventional histological grading.
- The more established biomarkers are as follows: DNA ploidy, microvessel density (Angiogenesis), KI-67, neuroendocrine differentiation, p53 $P27^{kip1}$, $p21^{WAF1}$, bcl-2, Her-2/neu, E-cadherin, CD44, Retinoblastoma (Rb) proteins, apoptotic index, androgen receptor status, PSA and PSAP expression and nuclear morphometry. None of them are actually incorporated to the clinic.

- It is important to recognize that these objective markers are subject to the same variability as more conventional histological parameters.

8.19 Pelvic Lymph Node Assessment

- The adverse prognosis of metastatic disease to the pelvic lymph nodes is universally accepted. The incidence of pelvic lymph node metastases at the time of radical prostatectomy has decreased over the last couple of decades.
- As a consequence of the declining incidence, concerns have been raised as to whether pelvic lymphadenectomy is necessary in all patients, especially those with a low risk of having positive lymph nodes based on pre-operative clinico-pathologic findings. The major factors contributing to this decrease are better patient selection as to who is a good candidate for surgery and the earlier detection of prostate cancer.

- In about 6% of the cases, the only lymph node metastasis is not in a grossly recognized lymph node, but in small lymph nodes embedded in the adipose tissue, a finding of uncertain significance that is not included in the current TNM. Figs 8.21–8.24

8.20 Isolated Tumor Cells

- Isolated tumor cells (ITC) are single cells or small clusters of cells not more than 0.2 mm in greatest dimension. Lymph nodes or distant sites with ITC found by either immunohistological examination or non-morphological techniques (e.g., flow cytometry, DNA analysis, polymerase chain reaction [PCR] amplification of a specific tumor marker) should be classified as N0 or M0, respectively. Specific denotation of the assigned N category is suggested for cases in which ITC are the only evidence of possible metastatic disease.

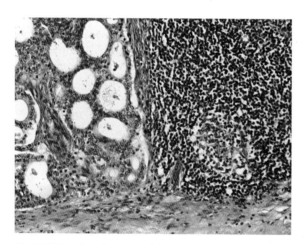

Fig 8.21 Lymph node metastasis by prostatic adenocarcinoma.

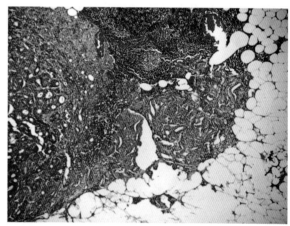

Fig 8.22 Lymph node metastasis by prostatic adenocarcinoma with extracapsular extension.

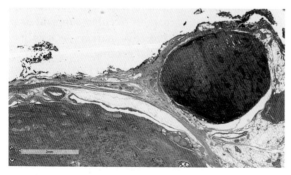

Fig 8.23 Lymph node metastasis by prostatic adenocarcinoma in a periprostatic lymph node.

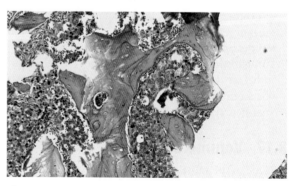

Fig 8.24 Bone metastasis by prostate cancer.

Suggested Reading

Berney DM, Algaba F, Camparo P, Compérat E, Griffiths D, Kristiansen G, Lopez-Beltran A, Montironi R, Varma M, Egevad L. Variation in Reporting of Cancer Extent and Benign Histology in Prostate Biopsies among European Pathologists. Virchows Arch. 2014 Mar 4. [Epub ahead of print].

McKenney JK, Wei W, Hawley S, Auman H, Newcomb LF, Boyer HD, Fazli L, Simko J, Hurtado-Coll A, Troyer DA, Tretiakova MS, Vakar-Lopez F, Carroll PR, Cooperberg MR, Gleave ME, Lance RS, Lin DW, Nelson PS, Thompson IM, True LD, Feng Z, Brooks JD. Histologic Grading of Prostatic Adenocarcinoma Can Be Further Optimized: Analysis of the Relative Prognostic Strength of Individual Architectural Patterns in 1275 Patients from the Canary Retrospective Cohort. Am J Surg Pathol. 2016 Nov; **40**(11): 1439–56.

Ayala GE, Muezzinoglu B, Hammerich KH, Frolov A, Liu H, Scardino PT, Li R, Sayeeduddin M, Ittmann MM, Kadmon D, Miles BJ, Wheeler TM, Rowley DR. Determining Prostate Cancer-specific Death through Quantification of Stromogenic Carcinoma Area in Prostatectomy Specimens. Am J Pathol. 2011 Jan; **178**(1): 79–87.

Berney DM, Algaba F, Camparo P, Compérat E, Griffiths D, Kristiansen G, Lopez-Beltran A, Montironi R, Varma M, Egevad L. The Reasons behind Variation in Gleason Grading of Prostatic Biopsies: Areas of Agreement and Misconception among 266 European Pathologists. Histopathology. 2014 Feb; **64**(3): 405–11. doi: 10.1111/his.12284. Epub 2013 Nov 6.

Yossepowitch O, Briganti A, Eastham JA, Epstein J, Graefen M, Montironi R, Touijer K. Positive Surgical Margins after Radical Prostatectomy: A Systematic Review and Contemporary Update. Eur Urol. 2014 Feb; **65**(2): 303–13. doi: 10.1016/j.eururo.2013.07.039. Epub 2013 Aug 3.

Schelling LA, Williamson SR, Zhang S, Yao JL, Wang M, Huang J, Montironi R, Lopez-Beltran A, Emerson RE, Idrees MT, Osunkoya AO, Man YG, Maclennan GT, Baldridge LA, Compérat E, Cheng L. Frequent TMPRSS2-ERG Rearrangement in Prostatic Small Cell Carcinoma Detected by Fluorescence in Situ Hybridization: The Superiority of Fluorescence in Situ Hybridization over ERG Immunohistochemistry. Hum Pathol. 2013 Oct; **44**(10): 2227–33. doi: 10.1016/j.humpath.2013.05.005. Epub 2013 Jul 12.

Montironi R, Cheng L, Lopez-Beltran A, Mazzucchelli R, Scarpelli M. Combined Handling of Prostate Base/Bladder Neck and Seminal Vesicles in Radical Prostatectomy Specimens: Our Approach with the Whole Mount Technique. Histopathology. 2013 Sep; **63**(3): 431–35. doi: 10.1111/his.12158. Epub 2013 Jun 24. No abstract available.

Montironi R, Lopez-Beltran A, Cheng L, Montorsi F, Scarpelli M. Central Prostate Pathology Review: Should It Be Mandatory? Eur Urol. 2013 Aug; **64**(2): 199–201. Discussion 202–03. doi: 10.1016/j.eururo.2013.04.002. Epub 2013 Apr 16. No abstract available.

Varinot J, Drouin S, Rouprêt M, Montironi R, Lopez-Beltran A, Compérat E. Prostate Cancer with Clear Cell Features and an Unusual Nested-like Pattern of Growth: A Case Report. Anal Quant Cytol Histol. 2012 Oct; **34**(5): 289–92.

Cheng L, MacLennan GT, Lopez-Beltran A, Montironi R. Anatomic, Morphologic and Genetic Heterogeneity of Prostate Cancer: Implications for Clinical Practice. Expert Rev Anticancer Ther. 2012 Nov; **12**(11): 1371–74. doi: 10.1586/era.12.127.

Egevad L, Ahmad AS, Algaba F, Berney DM, Boccon-Gibod L, Compérat E, Evans AJ, Griffiths D, Grobholz R, Kristiansen G, Langner C, Lopez-Beltran A, Montironi R, Moss S, Oliveira P, Vainer B, Varma M, Camparo P. Standardization of Gleason Grading among 337 European Pathologists. Histopathology. 2013 Jan; **62**(2): 247–56. doi: 10.1111/his.12008.

Varma M, Berney DM, Algaba F, Camparo P, Compérat E, Griffiths DF, Kristiansen G, Lopez-Beltran A, Montironi R, Egevad L. Prostate Needle Biopsy Processing: A Survey of Laboratory Practice across Europe. J Clin Pathol. 2013 Feb; **66**(2): 120–23. doi: 10.1136/jclinpath-2012-200993.

Brimo F, Montironi R, Egevad L, Erbersdobler A, Lin DW, Nelson JB, Rubin MA, van der Kwast T, Amin M, Epstein JI. Contemporary Grading for Prostate Cancer: Implications for Patient Care. Eur Urol. 2013 May; **63**(5): 892–901. doi: 10.1016/j.eururo.2012.10.015.

Mazzucchelli R, Scarpelli M, Lopez-Beltran A, Cheng L, Montironi R. Spectrum of Prostatic Nonepithelial Tumors and Tumorlike Conditions with Spindle Cell Features. Anal Quant Cytol Histol. 2012 Jun; **34**(3): 139–44.

Quick Charles M. MDa, Gokden Neriman MDa, Sangoi Ankur R. MDb, Brooks James D. MDc, McKenney Jesse K. MDa. The Distribution of PAX-2 Immunoreactivity in the Prostate Gland, Seminal Vesicle, and Ejaculatory Duct: Comparison with Prostatic Adenocarcinoma and Discussion of Prostatic Zonal Embryogenesis. Human Pathology. 2010; **41**: 1145–49.

Montironi R, Lopez Beltran A, Mazzucchelli R, Cheng L, Scarpelli M. Handling of Radical Prostatectomy Specimens: Total Embedding with Large-format Histology. Int J Breast Cancer. 2012; 2012: 932784. Epub 2012 Jul 10.

Montironi R, Scarpelli M, Cheng L, Lopez-Beltran A, Zhou M, Montorsi F. Do Not Misinterpret Intraductal Carcinoma of the Prostate as High-grade Prostatic Intraepithelial Neoplasia! Eur Urol. 2012 Sep; **62**(3): 518–22. Epub 2012 Jun 5.

Lopez-Beltran A, Cheng L, Blanca A, Montironi R. Cell Proliferation and Apoptosis in Prostate Needle Biopsies with Adenocarcinoma Gleason Score 6 or 7. Anal Quant Cytol Histol. 2012 Apr; **34**(2): 61–65.

Scarpelli M, Mazzucchelli R, Barbisan F, Santinelli A, Lopez-Beltran A, Cheng L, Montironi R. Is There a Role for Prostate Tumour Overexpressed-1 in the Diagnosis of HGPIN and of Prostatic Adenocarcinoma? A Comparison with Alpha-Methylacyl CoA Racemase. Int J Immunopathol Pharmacol. 2012 Jan–Mar; **25**(1): 67–74.

Camparo P, Egevad L, Algaba F, Berney DM, Boccon-Gibod L, Compérat E, Evans AJ, Grobholz R, Kristiansen G, Langner C, Lopez-Beltran A, Montironi R, Oliveira P, Vainer B, Varma M. Utility of Whole Slide Imaging and Virtual Microscopy in Prostate Pathology. APMIS. 2012 Apr; **120**(4): 298–304. doi: 10.1111/j.1600-0463.2011.02872.x. Review.

Montironi R, Scarpelli M, Mazzucchelli R, Cheng L, Lopez-Beltran A, Montorsi F. Extent of Cancer of Less than 50% in Any Prostate Needle Biopsy Core: How Many Millimeters Are There? Eur Urol. 2012 Apr; **61**(4): 751–56. Epub 2012 Jan 5. No abstract available.

Cheng L, Montironi R, Bostwick DG, Lopez-Beltran A, Berney DM. Staging of Prostate Cancer. Histopathology. 2012 Jan; **60**(1): 87–117. doi: 10.1111/j.1365-2559.2011.04025.x. Review.

Montironi R, Lopez-Beltran A, Scarpelli M, Mazzucchelli R, Cheng L. Handling of Radical Prostatectomy Specimens: Total Embedding with Whole Mounts, with Special Reference to the Ancona Experience (Letter). Histopathology. 2011 Nov; **59**(5): 1006–10.

Egevad L, Algaba F, Berney DM, Boccon-Gibod L, Compérat E, Evans AJ, Grobholz R, Kristiansen G, Langner C, Lockwood G, Lopez-Beltran A, Montironi R, Oliveira P, Schwenkglenks M, Vainer B, Varma M, Verger V, Camparo P. Interactive Digital Slides with Heat Maps: A Novel Method to Improve the Reproducibility of Gleason Grading. Virchows Arch. 2011 Aug; **459**(2): 175–82. Epub 2011 Jun 23.

Mazzucchelli R, Barbisan F, Santinelli A, Lopez-Beltran A, Cheng L, Scarpelli M, Montironi R. Immunohistochemical Expression of Prostate Tumor Overexpressed 1 in Cystoprostatectomies with Incidental and Insignificant Prostate Cancer. Further Evidence for Field Effect in Prostatic Carcinogenesis. Hum Pathol. 2011 Dec; **42**(12): 1931–36. Epub 2011 Jun 14.

Williamson SR, Zhang S, Yao JL, Huang J, Lopez-Beltran A, Shen S, Osunkoya AO, MacLennan GT, Montironi R, Cheng L. ERG-TMPRSS2 Rearrangement Is Shared by Concurrent Prostatic Adenocarcinoma and Prostatic Small Cell Carcinoma and Absent in Small Cell Carcinoma of the Urinary Bladder: Evidence Supporting Monoclonal Origin. Mod Pathol. 2011 Aug; **24**(8): 1120–27. doi: 10.1038/modpathol.2011.56.

Capitanio U, Cheng L, Lopez-Beltran A, Scarpelli M, Freschi M, Montorsi F, Montironi R. The Importance of Interaction between Urologists and Pathologists in Incidental Prostate Cancer Management. Eur Urol. 2011 Jul; **60**(1): 75–77.

Montironi R, Cheng L, Lopez-Beltran A, Mazzucchelli R, Scarpelli M. Editorial Comment to When Should We Expect no Residual Tumor (pT0) Once We Submit Incidental T1a-b Prostate Cancers to Radical Prostatectomy? Int J Urol. 2011 Feb; **18**(2): 153–54. doi: 10.1111/j.1442-2042.2010.02717.x.

Mazzucchelli R, Nesseris I, Cheng L, Lopez-Beltran A, Montironi R, Scarpelli M. Active Surveillance for Low-risk Prostate Cancer. Anticancer Res. 2010 Sep; **30**(9): 3683–92.

Montironi R, Mazzucchelli R, Lopez-Beltran A, Cheng L. Words of Wisdom. Re: Peripheral Zone Prostate Cancers: Location and Intraprostatic Patterns of Spread at Histopathology. Eur Urol. 2010 Jul; **58**(1): 180–82.

Montironi R, Cheng L, Lopez-Beltran A, Scarpelli M, Mazzucchelli R, Mikuz G, Kirkali Z, Montorsi F. Original Gleason System Versus 2005 ISUP Modified Gleason System: The Importance of Indicating Which System Is Used in the Patient's Pathology and Clinical Reports. Eur Urol. 2010 Sep; **58**(3): 369–73.

Montironi R, Vela Navarrete R, Lopez-Beltran A, Mazzucchelli R, Mikuz G, Bono AV. Histopathology Reporting of Prostate Needle Biopsies. 2005 Update. Virchows Arch. 2006; **449**(1): 1–13.

Lopez-Beltran A, Mikuz G, Luque RJ, Mazzucchelli R, Montironi R. Current Practice of Gleason Grading of Prostate Carcinoma. Virchows Arch. 2006 Feb; **448**(2): 111–18.

Marks RA, Koch MO, Lopez-Beltran A, Montironi R, Juliar BE, Cheng L. The Relationship between the Extent of Surgical Margin Positivity and Prostate Specific Antigen Recurrence in Radical Prostatectomy Specimens. Hum Pathol. 2007 Aug; **38**(8): 1207–11.

Cheng L, Bishop E, Zhou H, Maclennan GT, Lopez-Beltran A, Zhang S, Badve S, Baldridge LA, Montironi R. Lymphatic Vessel Density in Radical Prostatectomy Specimens. Hum Pathol. 2008 Apr; **39**(4): 610–15.

Mazzucchelli R, Lopez-Beltran A, Cheng L, Scarpelli M, Kirkali Z, Montironi R. Rare and Unusual Histological Variants of Prostatic Carcinoma: Clinical Significance. BJU Int. 2008 Nov; **102**(10): 1369–74.

Montironi R, Cheng L, Mazzucchelli R, Lopez-Beltran A. Pathological Definition and Difficulties in Assessing Positive Margins in Radical Prostatectomy Specimens. BJU Int. 2009 Feb; **103**(3): 286–88.

Lopez-Beltran A, Cheng L, Prieto R, Blanca A, Montironi R. Lymphoepithelioma-like Carcinoma of the Prostate. Hum Pathol. 2009 Jul; **40**(7): 982–87.

Montironi R, Cheng L, Lopez-Beltran A, Mazzucchelli R, Scarpelli M, Kirkali Z, Montorsi F. Joint Appraisal of the Radical Prostatectomy Specimen by the Urologist and the Uropathologist: Together, We Can Do It Better. Eur Urol. 2009 Dec; 56(6): 951–55.

Montironi R, Gasparrini S, Mazzucchelli R, Massari F, Cheng L, Lopez-Beltran A, Montorsi F, Scarpelli M. Re: Karim A. Touijer, James A. Eastham. The Sentinel Lymph Node Concept and Novel Approaches in Detecting Lymph Node Metastasis in Prostate Cancer. Eur Urol. 2016 Aug 24; pii: S0302-2838(16)30503-6. doi: 10.1016/j.eururo.2016.08.036. In press. www.dx.doi.org/10.1016/j.eururo.2016.02.047.

Conti A, Santoni M, Burattini L, Scarpelli M, Mazzucchelli R, Galosi AB, Cheng L, Lopez-Beltran A, Briganti A, Montorsi F, Montironi R. Update on Histopathological Evaluation of Lymphadenectomy Specimens from Prostate Cancer Patients. World J Urol. 2015 Dec 22; [Epub ahead of print]

Haki Yuksel O, Urkmez A, Verit A. Can Perineural Invasion Detected in Prostate Needle Biopsy Specimens Predict Surgical Margin Positivity in D'Amico Low Risk Patients? Arch Ital Urol Androl. 2016 Jul 4; 88(2): 89–92.

Bostwick DG, Day CE, Meiers I. Optimizing Prostate Specimen Handling for Diagnosis and Prognosis. Methods Mol Biol. 2014; 1180: 337–52.

Flood TA, Schieda N, Keefe DT, Morash C, Bateman J, Mai KT, Belanger EC, Robertson SJ, Breau RH. Perineural Invasion on Biopsy Is Associated with Upstaging at Radical Prostatectomy in Gleason Score 3 + 4 = 7 Prostate Cancer. Pathol Int. 2016 Nov; 66(11): 629–32.

Nunez AL, Giannico GA, Mukhtar F, Dailey V, El-Galley R, Hameed O. Frozen Section Evaluation of Margins in Radical Prostatectomy Specimens: A Contemporary Study and Literature Review. Ann Diagn Pathol. 2016 Oct; 24: 11–8.

Park YH, Kim Y, Yu H, Choi IY, Byun SS, Kwak C, Chung BH, Lee HM, Kim CS, Lee JY. Is Lymphovascular Invasion a Powerful Predictor for Biochemical Recurrence in pT3 N0 Prostate Cancer? Results from the K-CaP Database. Sci Rep. 2016 May 5; 6: 25419.

Fleshner K, Assel M, Benfante N, Lee J, Vickers A, Fine S, Carlsson S, Eastham J. Clinical Findings and Treatment Outcomes in Patients with Extraprostatic Extension Identified on Prostate Biopsy. J Urol. 2016 Sep; 196(3): 703–08.

Kim DK, Koo KC, Abdel Raheem A, Kim KH, Chung BH, Choi YD, Rha KH. Single Positive Lymph Node Prostate Cancer Can Be Treated Surgically without Recurrence. PLoS One. 2016 Mar 31; 11(3): e0152391.

Kang M, Oh JJ, Lee S, Hong SK, Lee SE, Byun SS. Perineural Invasion and Lymphovascular Invasion Are Associated with Increased Risk of Biochemical Recurrence in Patients Undergoing Radical Prostatectomy. Ann Surg Oncol. 2016 Aug; 23(8): 2699–706.

Meng Y, Liao YB, Xu P, Wei WR, Wang J. Perineural Invasion Is an Independent Predictor of Biochemical Recurrence of Prostate Cancer after Local Treatment: M meta-analysis. Int J Clin Exp Med. 2015 Aug 15; 8(8): 13267–74.

Pathology of the Prostate after Treatment

9.1 Non-neoplastic Prostate

- The appearance of hormonally-treated prostates is that of global senescence or involution of the gland. The transition zone shows simplification of the glandular lobules, although the lobular configuration is retained. The ducts and acini are small, ovoid, round or comma-shaped. There is no undulation of the epithelial border.

- The secretory cells have inconspicuous nucleoli, nuclear shrinkage, chromatin condensation and cytoplasmic clearing. The basal cell layer is prominent and focal "immature" squamous and basal cell hyperplasia is seen. Figs 9.1–9.4

- Within the peripheral and central zones, there is inconspicuous branching of the ducts and acini, which appear dilated, star-shaped and lined by flattened atrophic epithelium which is single-layered and seldom double-layered. Table 9.1

9.2 Prostatic Intraepithelial Neoplasia

- PIN is generally observed within scattered ducts with lower extent of PIN in treated glands. The cell lining shows a basal-cell layer which is marked and

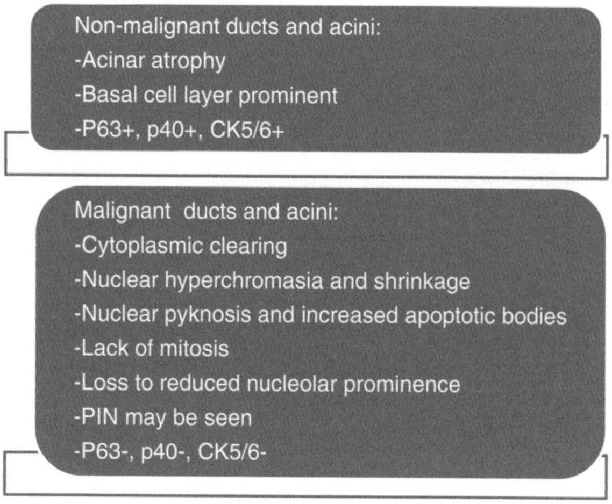

Non-malignant ducts and acini:
- Acinar atrophy
- Basal cell layer prominent
- P63+, p40+, CK5/6+

Malignant ducts and acini:
- Cytoplasmic clearing
- Nuclear hyperchromasia and shrinkage
- Nuclear pyknosis and increased apoptotic bodies
- Lack of mitosis
- Loss to reduced nucleolar prominence
- PIN may be seen
- P63-, p40-, CK5/6-

Fig 9.1 Features to suggest therapy related changes in prostate samples.

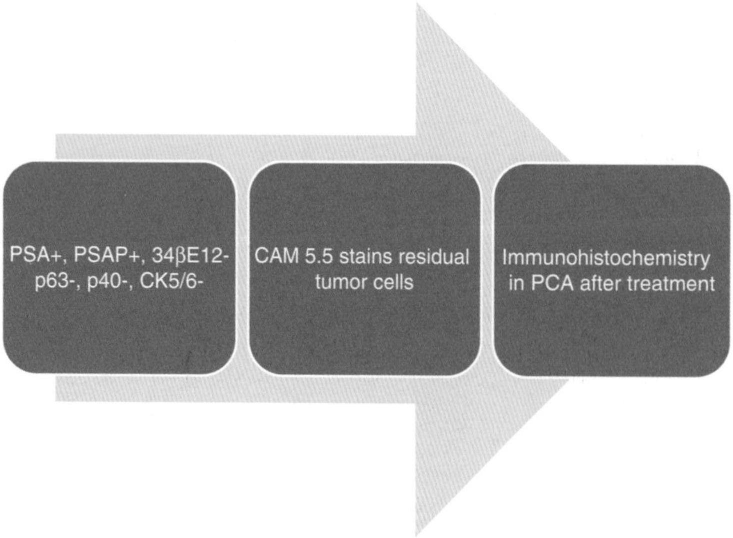

Fig 9.2 Immunohistochemistry may assist in the correct diagnosis of prostate specimens after anti-androgen therapy.

PSA+, PSAP+, 34βE12- p63-, p40-, CK5/6-

CAM 5.5 stains residual tumor cells

Immunohistochemistry in PCA after treatment

Table 9.1 Pathologic Findings in the Prostate Following Androgen Blockade (The Changes Affect Normal Prostate, PIN and Cancer)

Architecture

Prominent acinar atrophy with loss of hyperplastic glandular architecture in the transition zone

Basal cell prominence and hyperplasia in benign prostate

Squamous metaplasia, including the immature variant

Decrease in extent of PIN

Decrease in extent of prostatic adenocarcinoma with loss of luminal (acinar) architecture

Decreased frequency of intraluminal crystalloids in prostatic adenocarcinoma

Cytology

Cytoplasmic clearing and vacuolization

Nuclear shrinkage

Nuclear hyperchromasia

Nuclear pyknosis with increased frequency of apoptotic bodies

Lack of mitotic figures

Loss of nucleolar prominence

Stroma

Focal hypercellularity

Focal lymphocytic/histiocytic infiltrate (including foamy, lipid-laden histiocytes)

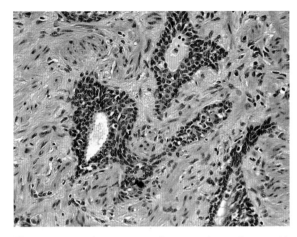

Fig 9.3 Non-neoplastic prostate after anti-androgen therapy with highlighted basal cell layer.

- The duct and acinar lumen are always rich in cells; some are macrophages, some are sloughed secretory cells with degenerative features, while others correspond to apoptotic cells. No post-treatment grading of PIN is possible.
- Blockade of 5-alpha-reductase with finasteride appears to have little or no effect on HGPIN, unlike other forms of androgen deprivation therapy.

9.3 Prostate Cancer

- Hormonal therapy results in a significant overall reduction in the volume of Pca when compared to untreated Pca in radical prostatectomy samples. Histological response seems to correlate with the tumor patterns and the Gleason grades observed before the androgen ablation therapy is started.
- Residual Pca invading the prostatic capsule, periprostatic soft tissue, seminal vesicle and metastatic to pelvic lymph nodes shows therapy-induced changes similar to adenocarcinomas confined within the prostate gland.
- The treated tumors, with acinar pattern (primary Gleason grade 1 to 3) in the biopsy before the androgen ablation therapy, show neoplastic acini which appear shrunken, a decreased frequency of intraluminal crystalloids and areas of individual infiltrating tumor cells separated by abundant connective tissue.

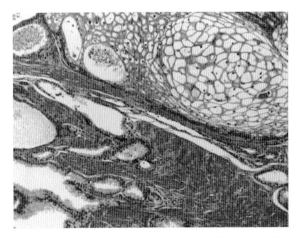

Fig 9.4 Non-keratinizing squamous metaplasia of the prostate after long term estrogen therapy.

recognizable in most instances. A certain degree of secretory cell type stratification is always present. However, crowding is less evident than in the untreated prostate. Fig 9.5

- The cells have nuclear shrinkage, chromatin condensation and pyknosis, inconspicuous nucleoli, and cytoplasmic clearing. Apoptotic cells are easily identifiable in all the cell type layers.

115

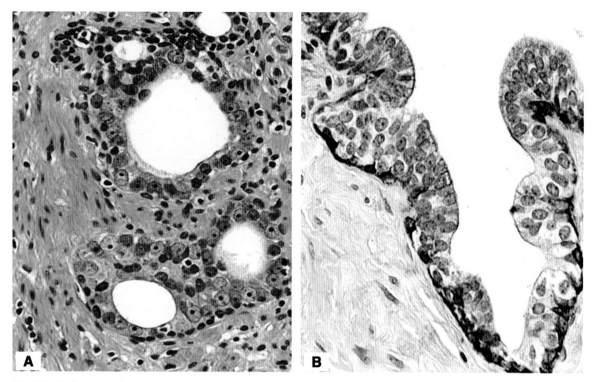

Fig 9.5 PIN after anti-androgen therapy (A). Anti-basal cell cytokeratin highlights basal cell layer (B).

- The epithelial tumor cells have cytoplasmic clearing and enlargement by coalescence of vacuoles and rupture of cell membranes. The nuclear chromatin shows different changes which range from a mild condensation – which barely allows the distinction between coarse chromatin granules (heterochromatin) and finely dispersed chromatin (euchromatin) – to a tightly condensed state close to that observed in apoptosis.
- Apoptotic bodies are easily identifiable in all epithelial cell layers, as well as macrophages and sloughed epithelial cells in the lumina.
- The hallmark of all the untreated adenocarcinomas is that the tumor nuclei are frequently multinucleolated, the nucleoli being prominent (mean diameter 1.47 μm), marginated and with a perinuclear halo. By contrary, in the treated cases, the nucleoli become inconspicuous, without margination, and have a decreased mean diameter of 1.09 μm, the nucleolar diameter being below 1.0 μm in 20% of the tumors. Figs 9.6–9.9
- The treated tumors with pre-treatment cribriform and solid/trabecular patterns (primary Gleason

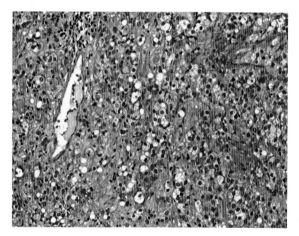

Fig 9.6 Microscopic features of prostate carcinoma after anti-androgen therapy (low power).

grade 4 and 5) show nuclear and cytoplasmic changes which appear less pronounced than in the acinar pattern.

- The stroma shows variable degrees of fibrosis, reduced capillary vascularity and variable density of lymphocytic infiltrates, often intermingled with mast cells, plasma cells, and eosinophils. Infiltrates

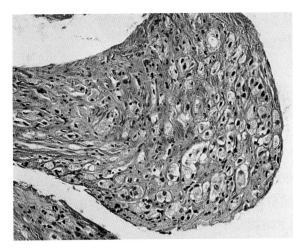

Fig 9.7 Microscopic features of prostate carcinoma after anti-androgen therapy (medium power).

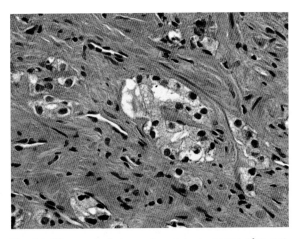

Fig 9.8 Microscopic features of prostate carcinoma after anti-androgen therapy (high power).

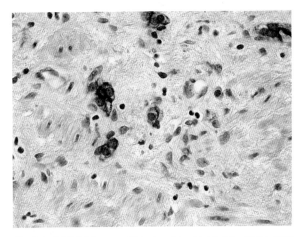

Fig 9.9 CAM 5.2 immunohistochemistry highlights cancer acini after anti-androgen therapy.

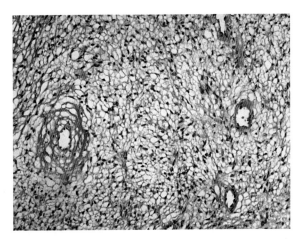

Fig 9.10 Stromal vacuolization after long-term treatment with finasteride.

of foamy histiocytes, difficult to distinguish from Pca cells with clear cytoplasm, are sometimes present. Periprostatic fibrosis, obscuring the normal cleavage plane and making the operation more difficult, is reported after hormonal therapy. The longer patients receive hormonal therapy prior to surgery, the more fibrosis is observed around the prostate.

- 5-alpha reductase inhibitors (5ARIs) are not likely to cause morphological changes in prostate cancer, particularly those associated with artifactually increased Gleason scores. There is currently no consensus on whether pathologists should avoid reporting Gleason scores in specimens obtained from patients treated with 5ARIs.

- Other novel drugs developed to manipulate BPH or prostate cancer produce morphologic changes that can be recognized by the practicing pathologist. This includes finasteride, dutasteride, and bicalutamida. Figs 9.10–9.17

9.4 Immunohistochemistry

- In some cases, residual tumors consist only of isolated cells or cell clusters within prostatic stroma. Significant difficulty may be encountered in separating minute clusters and single file ribbons of tumor cells from lymphocytes, myocytes and fibroblasts.
- Immunostaining with PSA and prostatic acid phosphatase can detect persisting tumor cells. Immunohistochemistry with a low-molecular-

weight cytokeratin, such as CAM 5.2 antibody, will stain residual Pca cells, but the same cells will lack reactivity for high-molecular-weight cytokeratin 34ßE12, which highlights basal cells.

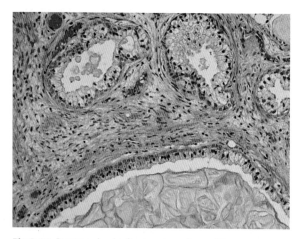

Fig 9.11 Prostate glands after long-term finasteride treatment.

9.5 Pathological "Grading" of Treated Prostate Cancer

- Because of therapy-induced morphologic changes, grading of residual Pca, based on Gleason criteria, is not accurate and, therefore, discouraged. However, it may be performed in situations of changes related to therapy that are not present in the prostate cancer. Fig 9.18

9.6 Pathologic Stage and Resection Margin Status of Treated Prostate Cancer

- There is conflicting evidence regarding pathological down staging, with some studies suggesting benefit and others no benefit of androgen manipulation before radical prostatectomy. Likewise, it seems like neoadjuvant therapy in clinical T2 tumors was associated with

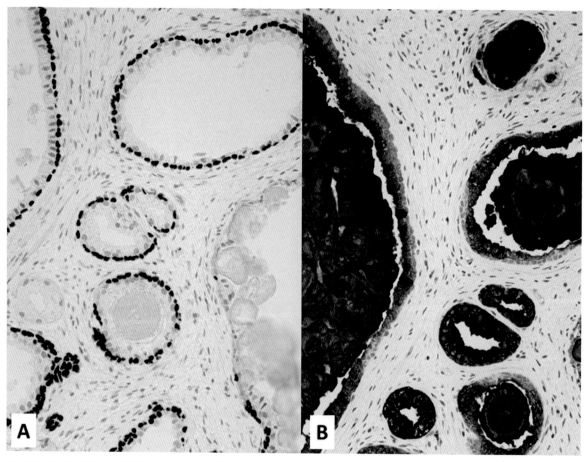

Fig 9.12 Basal cells (anti-p63) (A) and secretory cells (anti-PSA) (B) remained unchanged after long-term finasteride treatment.

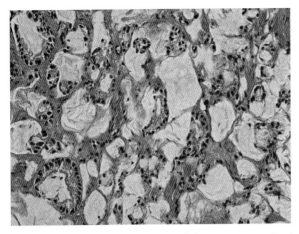

Fig 9.13 Mucinous adenocarcinoma of the prostate remained unchanged after long-term finasteride treatment.

20% decrease in positive margins in radical prostatectomy specimens.

9.7 Pathologic Changes after Radiation Therapy (RT)

Microscopically, radiation treated benign prostatic tissue shows extensive atrophy with frequent cytologic atypia and prominent or hyperplastic basal cell layer. Basal cells may show nuclear atypia in the form of nucleomegaly and/or nucleolomegaly. Variable nuclear size and shape account for the pleomorphism of the nuclei typically seen in these prostate samples. The atrophic glands show size reduction but also lower number of the glands. The luminal cells show a characteristic volume reduction. The prostatic stroma is fibrotic and may show chronic inflammation.

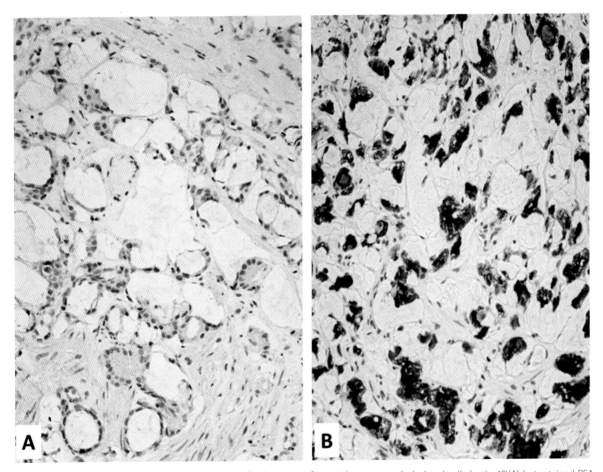

Fig 9.14 Mucinous adenocarcinoma of the prostate after long-term finasteride treatment lacks basal cells (anti-p40)(A) but retained PSA (anti-PSA) (B).

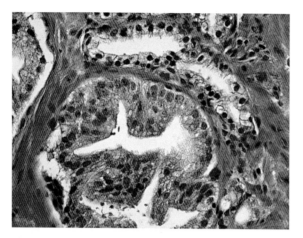

Fig 9.15 PIN after long-term dutasteride treatment.

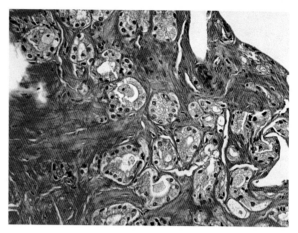

Fig 9.16 Acinar adenocarcinoma of prostate after long-term dutasteride treatment.

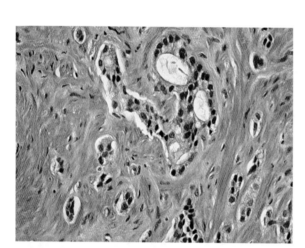

Fig 9.17 Acinar adenocarcinoma of prostate after bicalutamida treatment.

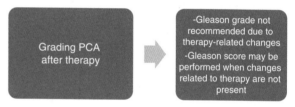

Grading PCA after therapy ⟹ -Gleason grade not recommended due to therapy-related changes
-Gleason score may be performed when changes related to therapy are not present

Fig 9.18 Grading criteria in the post-therapy setting.

9.8 Prostatic Intraepithelial Neoplasia

- PIN identified after RT usually retains the features characteristic of untreated PIN. It is readily recognized in the RP specimens. The salient pathologic features include nuclear crowding, nuclear overlapping and stratification, nuclear hyperchromasia and prominent nucleoli.
  The basal cell layer is still present, but fragmented. The most common patterns of PIN are tufting and micropapillary. Basal cell prominence and secretory cell cytoplasm vacuolization may be seen in PIN after RT. Fig 9.19
- In some cases, the use of immunostaining for high-molecular-weight keratin may be helpful in distinguishing atypical basal cell hyperplasia or other reparative changes from high-grade PIN. Figs 9.20–9.21

9.9 Prostatic Cancer

- The histological effects of RT on the cancer are identical. After radiation therapy, the prostate

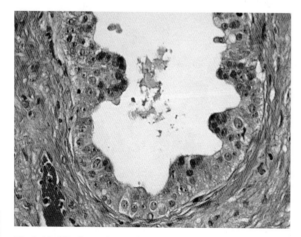

Fig 9.19 PIN after radiation therapy.

gland is usually small and hard. Radiation therapy affects prostate cancer variably with some glands showing marked radiation effect and others showing no evidence of radiation damage.

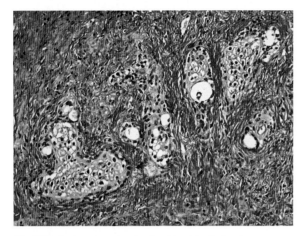

Fig 9.20 Benign prostate glands with metaplastic changes seen after external radiation therapy.

Architecturally, carcinoma showing treatment effects typically loses their glandular pattern, resulting in clustered cells or individual cells.

- Cytologically, the cytoplasm of the tumor cells is pale, increased in volume and often vacuolated. There is often a greater variation of nuclear size than in non-irradiated prostate cancer and the nuclei may be pyknotic or large with clumped chromatin. Nucleoli are often lost. The stroma is often sclerosed or hyalinized. Figs 9.22–9.23

9.10 Immunohistochemistry

- By immunohistochemistry, tumor cells with treatment effect are usually positive for PAP and PSA. These antibodies, along with pan-cytokeratins, are very helpful to detect isolated residual tumor cells, which can be overlooked in H&E stained sections. Immunohistochemistry with antibodies against 34βE12 or p63 is useful to distinguish cancer from normal cells with effects

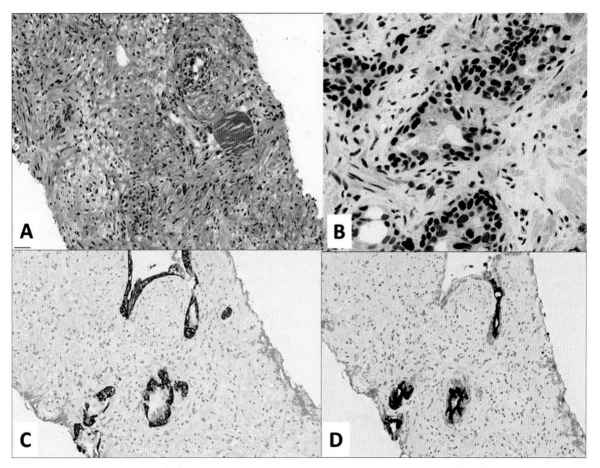

Fig 9.21 Benign prostate glands with changes seen after external radiation therapy (A) with retained p63 (B), 34βE12 (C) and PSA (D).

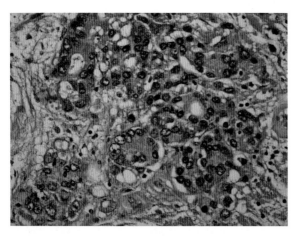

Fig 9.22 Microscopic features of prostate carcinoma after radiation therapy (high power).

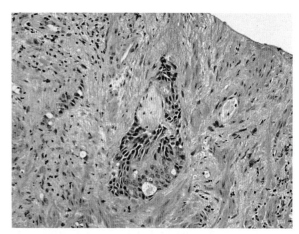

Fig 9.23 Perineural invasion in prostate carcinoma after radiation therapy.

due to radiation therapy. Racemase expression may be preserved in some cases.

9.11 Pathologic "Grading" of Treated Adenocarcinoma

- Following radiation therapy, prostatic biopsy should be diagnosed as no evidence of cancer, cancer showing no or minimal radiation effect, cancer showing significant radiation effect or a combination of the above. Although there are different systems to grade radiation effects in cancer, these are not recommended for routine clinical practice.

9.12 Chemotherapy

- The agents used to treat prostate cancer include cisplatin, mitoxantrone, etoposide, estramustine, vinblastine, docetaxel and paclitaxel. There is little information on the effects of such compounds on the morphology of prostatic carcinoma.
- A recent neoadjuvant trial using docetaxel and mitoxanthrone described some interesting morphological changes in the cancer, including inconspicuous collapsed glands, small inconspicuous individual tumor cells, prominently vacuolated tumor cells and intraductal and cribriform architectural growth patterns.

9.13 Emerging Ablative Therapies

- The concept that many men with low risk prostate cancer are being either over-treated by radical prostatectomy or under-treated by active

surveillance has provided a stimulus to develop minimally invasive, focal therapies that attempt to ablate the entire gland or only a portion of it. These approaches include high-intensity focused ultrasound (HIFU), cryotherapy and laser therapy. Figs 9.24–9.25

- Post-treatment tissue samples show well-circumscribed areas of coagulative necrosis, granulation tissue, inflammatory and histiocytic infiltrates and fibrosis. Ghosts of neoplastic glands can be seen in areas showing coagulative necrosis. Biopsies obtained from areas where the treatment was sub-optimal and from untreated zones show normal prostate tissue and/or adenocarcinoma with no apparent morphological alterations. In areas of viable tumor, there are generally no treatment-induced histological changes that would preclude the use of Gleason scoring. One must be aware of any history of pre-treatment anti-androgen therapy that may have been used to shrink the gland prior to treatment, in which case Gleason scoring may not be applicable.

9.14 Targeted Molecular Therapies and Newer Treatments

- There are many new compounds at various stages of development that target apoptosis and differentiation, growth factor and signal transduction pathways, and angiogenesis, as well as novel cytotoxic agents and immunologic therapies.
- Several newer forms of hormone therapy have been developed. Some of these may be helpful

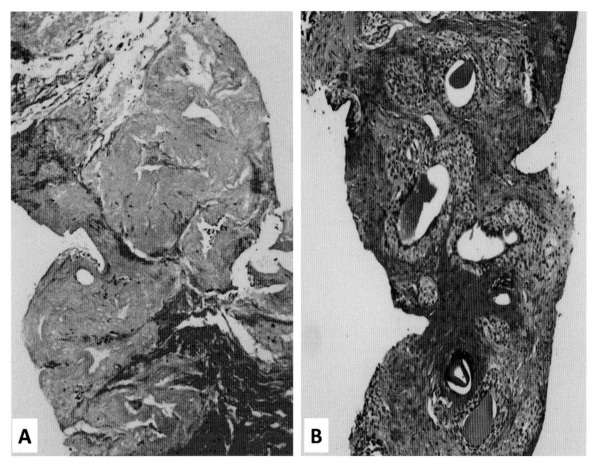

Fig 9.24 Pathologic changes after cryotherapy with stromal hyalinization (A) and urothelial metaplasia of the prostate glands (B).

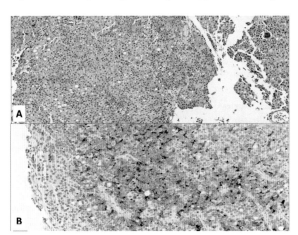

Fig 9.25 Recurrent high grade prostate cancer (A) with retained PSA expression (B) after laser therapy.

when the standard forms of hormone therapy are no longer effective. For instance, enzalutamide and abiraterone are novel hormonal agents approved for the treatment of metastatic castration-resistant prostate cancer (mCRPC) after taxane–based chemotherapy. Another new drug being studied, known as orteronel, works in a similar way to abiraterone. This drug may target CYP17 more precisely, which may do away with the need for taking a steroid drug such as prednisone along with treatment.

• Recently, also several types of vaccines for boosting the body's immune response to prostate cancer cells are being tested in clinical trials. These vaccines are designed to help treat, not prevent, prostate cancer. One possible advantage of these types of treatments is that they seem to have very limited side effects. An example of this type of vaccine is sipuleucel-T (Provenge), which has received FDA approval. Another prostate cancer vaccine (PROSTVAC-VF) uses a virus that has been genetically modified to contain prostate-specific antigen (PSA). The patient's immune system should respond to the virus and begin to recognize and destroy cancer cells containing PSA. Early results with this vaccine have been promising. Several other prostate cancer vaccines are also in development.

- A drug called ipilimumab (Yervoy) targets certain white blood cells that help control the immune system. This drug is used to treat advanced melanoma, and is being tested in men with advanced prostate cancer.

- Targeted therapy is a newer type of cancer treatment that uses drugs or other substances to identify and attack cancer cells while doing little damage to normal cells. Each type of targeted therapy works differently, but all alter the way a cancer cell grows, divides, repairs itself or interacts with other cells. Cabozantinib is a new drug that has as targets both MET and VEGFR protein. In early studies, this drug was found to be able to reduce the size of or eliminate bone tumors on imaging scans in many men whose prostate cancer was no longer responding to hormones.

- At present, several anti-angiogenic drugs have been tested in clinical trials. One of these is thalidomide, which has been approved by the FDA to treat patients with multiple myeloma. It was combined with chemotherapy in an early phase study of men with advanced prostate cancer.

- Data on the effects of these therapies on cancer morphology will be available in the coming years and pathologists will have a central role in this process.

9.15 Nutritional Supplements

- The vitamins E and D, and nutritional supplements such as selenium, green tea, tomato products and soy used as potential preventative agents for prostate cancer are currently under investigation.

- No significant histological changes in either normal prostate tissue or prostate cancer have been described to date and the use of these agents will likely have no impact on the ability of histopathologists to diagnose and grade prostate cancer. The same would appear to apply to herbal supplements used to promote prostate health, such as saw palmetto berry extract.

Suggested Reading

Evans AJ, Ryan P, van der Kwast T. Treatment Effects in the Prostate Including Those Associated with Traditional and Emerging Therapies. Adv Anat Pathol. 2011; **18**(4): 281–93.

Srigley JR, Delahunt B, Evans AJ. Therapy-associated Effects in the Prostate Gland. Histopathology. 2012; **60**(1): 153–65.

Bono AV, Mazzucchelli R, Ferrari I, et al. Bicalutamide 50 mg Monotherapy in Patients with Isolated High-grade PIN: Findings in Repeat Biopsies at 6 Months. J Clin Pathol. 2007; **60**(4): 443–46.

Zattoni F. Prostate Cancer: What Are the News in Hormonal Therapy? The Role of GnRH Antagonists. Arch Ital Urol Androl. 2012; **84** (3): 111–16.

Humphrey PA. Treatment Effects. In: Prostate Pathology. Humphrey PA (Ed.), ASCP PRESS. Chicago, USA. 2003; 456–76.

Montironi R, Schulman CC. Pathological Changes in Prostate Lesions after Androgen Manipulation. J Clin Pathol. 1998; **51** (1): 5–12.

Petraki CD, Sfikas CP. Histopathological Changes Induced by Therapies in the Benign Prostate and Prostate Adenocarcinoma. Histol Histopathol. 2007; **22** (1): 107–18.

Têtu B. Morphological Changes Induced by Androgen Blockade in Normal Prostate and Prostatic Carcinoma. Best Pract Res Clin Endocrinol Metab. 2008; **22**(2): 271–83.

Brawer MK. Hormonal therapy for prostate cancer. Rev Urol. 2006; **8**(2): S35–S47.

Crawford ED. Hormonal Therapy of Prostate Cancer: Historical Approaches. Rev Urol. 2006; **6**(7): S3–S11.

Civantos F, Marcial MA, Banks ER, et al. Pathology of Androgen Deprivation Therapy in Prostate Carcinoma: A Comparative Study of 173 Patients. Cancer. 1995; **75**(7): 1634–41.

Têtu B, Srigley JR, Boivin JC, et al. Effect of Combination Endocrine Therapy (LHRH Agonist and Flutamide) on Normal Prostate and Prostatic Adenocarcinoma. A Histopathologic and Immunohistochemical Study. Am J Surg Pathol. 1991; **15**(2): 111–20.

Andriole G, Bostwick D, Civantos F, et al. The Effects of 5alpha-Reductase Inhibitors on the Natural History, Detection and Grading of Prostate Cancer: Current State of Knowledge. J Urol. 2005; **174**(6): 2098–104.

Thompson IM, Goodman PJ, Tangen CM, et al. The Influence of Finasteride on the Development of Prostate Cancer. N Engl J Med. 2003; **349**(3): 215–24.

Wilt TJ, Macdonald R, Hagerty K, et al. 5-α-Reductase Inhibitors for Prostate Cancer Chemoprevention: An updated Cochrane Systematic Review. BJU Int. 2010; **106**(10): 1444–51.

Bostwick DG, Qian J. Effect of Androgen Deprivation Therapy on Prostatic Intraepithelial Neoplasia. Urology. 2001; **58**(2): 91–93.

Ferguson J, Zincke H, Ellison E, Bergstrahl E, Bostwick DG. Decrease of Prostatic Intraepithelial Neoplasia (PIN) Following Androgen Deprivation Therapy in Patients with Stage T3 Carcinoma Treated by Radical Prostatectomy. Urology. 1994; **44**(1): 91–95.

Vaillancourt L, Tetu B, Fradet Y, et al. Effect of Neoadjuvant Endocrine Therapy (Combined Androgen Blockade) on Normal Prostate and Prostatic Carcinoma. J Surg Pathol. 1996; **20**: 86–93.

Montironi R, Magi Galluzzi C, Muzzonigro G, Prete E, Polito M, Fabris G. Effect of Combination Endocrine Therapy (LHRH Agonist and Flutamide) on Normal Prostate, Prostatic Intraepithelial Neoplasia and Prostatic Adenocarcinoma. J Clin Pathol. 1994; **47**(10): 906–13.

Dhom G, Degro S. Therapy of Prostatic Cancer and Histopathologic Follow-up. Prostate. 1982; **3**(6): 531–42.

Selli C, Montironi R, Bono A, et al. PROSIT Study Group. Effects of Complete Androgen Blockade for 12 and 24 Weeks on the Pathological Stage and Resection Margin Status of Prostate Cancer. J Clin Pathol. 2002; **55**(7): 508–13.

Armas OA, Aprikian A, Melamed J, et al. Clinical and Pathobiological Effects of Neoadjuvant Total Androgen Ablation Therapy in Clinically Localized Prostatic Carcinoma. Am J Surg Pathol. 1994; **18**(10): 979–91.

Magi Galluzzi C, Montironi R, Giannulis I, Diamanti L, Scarpelli M. Prostatic Invasive Adenocarcinoma. Effect of Combination Endocrine Therapy (LHRH Agonist and Flutamide) on the Expression and Location of Proliferating Cell Nuclear Antigen (PCNA). Pathol Res Pract. 1993; **189**(10): 1154–60.

Minardi D, Galosi AB, Giannulis I, Montironi R, Polito M, Muzzonigro G. Comparison of Proliferating Cell Nuclear Antigen Immunostaining in Lymph Node Metastases and Primary Prostate Adenocarcinoma after Neoadjuvant Androgen Deprivation Therapy. Scand J Urol Nephrol. 2004; **38**(1): 19–25.

Montironi R, Magi Galluzzi C, Fabris G. Apoptotic Bodies in Prostatic Intraepithelial Neoplasia and Prostatic Adenocarcinoma Following Total Androgen Ablation. Pathol Res Pract. 1995; **191**(9): 873–80.

Murphy WM, Soloway MS, Barrows GH. Pathologic Changes Associated with Androgen Deprivation Therapy for Prostate Cancer. Cancer. 1991; **68**(4): 821–28.

Reuter VE. Pathological Changes in Benign and Malignant Prostatic Tissue Following Androgen Deprivation Therapy. Urology. 1997; **49**(3A): 16–22.

Smith DM, Murphy WM. Histologic Changes in Prostate Carcinomas Treated with Leuprolide (Luteinizing Hormone-releasing Hormone Effect). Distinction from Poor Tumor Differentiation. Cancer. 1994; **73**(5): 1472–77.

Van de Voorde WM, Elgamal AA, Van Poppel HP, Verbeken EK, Baert LV, Lauweryns JM. Morphologic and Immunohistochemical Changes in Prostate Cancer after Preoperative Hormonal Therapy. Cancer. 1994; **74**(12): 3164–75.

Akakura K, Bruchovsky N, Goldenberg SL, Rennie PS, Buckley AR, Sullivan LD. Effects of Intermittent Androgen Suppression on Androgen-dependent Tumors. Cancer. 1993; **71**(9): 2782–90.

Efstathiou E, Abrahams NA, Tibbs RF, et al. Morphologic Characterization of Preoperatively Treated Prostate Cancer: Toward a Post-therapy Histologic Classification. Eur Urol. 2010; **57**(6): 1030–38.

Lucia MS, Epstein JI, Goodman PJ, et al. Finasteride and High-grade Prostate Cancer in the Prostate Cancer Prevention Trial. J Natl Cancer Inst. 2007; **99**(18): 1375–83.

Rubin MA, Allory Y, Molinie′ V, et al. Effects of Long-term Finasteride Treatment on Prostate Cancer Morphology and Clinical Outcome. Urology. 2005; **66**(5): 930–34.

Scattoni V, Montironi R, Mazzucchelli R, et al. Pathological Changes of High-grade Prostatic Intraepithelial Neoplasia and Prostate Cancer after Monotherapy with Bicalutamide 150 mg. BJU Int. 2006. **98**(1): 54–58.

Bullock MJ, Srigley JR, Klotz LH, Goldenberg SL. Pathologic Effects of Neoadjuvant Cyproterone Acetate on Nonneoplastic Prostate, Prostatic Intraepithelial Neoplasia, and Adenocarcinoma. A Detailed Analysis of Radical Prostatectomy Specimens from a Randomized Trial. Am J Surg Pathol. 2002; **26**(11): 1400–13.

Schulman CC, Wildschutz T, Zlotta AR. Neoadjuvant Hormonal Treatment Prior to Radical Prostatectomy: Facts and Questions. Eur Urol. 1997; **32**(3): 41–47.

Gleave ME, Goldenberg SL, Jones EC, Bruchovsky N, Kinahan J, Sullivan LD. Optimal Duration of Neoadjuvant Androgen Withdrawal Therapy before Radical Prostatectomy in Clinically Confined Prostate Cancer. Sem Urol Oncol. 1996; **14**(2): 39–47.

Bazinet M, Zheng W, Begin LR, Aprikian AG, Karakiewicz PI, Elhilali MM. Morphologic Changes Induced by Neoadjuvant Androgen Ablation May Result in Underdetection of Positive Surgical Margins and Capsular Involvement by Prostatic Adenocarcinoma. Urology. 1997; **49**(5): 721–25.

Gould VE, Doljanskaia V, Gooch GT, Bostwick DG. Stability of the Glycoprotein A-80 in Prostatic Carcinoma Subsequent to Androgen Deprivation Therapy. Am J Surg Pathol. 1997; **21**(3): 319–26.

Abbas F, Scardino PT. Why Neoadjuvant Androgen Deprivation Prior to Radical Prostatectomy is Unnecessary. Urol Clin North Am. 1996; **23**(4): 587–604.

Schulman CC. Neoadjuvant Androgen Blockade Prior to Prostatectomy: A Retrospective Study and Critical Review. Prostate. 1994; **5**: 9–13.

Watson RB, Soloway MS. Neoadjuvant Hormonal Treatment before Radical Prostatectomy. Sem Urol Oncol. 1996; **14**(2): 48–56.

Heidenreich A, Richter S, Thuer D. Prognostic Parameters, Complications, and Oncologic and Functional Outcome of Salvage Radical Prostatectomy for Locally Recurrent Prostate Cancer after 21st-century Radiotherapy. Eur Urol. 2010; **57**(3): 437–43.

Böcking A, Auffermann W. Cytological Grading of Therapy-induced Tumor Regression in Prostatic Carcinoma: Proposal of a New System. Diagn Cytopathol. 1987; **3**(2): 108–11.

Crook JM, Bahadur YA, Robertson SJ, Perry GA, Esche BA. Evaluation of Radiation Effect, Tumor Differentiation and Prostate Specific Antigen Staining in Sequential Prostate Biopsies after External Beam Radiotherapy for Patients with Prostate Carcinoma. Cancer. 1997; **79**(1): 81–89.

Crook JM, Malone S, Perry G, et al. Twenty-four Month Postradiation Prostate Biopsies are Strongly Predictive of 7-year Disease Free Survival: Results from a Canadian Randomized Trial. Cancer. 2009; **115**(3): 673–79.

O'Brien C, True LD, Higano CS, Rademacher BL, Garzotto M, Beer TM. Histologic Changes Associated with Neoadjuvant Chemotherapy Are Predictive of Nodal Metastases in Patients with High-risk Prostate Cancer. Am J Clin Pathol. 2010; **133**(4): 654–61.

Falconieri G, Lugnani F, Zanconati F, Signoretto D, Di Bonito L. Histopathology of the Frozen Prostate. The Microscopic Bases of Prostatic Carcinoma Cryoablation. Pathol Res Pract. 1996; **192**(6): 579–87.

Galosi AB, Lugnani F, Muzzonigro G. Salvage Cryosurgery for Recurrent Prostate Carcinoma after Radiotherapy. J Endourol. 2007; **21**(1): 1–7.

Morgenstern N, Ro JY, Batts P, et al. Prostate Cryotherapy: Chronological Post-therapy Histologic Changes with Clinical Correlation. Mod Pathol. 1997; **10**: 83A.

Shabaik A, Wilson S, Bidair M, et al. Pathologic Changes in Prostate Biopsies Following Cryoablation Therapy of Prostate Carcinoma. J Urol Pathol. 1995; **3**: 183–93.

Armstrong AJ, George DJ. New Drug Development in Metastatic Prostate Cancer. Urol Oncol. 2008; **26** (4): 430–37.

Gerritsen WR. The Evolving Role of Immunotherapy in Prostate Cancer. Ann Oncol. 2012; **2**(8): viii22–7.

Cheng ML, Fong L. Beyond Sipuleucel-T: Immune Approaches to Treating Prostate Cancer. Curr Treat Options Oncol. 2014 Jan 10; [Epub ahead of print].

Nguyen HM, Ruppender N, Zhang X, et al. Cabozantinib Inhibits Growth of Androgen-sensitive and Castration-resistant Prostate Cancer and Affects Bone Remodeling. PLoS One. 2013; **8**(10): e78881.

Chapter 10

Basic Molecular Pathology of Prostate Cancer

10.1 Inherited Susceptibility

- Currently, the evidence for a strong genetic basis in prostatic carcinoma is compelling; about 9% of all cases of Pca are thought to have a genetic basis.
- The identification of highly penetrant Pca genes, i.e., genes that markedly increase the risk of cancer, has been particularly difficult for two main reasons. First, due to the advanced age of onset (median 60 years), availability of more than two generations to perform molecular studies on is difficult.
- Second, given the high frequency of Pca, it is likely that cases considered to be hereditary during segregation studies actually represent phenocopies, i.e., sporadic cases in families with high rates of Pca. In addition, hereditary prostate cancer (HPC) does not occur in any of the known cancer syndromes and does not have any clinical (other than a somewhat early age of onset at times) or pathologic characteristics to allow researchers to distinguish it from sporadic Pca. Rearrangement in chromosome 22 between TMPRSS2 and ERG is seen in about 50% of Pca. Figs 10.1–10.2
- Hereditary Pca is characterized by Mendelian autosomal dominant or X-linked modes of inheritance, and an early onset of the disease. Based on the family clustering of Pca, a number of groups have worked to identify the genes involved. Generally, they have used linkage analysis of large families affected by Pca. Work over the past decade using genome-wide scans in Pca families has identified high-risk loci.

10.2 Susceptibility Loci

- There are at least seven susceptibility loci for Pca identified on different chromosomes. Chromosome 1 is of particular interest, with three proposed loci. The chromosomal region 1q24-25,

designated the locus of the hereditary prostate cancer (HPC1) gene, has been the most thoroughly investigated. Some analyses have confirmed a link between HPC1 and Pca, while others have failed to detect an association. The other two proposed susceptibility loci are 1q42.2-q43 and 1p36.

- Additional loci have been identified on chromosome 16 (16q23.2), chromosome 17 (17p11, or HPC2, i.e., hereditary prostate cancer 2,

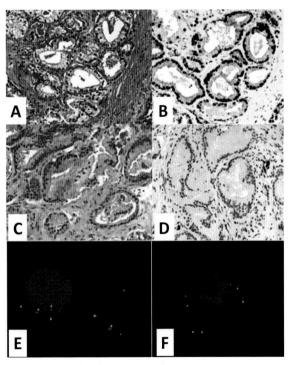

Fig 10.1 Prostate cancer and ERG status as seen by immunohisto-chemistry and ERG FISH analysis. Prostate cancer (A) that exhibited ERG protein expression by immunohistochemistry (B), and prostate cancer (C) that demonstrated negative ERG expression by immuno-histochemistry (D). ERG rearrangement by FISH. In each nucleus, one red-green-aqua signal triplet is closely juxtaposed, whereas the other copy exhibits a widely separated green signal (E). No ERG rearrangement was present as evidenced by two copies of closely juxtaposed red-green-aqua signals (F).

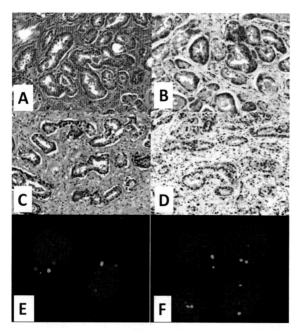

Fig 10.2 Prostate cancer (A) with normal PTEN immunohistochemistry (B) and prostate cancer (C) showing loss of PTEN (D). Normal PTEN copy number (E) as indicated by two red (PTEN) and two green (CEP10) signals. Hemizygous PTEN deletion as indicated by the loss of one red signal (PTEN) and two normal green signals (CEP10).

also called ELAC2), chromosome 20 (20q13 or HPC20) and chromosome X (Xq27-28 or HPCX).

10.3 Candidate HPC genes

- Mutations in a growing number of candidate HPC loci and genes have been detected, suggesting that defects in critical pathways involving DNA damage response, apoptosis and innate immunity may have a particularly important role in the initiation of Pca. The types of alterations associated with such genes are basically represented by base substitutions, deletions and insertions. The following highly penetrant genes probably account for 10% or less of hereditary Pca cases: RNASEL (a candidate tumor suppressor gene within the HPC1 locus located on 1q24-25), MSR1 (located on 8p22, encodes subunits of class A macrophage-scavenger receptor 1), CYP17 (located on 10q24.3, encodes cytochrome P-450c17, an enzyme that catalyzes key reactions in sex-steroid biosynthesis), HPC2/ELAC2 (located on 17p11 and is considered a tumor suppressor gene), BRCA2 (located on chromosome 13q) and CHEK2 (encodes an upstream regulator of p53 in the DNA damage signaling pathway). A number of germline variants and mutations of these genes have been associated with increased risk of Pca.

- An increased risk of Pca has been associated with sexually transmitted infections, regardless of the pathogen, suggesting that inflammation, rather than infection, initiates prostatic carcinogenesis. Inflammatory cells elaborate numerous microbiological oxidants than might cause cellular or genomic damage in the prostate. Two of the candidate Pca susceptibility genes identified thus far, RNASEL and MRS1, encode proteins with critical functions in host response to infections. Mutations in these genes might reduce the ability to eradicate infectious agents, thus resulting in chronic inflammation. RNASEL is believed to regulate cellular proliferation and apoptosis through the interferon-inducible 2',5'-oligoadenylate dependent RNA decay pathway. At least two mutations inactivating RNASEL have been identified that are potentially responsible for Pca cases in families showing linkage to HPC1. Germline MSR1 mutations have been linked to Pca in some families with early-onset hereditary Pca.

- One of the strongest risk factors for prostate cancer is a family history of the disease. Germline mutations in the breast cancer predisposition gene 2 (BRCA2) are the genetic events known to date that confer the highest risk of prostate cancer (8.6-fold in men of 65 years). Although the role of BRCA2 and BRCA1 in prostate tumorigenesis remains unrevealed, deleterious mutations in both genes have been associated with more aggressive disease and poor clinical outcomes. BRCA germline mutations, mainly in the BRCA2 gene, are one of those predictive factors.

- BRCA2, located on chromosome 13q, is a gene that has been implicated as a prostate cancer susceptibility locus primary due to its analysis in breast cancer families. Studies of families with breast cancer suggest that male carriers of BRCA2 mutations are at increased risk for Pca, particularly at an early age. Inactivating mutations in BRCA2 have been reported in approximately 2% of men with early onset Pca, thus confirming the relevance of this gene to Pca susceptibility. Inherited mutations in

DNA-repair genes such as BRCA2 are associated with increased risks of lethal prostate cancer.

- A recent report related BRCA2 somatic mutation to targeted therapy. Although the prevalence of germline mutations in DNA-repair genes among men with localized prostate cancer who are unselected for family predisposition is insufficient to warrant routine testing, the frequency of such mutations in patients with metastatic prostate cancer has not been established. A recent study based on 692 men with documented metastatic prostate cancer who were unselected for family history of cancer or age at diagnosis, showed germline DNA using multiplex sequencing assays to assess mutations in 20 DNA-repair genes associated with autosomal dominant cancer-predisposition syndromes.

- A total of 84 germline DNA-repair gene mutations that were presumed to be deleterious were identified in 82 men (11.8%); mutations were found in 16 genes, including BRCA2 (37 men [5.3%]), ATM (11 [1.6%]), CHEK2 (10 [1.9% of 534 men with data]), BRCA1 (6 [0.9%]), RAD51D (3 [0.4%]) and PALB2 (3 [0.4%]). Mutation frequencies did not differ according to whether a family history of prostate cancer was present or according to age at diagnosis. Overall, the frequency of germline mutations in DNA-repair genes among men with metastatic prostate cancer significantly exceeded the prevalence of 4.6% among 499 men with localized prostate cancer ($P<0.001$), including men with high-risk disease, and the prevalence of 2.7% in the Exome Aggregation Consortium, which includes 53,105 persons without a known cancer diagnosis ($P<0.001$).

- The incidence of germline mutations in genes mediating DNA-repair processes among men with metastatic prostate cancer was 11.8%, which was significantly higher than the incidence among men with localized prostate cancer. The frequencies of germline mutations in DNA-repair genes among men with metastatic disease did not differ significantly according to age at diagnosis or family history of prostate cancer.

- These observations provide potential new therapeutic opportunities for the use of poly (ADP-ribose) polymerase inhibitors and other therapies, especially in advanced forms of the disease. Of note is the recent U.S. Food and Drug Administration breakthrough therapy designation of olaparib for the treatment of BRCA1/2- or ATM-mutated metastatic castration-resistant prostate cancer. The implications of this new knowledge for clinical practice now and in the future are discussed.

10.4 Genetic Polymorphisms

- Perhaps even more important in terms of inherited susceptibility for Pca are common polymorphisms in a number of low penetrance alleles of other genes – the so-called genetic modifier alleles. The major pathways currently under examination include those involved in androgen action, DNA repair, carcinogen metabolism and inflammation pathways. It is widely assumed that the specific combinations of these variants, in the proper environmental setting, can profoundly affect the risk of developing Pca.

- The androgen receptor (AR) gene, a member of the steroid and thyroid hormone receptor gene superfamily, is a transcription factor that mediates the action of androgens in prostate cells. It is located on Xq11–12. The amino-terminal domain encoded by exon 1 contains a variable number of trinucleotide repeats. Decreased transactivation activity and binding affinity for androgens is associated with an increased number of trinucleotide repeats. Shorter CAG repeat lengths have been associated with a greater risk of developing Pca.

- Additional examples of genetic polymorphisms are related to SRD5A2 – a gene located on 2p23 that encodes a polypeptide that catalyzes the conversion of testosterone to dihydrotestosterone – and to Vitamin D Receptor. Polymorphisms in the former have been reported to confer an increased risk of Pca, particularly in African Americans and Hispanics. The contribution of the Vitamin D Receptor gene polymorphisms to Pca susceptibility remains controversial.

10.5 Somatic Gene Alterations

- Many somatic mutations, gene deletions, gene amplifications, chromosomal rearrangements and changes in DNA methylation are detectable in Pca cells at the time of diagnosis. These alterations probably accumulate over a period of several decades and the number of changes increases with the stage of the disease. Telomerase activity is frequently upregulated in Pca. This may contribute to genetic instability and promote neoplastic transformation. Although multiple alterations that appear to contribute to disease progression have been suggested, no single key change has been detected. Perhaps the exception is the description of rearrangements in chromosome 22 between TMPRSS2 and ERG seen in about 50% of Pca. Fig 10.1

10.6 Gene Pathway Alterations

- The roles of PTEN, CDKN1B, AMACR and TMPRSS2-ERG fusion genes have been investigated in several recent publications.
- PTEN (phosphatase and tensin homologue) is a tumor-suppressor gene encoding a phosphatase active against both protein and lipid substrates. PTEN induces G1 cell cycle arrest via negative regulation of the phosphatidylinositol 3'-kinase/protein kinase B (PI3/Akt) signaling pathway that is essential for cell-cycle progression and cell survival. By inhibiting PI3 K/Akt, PTEN can increase the levels of CDKN1B messenger RNA and p27 protein (see below). PTEN is frequently mutated or deleted in Pca cell lines and human tumors. PTEN alterations are more common in metastatic deposits than in primary carcinomas. By immunohistochemistry, PTEN is present in normal epithelial cells and PIN. The level of PTEN is frequently reduced in Pca of high grade or stage. Somatic allelic losses (i.e., haploinsufficiency) in both PTEN and NKX3.1 appear to be common in prostate carcinoma and may promote an abnormal proliferation of prostate cells. Fig 10.2
- CDKN1B encodes p27kip1, a cyclin-dependent kinase inhibitor. The p27kip1 protein regulates cell cycle progression from G1 to S phase by its inhibitory interaction with the cyclin E/cdk2 complex. In Pca, p27kip1 expression progressively decreases with increasing tumor grade and stage. Low levels of p27kip1 may be as much a result of CDKN1B alterations as of the PTEN loss whose function is mediated by the PI3 K-Akt signaling pathway. A recent paper by Dreher et al. dealt with a combined analysis of PTEN and p27kip1 expression in Pca and greatly contributed to the

knowledge that activated Akt blocks p27kip1 entry into the nucleus by phosphorylating a residue within the nuclear localization signal of p27kip1.
- AMACR (Alpha-methylacyl-CoA racemase) encodes an enzyme that plays an important role in the β-oxidation of branched-chain fatty acids and serves as a "caretaker" gene. It has been found consistently upregulated in Pca and high grade prostatic intraepithelial neoplasia (HGPIN), a direct precursor of Pca.

10.7 TMPRSS2 Gene Fusion in Prostate Cancer

- About 50% of PCa shows fusion of the TMPRSS2 and ETS gene family, a change that is specific for prostate cancer. ETS transcription factors include ERG, ETV1, ETV4 and ETV5 as 3' end fusion. ERG is the most common fused gene at 5' end with TMPRSS2 comprising about 90% of cases. Fused ERG is under the control of an androgen-regulated promoter, thus causing overexpression. Fusion of these two genes occurs via genetic rearrangements or more rarely by translocation. The most common reported fusion is between exon 1 of TMPRSS2 and exon 4.
- Histologic characteristics of Pca associated with TMPRSS2:ERG include aggressive features like cribriform pattern, intraductal spread, macronucleoli and signet-ring cells.
- The clinical significance of this gene fusion remains unclear due to conflicting reports by different studies. Most reports support aggressive behavior of Pca cases bearing TMPRSS2:ERG fusion.
- The fusion of TMPRSS2 and ERG loci at the chromosomal level and the subsequent overexpression of the TMPRSS2:ERG transcript and truncated ERG protein product is specific (100%) for Pca in tissue specimens.
- RT-PCR based assays to detect urinary TMPRSS2: ERG are usually associated with indicators of clinically significant Pca at biopsy/histology, including tumor volume and high Gleason score.

10.8 DNA Methylation

- Epigenetic events that can affect gene expression without altering the actual sequence of DNA include phenomena such as DNA methylation, chromatin remodeling, histone modification and

RNA interference. Many gene promoters are associated with GC rich regions of the DNA known as CpG islands. Abnormal methylation of CpG islands located within gene promoters is associated with decreased transcriptional activity and it occurs in many types of cancers. Abnormal methylation of genes such as those involved with control of cellular growth or detoxification is believed to have a critical role in early stages of Pca progression. A certain number of genes, such as GSTP1 and E-Cadherin, are commonly methylated in human Pca.

- GSTP1 (pi-class of Glutathione S-transferase), located on 11q13, probably serves as a caretaker gene. It defends prostate cells against genomic damage mediated by carcinogens or various oxidants. GSTP1 demonstrates hypermethylation in more than in 90% of prostate carcinomas, thus preventing expression of this protective gene.
- E-Cadherin, located on 16q22.1, encodes a Ca2+-dependent cell adhesion molecule that is important in normal cell growth and development and is considered a suppressor of neoplastic invasion. E-Cadherin is methylated in approximately 50% of cases. Decreased expression of E-cadherin has been detected in several primary and metastatic prostate carcinomas.

10.9 Androgen Receptors

- Many somatic alterations of androgen receptors (AR) have been detected in those Pcas that progress despite hormonal treatment. At the same time, prostate tumor cells appear to have several possible mechanisms by which they could become androgen refractory.
- Mutations of the AR could allow it to respond to other steroids or even to anti-androgens. In particular, mutations in the ligand-binding domain of AR could not only increase sensitivity to normal ligands, such as adrenal androgens, which are present at low levels, but also may cause the AR to be responsive to other molecules, such as antiandrogens, which are not normal ligands.
- Mutations in the AR hormone-binding domain or amplification of the AR gene could also increase tumor cell sensitivity to androgens. In fact, the increased levels of AR DNA are associated with an increase in AR messenger RNA. Increased levels of AR protein associated with AR gene amplification have been implicated in the ability of cells to more

effectively use the low levels of androgens that are produced by the adrenal glands and that are still available during androgen deprivation therapy.

- Alterations in the expression or function of genes in regulatory pathways involving peptide growth factors or cytokines could cause inappropriate activation of the AR. For instance, growth factors serve as ligands for receptor tyrosine kinases and activate downstream intracellular kinase cascades. Receptor tyrosine kinases may also be involved in the progression to androgen-refractory Pca through an interaction with the AR. The receptor tyrosine kinase Her2/Neu is expressed at low levels in normal epithelial cells. Several studies have demonstrated Her2/Neu protein overexpression and/or gene amplification in a subset of Pca patients.
- The AR could be bypassed entirely, possibly as a result of constitutive activation of regulatory molecules downstream of the AR. For instance, PTEN inactivation, p53 mutations, bcl-2 pathway alterations, neuroendocrine factors and alternative growth factor regulation and utilization could potentially bypass the need for activation of the AR in some tumors.

10.10 Genomic Heterogeneity of Prostate Cancer

- Genetic diversity among prostate cancers suggests that information from a single cancer biopsy might not be sufficient to guide treatment decisions. Next-generation sequencing is revealing genomic heterogeneity in localized prostate cancer (CaP). Incomplete sampling of CaP multiclonality has limited the implications for molecular subtyping, stratification and systemic treatment.
- Somatic mutations, copy number alternations, gene expression, gene fusions and phylogeny were defined. The impact of genomic alterations on CaP molecular classification, gene sets measured in Oncotype DX, Prolaris and Decipher assays, and androgen receptor activity among CaP cores were determined. There was considerable variability in genomic alterations among CaP cores, and between RNA- and DNA-based platforms. Table 10.1
- Heterogeneity was found in molecular grouping of individual CaP foci and the activity of gene sets

131

Table 10.1 Key Features of Three Commercialized Genomic Tests for Prostate Cancer

	Decipher	Oncotype Dx	Prolaris
Gene panel	22 RNAs from different regions of genome	12 cancer-related to different pathways, plus five reference genes	46 RNAs expression signature
Tissue tested	RP (pT3, margin+ or rising PSA)	Biopsy, very-low-to-intermediate risk	Biopsy or RP
Utility	Predicts probability of metastasis five years after RP	Predicts likelihood of favorable pathology	Cell cycle progression score for mortality or biochemical recurrence
Tissue requirements	1 × 1.0-mm diameter punch of highest Gleason grade in FFPE block	6 × 5-µ sections (1.0 mm length) + two H&Es	5 × 5-µ sections (0.5 mm length) + two H&Es

RP: radical prostatectomy; PSA: prostate specific antigen; FFPE: formalin fixed paraffin embedded

underlying the assays for risk stratification and androgen receptor activity, and was validated in independent genomic data sets.

- Determination of the implications for clinical decision-making requires follow-up studies. Genomic make-up varies widely among CaP foci, so care should be taken when making treatment decisions based on a single biopsy or index lesion.

Suggested Reading

Davis JW. Novel Commercially Available Genomic Tests for Prostate Cancer: A Roadmap to Understanding Their Clinical Impact. BJU Int. 2014; **114**: 320–22.

Dhawan M, Ryan CJ, Ashworth A. DNA Repair Deficiency Is Common in Advanced Prostate Cancer: New Therapeutic Opportunities. Oncologist. 2016 Jun 17; **pii**: The Oncologist. 2016–0135. [Epub ahead of print].

Pritchard CC, Mateo J, Walsh MF, De Sarkar N, Abida W, Beltran H, Garofalo A, Gulati R, Carreira S, Eeles R, Elemento O, Rubin MA, Robinson D, Lonigro R, Hussain M, Chinnaiyan A, Vinson J, Filipenko J, Garraway L, Taplin ME, AlDubayan S, Han GC, Beightol M, Morrissey C, Nghiem B, Cheng HH, Montgomery B, Walsh T, Casadei S, Berger M, Zhang L, Zehir A, Vijai J, Scher HI, Sawyers C, Schultz N, Kantoff PW, Solit D, Robson M, Van Allen EM, Offit K, de Bono J, Nelson PS. Inherited DNA-Repair Gene Mutations in Men with Metastatic Prostate Cancer. N Engl J Med. 2016 Jul 6. [Epub ahead of print].

Cheng L, Davidson DD, Maclennan GT, Lopez-Beltran A, Montironi R, Wang M, Tan PH, Baldridge LA, Zhang S. Atypical Adenomatous Hyperplasia of Prostate Lacks TMPRSS2-ERG Gene Fusion. Am J Surg Pathol. 2013 Oct; **37**(10): 1550–54. doi: 10.1097/PAS.0b013e318294e9bc.

Castro Elena, Eeles Rosalind. The Role of BRCA1 and BRCA2 in Prostate Cancer. Asian Journal of Andrology. 2012; **14**: 409–14.

Schelling LA, Williamson SR, Zhang S, Yao JL, Wang M, Huang J, Montironi R, Lopez-Beltran A, Emerson RE, Idrees MT, Osunkoya AO, Man YG, Maclennan GT, Baldridge LA, Compérat E, Cheng L. Frequent TMPRSS2-ERG Rearrangement in Prostatic Small Cell Carcinoma Detected by Fluorescence in Situ Hybridization: The Superiority of Fluorescence in Situ Hybridization over ERG Immunohistochemistry. Hum Pathol. 2013 Oct; **44**(10): 2227–33. doi: 10.1016/j.humpath.2013.05.005. Epub 2013 Jul 12.

Rao Q, Williamson SR, Lopez-Beltran A, Montironi R, Huang W, Eble JN, Grignon DJ, Koch MO, Idrees MT, Emerson RE, Zhou XJ, Zhang S, Baldridge LA, Cheng L. Distinguishing Primary Adenocarcinoma of the Urinary Bladder from Secondary Involvement by Colorectal Adenocarcinoma: Extended Immunohistochemical Profiles Emphasizing Novel Markers. Mod Pathol. 2013 May; **26**(5): 725–32. doi: 10.1038/modpathol.2012.229. Epub 2013 Jan.

Rubin MA. ETS Rearrangements in Prostate Cancer. Asian Journal of Andrology. 2012; **14**: 393–99.

Mazzucchelli R, Scarpelli M, Barbisan F, Santinelli A, Lopez-Beltran A, Cheng L, Montironi R. Immunohistochemical Expression of Prostate Tumour Overexpressed 1 (PTOV1) in Atypical Adenomatous Hyperplasia (AAH) of the Prostate: Additional Evidence Linking (AAH) to Adenocarcinoma. Cell Oncol (Dordr). 2013 Feb; **36**(1): 37–42. doi: 10.1007/s13402-012-0111-7.

Quick Charles M. MDa, Gokden Neriman MDa, Sangoi Ankur R. MDb, Brooks James D. MDc, McKenney Jesse K. MD. The Distribution of PAX-2 Immunoreactivity in the Prostate Gland, Seminal Vesicle, and Ejaculatory Duct: Comparison with Prostatic Adenocarcinoma and Discussion of Prostatic Zonal Embryogenesis. Human Pathology. 2010; **41**: 1145–49.

Harvey Aaron M. MD, Grice Beverly HTL, Hamilton Candice HTL, Truong Luan D. MD, Ro Jae Y. MD, Ayala Alberto G. MD, Zhai Qihui "Jim" MD. Diagnostic Utility of P504S/p63 Cocktail Prostate-specific Antigen, and Prostatic Acid Phosphatase in Mazzucchelli R, Barbisan F, Santinelli A, Lopez-Beltran A, Cheng L, Scarpelli M, Montironi R. Immunohistochemical Expression of Prostate Tumor Overexpressed 1 in Cystoprostatectomies with Incidental and Insignificant Prostate Cancer. Further Evidence for Field Effect in Prostatic Carcinogenesis. Hum Pathol. 2011 Dec; **42**(12): 1931–36. Epub 2011 Jun 14.

Williamson SR, Zhang S, Yao JL, Huang J, Lopez-Beltran A, Shen S, Osunkoya AO, MacLennan GT, Montironi R, Cheng L. ERG-TMPRSS2 Rearrangement Is Shared by Concurrent Prostatic Adenocarcinoma and Prostatic Small Cell Carcinoma and Absent in Small Cell Carcinoma of the Urinary Bladder: Evidence Supporting Monoclonal Origin. Mod Pathol. 2011 Aug; **24**(8): 1120–27. doi: 10.1038/modpathol.2011.56.

Zhang C, Montironi R, MacLennan GT, Lopez-Beltran A, Li Y, Tan PH, Wang M, Zhang S, Iczkowski KA, Cheng L. Is Atypical Adenomatous Hyperplasia of the Prostate a Precursor Lesion? Prostate. 2011 Dec; **71**(16): 1746–51. doi: 10.1002/pros.21391. Epub 2011 Apr 7.

Wang X, Jones TD, Zhang S, Eble JN, Bostwick DG, Qian J, Lopez-Beltran A, Montironi R, Harris JJ, Cheng L. Amplifications of EGFR Gene and Protein Expression of EGFR, Her-2/Neu, c-kit, and Androgen Receptor in Phyllodes Tumor of the Prostate. Mod Pathol. 2007 Feb; **20**(2): 175–82.

Hodges KB, Abdul-Karim FW, Wang M, Lopez-Beltran A, Montironi R, Easley S, Zhang S, Wang N, MacLennan GT, Cheng L. Evidence for Transformation of Fibroadenoma of the Breast to Malignant Phyllodes Tumor. Appl Immunohistochem Mol Morphol. 2009 Jul; **17**(4): 345–50.

Smith SC- Palanisamy N, Zuhlke KA, Johnson AM, Siddiqui J, Chinnaiyan AM, Kunju LP, Cooney KA, Tomlins SA. HOXB13 G84E-related Familial Prostate Cancers: A Clinical, Histologic, and Molecular Survey. Am J Surg Pathol. 2014 May; **38**(5): 615–26.

Fisher KW, Zhang S, Wang M, Montironi R, Wang L, Baldrige LA, Wang JY, MacLennan GT, Williamson SR, Lopez-Beltran A, Cheng L. TMPRSS2-ERG Gene Fusion Is Rare Compared to PTEN Deletions in Stage T1a Prostate Cancer. Mol Carcinog. 2016 Aug 8; doi: 10.1002/mc.22535.

Buti S, Ciccarese C, Iacovelli R, Bersanelli M, Scarpelli M, Lopez-Beltran A, Cheng L, Montironi R, Tortora G, Massari F. Inside the 2016 American Society of Clinical Oncology Genitourinary Cancers Symposium: Part 2 – Prostate and Bladder Cancer. Future Oncol. 2016 Sep; **12**(17): 1971–74. doi: 10.2217/fon-2016-0166.

M. Francesca Monn1, Rodolfo Montironi2, Antonio Lopez-Beltran3,4, Liang Cheng1,5. Emerging Molecular Pathways and Targets in Neuroendocrine Prostate Cancer. Translational Cancer Research. doi 10.21037/tcr.2016.07.36

Wei L, Wang J, Lampert E, Schlanger S, DePriest AD, Hu Q, Gomez EC, Murakam M, Glenn ST, Conroy J, Morrison C, Azabdaftari G, Mohler JL, Liu S, Heemers HV. Intratumoral and Intertumoral Genomic Heterogeneity of Multifocal Localized Prostate Cancer Impacts Molecular Classifications and Genomic Prognosticators. Eur Urol. 2016 Jul 20. **pii**: S0302–2838 (16) 30406–7. doi: 10.1016/j.eururo.2016.07.008. [Epub ahead of print]

Roberta Mazzucchelli, Silvia Gasparrini, Andrea B. Galosi, Francesco Massari, Maria Rosaria Raspollini, Marina Scarpelli, Antonio Lopez-Beltran, Liang Cheng, Rodolfo Montironi Genitourinary Cancers: Molecular Determinants for Personalized Therapies. Urologia. 2016; **83** (3): 107–109.

Packer JR, Maitland NJ. The Molecular and Cellular Origin of Human Prostate Cancer. Biophys Acta. 2016 Jun; **1863** (6 Pt A): 1238–60.

Fisher KW, Zhang S, Wang M, Montironi R, Wang L, Baldrige LA, Wang JY, MacLennan GT, Williamson SR, Lopez-Beltran A, Cheng L. TMPRSS2-ERG Gene Fusion Is Rare Compared to PTEN Deletions in Stage T1a Prostate Cancer. Mol Carcinog. 2016 Aug 8. doi: 10.1002/mc.22535. [Epub ahead of print]

Rare Forms of Prostatic Carcinomas

Chapter 11

11.1 Basal Cell Carcinoma and Basal Cell Proliferations of the Prostate

- Basal cell proliferations in the prostate gland exhibit a morphologic continuum ranging from basal cell hyperplasia in the setting of nodular hyperplasia to malignant basal cell lesions that resemble, to a certain degree, basal cell carcinoma of the skin and adenoid cystic carcinoma of the salivary glands. A large number of terms have been used for these neoplasms and related growths. Table 11.1
- A spectrum of basal cell proliferations ranging from hyperplasia to carcinoma exists in the prostate. These are usually located in the transition zone. Figs 11.1–11.8

11.2 Ordinary (Usual, Typical or Classical) Basal Cell Hyperplasia (BCH)

- Consists of numerous small- to normal-sized, round basophilic acini with several layers of basal cells (glandular architectural type) or solid nests either arranged in a lobular configuration or seldom "infiltrating" the stroma.
- None of the cases of ordinary BCH, by definition, contain either prominent nucleoli (their mean

diameter is less than 1 μm) or polymorphism; however, rare cases may show the presence of hyper-chromatic nuclei, enlarged nuclei and rare mitotic figures. BCH resembles prostate acini seen in the fetus. BCH may be composed of basal cell nests with areas of luminal differentiation resembling similar lesions of the salivary gland. This is denoted as the adenoid basal form of BCH.

- Histologic features may include intra-cytoplasmic globules (these stain for alpha-fetoprotein and alpha-1 antitrypsin), calcifications, squamous features and cribriform morphology; these are changes not seen in other prostatic lesions and therefore useful in differential diagnosis.
- BCH may have a florid appearance (i.e., florid basal cell hyperplasia) showing compact glandular proliferation with solid nests; the cytology in some areas looks disturbing because the cells have a moderately enlarged nucleus, often with a prominent nucleolus; a few mitotic figures are present; the intervening stroma is scant and cellular; the lesions are not well circumscribed and are intermingled with the surrounding glands, giving the false impression of "infiltration." Florid basal cell hyperplasia is also being defined as

Table 11.1 Basal Cell Proliferations of the Prostate

Subtypes
- Ordinary (usual) basal cell hyperplasia (including basal cell adenoma and adenomatosis)
- Florid basal cell hyperplasia
- Basal cell hyperplasia with prominent nucleoli (or atypical basal cell hyperplasia)
- Basal cell carcinoma (adenoid cystic carcinoma)

Differential Diagnosis
- High-grade PIN
- Acinar adenocarcinoma
- Sclerosing adenosis
- Benign seminal vesicle/ejaculatory duct epithelium
- Squamous metaplasia
- Transitional cell metaplasia

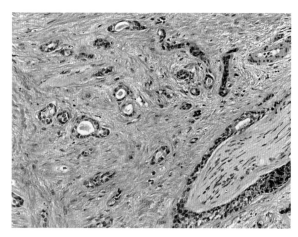

Fig 11.1 Basal cell carcinoma with perineural invasion.

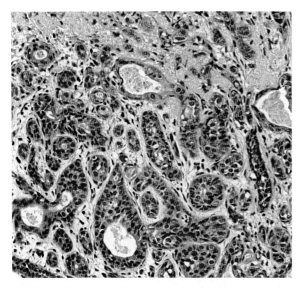

Fig 11.2 Solid acinar pattern of basal cell carcinoma.

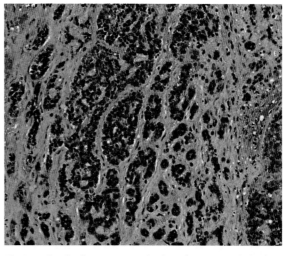

Fig 11.3 Basal cell carcinoma with adenoid cystic morphology.

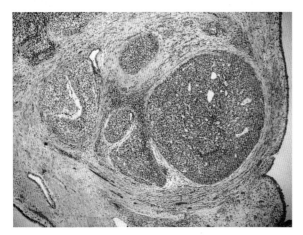

Fig 11.4 Nodular basal cell carcinoma.

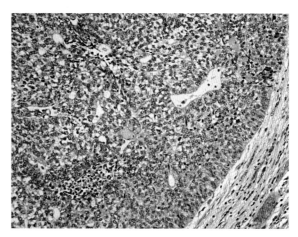

Fig 11.5 High power view of basal cell carcinoma with peripheral palisading.

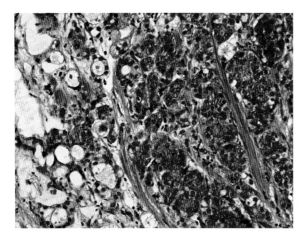

Fig 11.6 Basal cell carcinoma admixed with acinar adenocarcinoma.

extensive proliferation of basal cells involving more than 100 small crowded acini (in a given section) forming a nodule.

- BCH may have prominent nucleoli (i.e., basal cell hyperplasia with prominent nucleoli; basal cell hyperplasia with atypia), but is otherwise identical to ordinary BCH. The nucleoli are round to oval and lightly eosinophilic, similar to those seen in acinar adenocarcinoma of the prostate (their mean diameter is 1.96 μm). There is chronic inflammation in most cases, suggesting that prominent nucleoli are a reflection of reactive atypia.
- BCH with prominent nucleoli may be mistaken for high-grade prostatic intraepithelial neoplasia

135

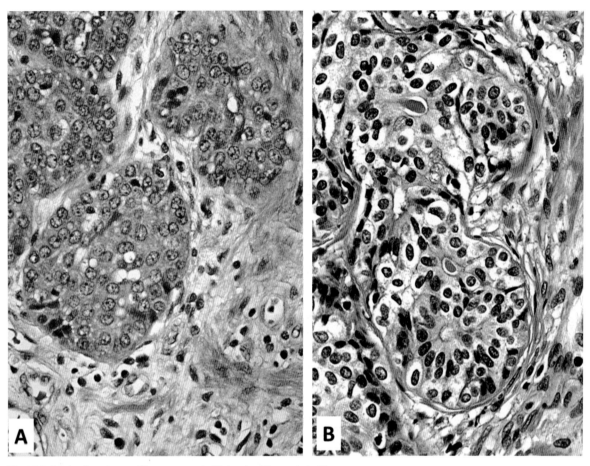

Fig 11.7 Basal cell carcinoma (A) as compared with basal cell hyperplasia (B).

Fig 11.8 Differential diagnosis of basal cell carcinoma.

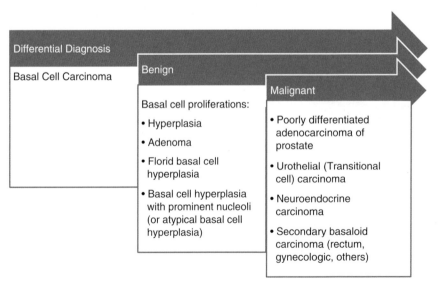

Differential Diagnosis	Benign	Malignant
Basal Cell Carcinoma	Basal cell proliferations: • Hyperplasia • Adenoma • Florid basal cell hyperplasia • Basal cell hyperplasia with prominent nucleoli (or atypical basal cell hyperplasia)	• Poorly differentiated adenocarcinoma of prostate • Urothelial (Transitional cell) carcinoma • Neuroendocrine carcinoma • Secondary basaloid carcinoma (rectum, gynecologic, others)

(PIN). Although occasionally the distinction between these two entities may be difficult, usually they are distinct. The nuclei in BCH tend to be round, whereas, at times, the cells form small solid basal cell nests. In contrast, the cells in PIN tend to be more pseudo-stratified and columnar and do not occlude the glandular lumina. Within areas of BCH, atypical looking basal cells can be seen underling the overlying benign appearing secretory cells. PIN has full thickness cytological atypia with the nuclei oriented perpendicular to the basement membrane. The use of antibodies against either 34betaE12 or p63 can help in difficult cases. In BCH, immunohistochemistry shows multilayered staining of the basal cells, whereas an interrupted immuno-reactive basal cell layer is seen in PIN. Immunostaining for alpha-methylacyl-coenzyme racemase (i.e., P504S) is negative in florid BCH and positive in HGPIN and adenocarcinoma. Immunostaining for glutathione-s-transferase pi (GST-pi) is positive in florid BCH and negative in adenocarcinoma.

- BCH, mainly with a glandular architecture or when florid, may be confused with adenocarcinoma. BCH can be distinguished from adenocarcinoma by its very basal cell appearance. The glands appear basophilic at low power due to multilayering of basal cells which have scant cytoplasm. In contrast, gland-forming adenocarcinoma of the prostate almost always has more abundant cytoplasm, resulting in a more eosinophilic appearance to the glands. Utilization of immunohistochemistry with basal cell specific antibodies (34betaE12 or p63) can differentiate between these two lesions.
- Whether florid BCH is the direct precursor of basal cell carcinoma remains as an open question.

11.3 Basal Cell Adenoma

- Is identical to ordinary BCH, although the proliferating basal cell masses are usually large and circumscribed, with nodular or adenoma-like patterns. In contrast to basal cell carcinoma, basal cell adenoma is well circumscribed, lacks necrosis, and the stroma between the basal cell nests is similar to that of the surrounding normal prostatic stroma. Occasionally, BCH is multifocal (also known as adenomatosis). The terms basal cell adenoma and adenomatosis are very rarely used.

Table 11.2 Pathology of Basal Cell Carcinoma

Diagnostic Criteria for Malignancy
- Extensive infiltration between normal prostate glands
- Extension out of the prostate
- Perineural invasion
- Necrosis

Differential Diagnosis
- Poorly differentiated adenocarcinoma (mostly Gleason's grade 5)
- Transitional cell (urothelial) carcinoma
- Neuroendocrine carcinoma
- Basaloid carcinoma of the rectum

11.4 Basal Cell Carcinoma (Basal Cell Carcinoma/Adenoid Cystic Carcinoma)

- It is characterized by proliferation of cells arranged in various architectural patterns. Two morphological variants of basal cell carcinomas can be recognized in the prostate. Similar to basal cell carcinoma of the skin, it is characterized by islands and cords of basaloid cells with peripheral palisading. The second type, also called adenoid cystic carcinoma-like, is composed of nests of infiltrating tumor cells with an adenoid cystic pattern, morphologically similar to the adenoid cystic carcinoma of the salivary glands. Focal squamous differentiation and clear cell change may be focally present. Table 11.2
- The diagnostic criteria for malignancy in basal cell carcinoma include:

1 Extensive infiltration between normal prostate glands
2 Extension out of the prostate
3 Perineural invasion
4 Variable tumor necrosis

- The differential diagnosis of basal cell carcinoma includes poorly differentiated (mostly Gleason's grade 5) adenocarcinoma (basal cell carcinoma may occur, rarely, in combination with conventional adenocarcinoma) and urothelial carcinoma. Poorly differentiated adenocarcinoma may grow in solid nests and, similarly to basal cell carcinoma, is not reactive for PSA. Lack of immuno-reactivity for p63 and 34betaE12, however, is helpful in recognizing conventional adenocarcinoma, though it has been reported that this tumor may occasionally express p63. Most basal cell carcinomas express diffusely bcl-2 by immunohistochemistry.

- Similarly to basal cell carcinoma, urothelial carcinoma may exhibit a solid growth pattern with peripheral palisading and central necrosis, and may express high level of p63. However, urothelial carcinoma expresses CK20 and CK7 in most cases. Basal cell carcinoma is positive for CK7 and negative for CK20.
- There is limited information regarding basal cell carcinoma. Patients are generally elderly, presenting with urinary obstruction, TURP being the most common tissue source of diagnosis. Rare cases may occur in younger patients.
- The outcome for patients diagnosed with basal cell carcinoma of the prostate is uncertain, since most cases have been reported with a short follow-up. Overall, basal cell carcinoma of the prostate is viewed as a low grade carcinoma with a 20% rate of metastases.

11.5 Immunohistochemistry of Basal Cell Proliferations

- Immunohistochemistry clearly indicates that they have the same immuno-phenotype of the basal cells present in normal ducts and acini. The cells are positively and strongly stained with 34betaE12, p63 or p40. These are the two consolidated markers for the basal cells in the prostate, and their absence is in favor of prostate adenocarcinoma.
- The cells that are located in the center of the nests and those lining the small luminal stain positively with AE1/AE3, whereas the basaloid cells are negative, but positive for basal cell markers.
- Another interesting feature is that the basal cell proliferations express two markers usually seen in neoplasias of other sites and organs. The first is the demonstration of laminin both in the stroma surrounding the cell nests and in small eosinophilic globules surrounded by the cells. This feature is usually seen in tumors of the salivary glands. The other is represented by the expression of HER2-neu onco-protein, similar to that seen in breast cancer. The presence of a small proportion of cells with neuroendocrine differentiation, as documented by chromogranin immunostaining, has also been reported.

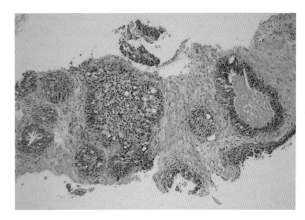

Fig 11.9 Urothelial carcinoma of the prostate.

11.6 Urothelial Carcinoma of the Prostate

- The frequency of primary urothelial carcinoma ranges from 0.7 to 2.8% of prostatic tumors in adults. In patients with invasive bladder carcinoma, there is involvement of the prostate gland in up to 45% of cases.
- Primary urothelial carcinoma is usually located within the proximal prostatic ducts. Many cases are locally advanced at diagnosis and replace the prostate gland. Primary urothelial carcinoma presents like other prostatic masses, including urinary obstruction and hematuria. Most cases are diagnosed by transurethral resection or by needle biopsy. Fig 11.9
- Digital rectal examination is abnormal in the majority of cases.
- In situ urothelial carcinoma can spread along ducts and involve acini or may spread along ejaculatory ducts and into seminal vesicles. Invasion of prostatic stroma (subepithelial connective tissue as pT1 or with established stromal invasion as pT2) is the most relevant feature.
- Local spread beyond the confines of the prostate may occur. Metastases are to regional lymph nodes and bone. Bone metastases are osteolytic. These tumors are staged as urethral tumors. The full range of histological types and grades of urothelial neoplasia can be seen in primary and secondary urothelial neoplasms of the prostate.
- The single most important prognostic parameter is the presence of prostatic stromal invasion. With

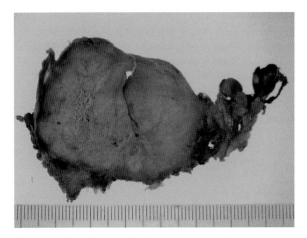

Fig 11.10 Gross features of adeno-squamous carcinoma.

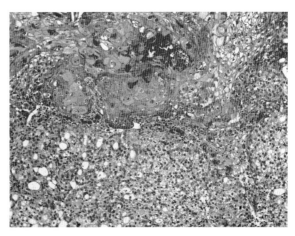

Fig 11.11 Histologic features of adeno-squamous carcinoma.

stromal invasion or extension beyond the confines of the prostate, prognosis is poor.

11.7 Squamous Cell Neoplasms of the Prostate

- Squamous cell carcinomas may originate either in the periurethral glands or in the prostatic glandular acini. Approximately 50% of adenosquamous carcinomas may arise in prostate cancer patients subsequent to endocrine therapy or radiotherapy. The incidence of squamous cell carcinoma of the prostate is less than 0.6% of all prostate cancers. Adenosquamous carcinoma of the prostate is even less frequent. Figs 11.10–11.11
- Most, if not all, pure squamous cell carcinomas become clinically manifest by local symptoms such as urinary outflow obstruction, occasionally in association with bone pain and hematuria. Adenosquamous carcinomas may be detected by increased serum PSA, but more typically by obstruction of the urinary outflow, requiring transurethral resection. Both squamous cell carcinomas and adenosquamous carcinomas tend to metastasize rapidly with a predilection for the skeletal bones.
- By definition, pure squamous cell carcinomas do not contain glandular features and they are identical to squamous cell carcinomas of other organs. Primary prostatic squamous cell carcinomas must be distinguished on clinical grounds from secondary involvement of the gland by bladder or urethral squamous carcinomas.

Histologically, squamous cell carcinoma must be distinguished from squamous metaplasia as may occur in infarction or after hormonal therapy. Histologically, squamous metaplasia associated to prostatic infarction may be very atypical and therefore a challenging diagnosis. One must pay attention to necrotic or fibrotic background. Usually, squamous metaplasia associated to infarction is frequently associated with basal cell proliferation and has a lobular configuration, a rare finding in squamous carcinoma which shows an infiltrative appearance.
- Adenosquamous carcinomas are defined by the presence of both glandular (acinar) and squamous carcinoma components. The glandular tumor component generally expresses PSA and PAP, whereas the squamous component displays high molecular weight cytokeratins.

11.8 Sarcomatoid Carcinoma (Carcinosarcoma) of the Prostate

- Sarcomatoid carcinoma is composed of a glandular component showing a variable Gleason score. The sarcomatoid component often consists of a non-specific malignant spindle-cell proliferation. Epithelial elements react with antibodies against PSA and/or pan-cytokeratins, whereas spindle-cell elements react with markers of soft tissue tumors and variably express cytokeratins or CD10.
- Osteosarcoma, chondrosarcoma, rhabdomyosarcoma, leiomyosarcoma,

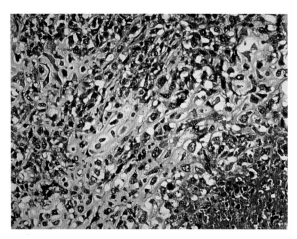

Fig 11.12 Sarcomatoid carcinoma with osteosarcoma.

liposarcoma, angiosarcoma or multiple types of heterologous differentiation may be seen. Sarcomatoid carcinoma should be distinguished from the rare carcinoma with metaplastic, benign-appearing bone or cartilage in the stroma. Fig 11.12

Suggested Reading

Bachurska SY, Staykov DG, Ivanov GP, Belovezhdov VT. Lack of ERG-antibody in Benign Mimickers of Prostate Cancer. Folia Med (Plovdiv). 2016 Mar 1; **58**(1): 48–53.

Simper NB, Jones CL, MacLennan GT, Montironi R, Williamson SR, Osunkoya AO, Wang M, Zhang S, Grignon DJ, Eble JN, Tran T, Wang L, Baldrige LA, Cheng L. Basal Cell Carcinoma of the Prostate Is an Aggressive Tumor with Frequent Loss of PTEN Expression and Overexpression of EGFR. Hum Pathol. 2015 Jun; **46**(6): 805–12. doi: 10.1016/j.humpath.2015.02.004.

Arista-Nasr J, Martinez-Benitez B, Bornstein-Quevedo L, Aguilar-Ayala E, Aleman-Sanchez CN, Ortiz-Bautista R. Low Grade Urothelial Carcinoma Mimicking Basal Cell Hyperplasia and Transitional Metaplasia in Needle Prostate Biopsy. Int Braz J Urol. 2016 Mar–Apr; **42**(2): 247–52.

Smith BA, Sokolov A, Uzunangelov V, Baertsch R, Newton Y, Graim K, Mathis C, Cheng D, Stuart JM, Witte ON. A Basal Stem Cell Signature Identifies Aggressive Prostate Cancer Phenotypes. Proc Natl Acad Sci USA. 2015 Nov 24; **112**(47): E6544–52.

Zhang M, Pettaway C, Vikram R, Tamboli P. Adenoid Cystic Carcinoma of the Urethra/Cowper's Gland with Concurrent High-grade Prostatic Adenocarcinoma: A Detailed Clinico-Pathologic Case Report and Review of the Literature. Hum Pathol. 2016 Aug 20. **pii**; S0046–8177 (16): 30181–2. doi: 10.1016/j.humpath.2016.07.027.

Bishop JA, Yonescu R, Epstein JI, Westra WH. A Subset of Prostatic Basal Cell Carcinomas Harbor the MYB Rearrangement of Adenoid Cystic Carcinoma. Hum Pathol. 2015 Aug; **46**(8): 1204–08. doi: 10.1016/j.humpath.2015.05.002.

Wu A, Kunju LP. Prostate Cancer with Aberrant Diffuse p63 Expression: Report of a Case and Review of the Literature and Morphologic Mimics. Arch Pathol Lab Med. 2013 Sep; **137**(9): 1179–84. doi: 10.5858/arpa.2013-0254-CR. Review.

Chang K, Dai B, Kong Y, Qu Y, Wu J, Ye D, Yao X, Zhang S, Zhang H, Zhu Y, Yao W. Basal Cell Carcinoma of the Prostate: Clinicopathologic Analysis of Three Cases and a Review of the Literature. World J Surg Oncol. 2013 Aug 13; **11**(1): 193. doi: 10.1186/1477-7819-11-193. Review.

Rodriguez-Carlin A, Arellano L, López-Fontana G, Bolufer E, Castillo OA. Basaloid Carcinoma of the Prostate: An Extremely Rare Tumor. Arch Esp Urol. 2013 May; **66**(4): 380–84. English, Spanish.

Tuan J, Pandha H, Corbishley C, Khoo V. Basaloid Carcinoma of the Prostate: A Literature Review with Case Report. Indian J Urol. 2012 Jul; **28**(3): 322–24. doi: 10.4103/0970-1591.102714.

Komura K, Inamoto T, Tsuji M, Ibuki N, Koyama K, Ubai T, Azuma H, Katsuoka Y. Basal Cell Carcinoma of the Prostate: Unusual Subtype of Prostatic Carcinoma. Int J Clin Oncol. 2010 Dec; **15**(6): 594–600. doi: 10.1007/s10147-010-0082-5.

Bauer R. Cylindroma of the Prostate. Am J Surg Pathol. 2007 Aug; **31**(8): 1288–91.

Ali TZ, Epstein JI. Basal Cell Carcinoma of the Prostate: A Clinicopathologic Study of 29 Cases. Am J Surg Pathol. 2007 May; **31**(5): 697–705.

Begnami MD, Quezado M, Pinto P, Linehan WM, Merino M. Adenoid Cystic/Basal Cell Carcinoma of the Prostate: Review and Update. Arch Pathol Lab Med. 2007 Apr; **131**(4): 637–40.

Cheng L, MacLennan GT, Lopez-Beltran A, Montironi R. Anatomic, Morphologic and Genetic Heterogeneity of Prostate Cancer: Implications for Clinical Practice. Expert Rev Anticancer Ther. 2012 Nov; **12**(11): 1371–74. doi: 10.1586/era.12.127.

Lopez-Beltran A, Cheng L, Prieto R, Blanca A, Montironi R. Lymphoepithelioma-like Carcinoma of the Prostate. Hum Pathol. 2009 Jul; **40**(7): 982–87.

Morichetti D, Mazzucchelli R, Lopez-Beltran A, Cheng L, Scarpelli M, Kirkali Z, Montorsi F, Montironi R. Secondary Neoplasms of the Urinary System and Male Genital Organs. BJU Int. 2009 Sep; **104**(6): 770–76.

Chapter 12

Tumors and Tumor-like Conditions of the Prostate Stroma

- A wide variety of soft tissue lesions occur in the prostate, including reactive stromal proliferations, benign neoplasms and sarcomas. Although many of these tumors are distinguished easily, considerable diagnostic difficulty may be encountered with some of the rare lesions. Patient age and clinical history are essential in this setting. The serum PSA concentration is usually not significantly elevated.
- The most common lesion is represented by benign prostatic hyperplasia, which is easy to recognize because of the usual association with areas of glandular proliferation. Pure stromal nodules may be challenging because of the presence of myxoid stroma with spindle cells. They lack mitosis and infiltrative borders. Figs 12.1–12.2
- Inflammatory myofibroblastic tumor may arise in the prostate, mimicking sarcomas. Sarcomas in the prostate are rarely reported and represent 0.1% of prostatic malignant neoplasms and are discussed in Chapter 1.13.
- The most common sarcomas are rhabdomyosarcoma and leiomyosarcoma. The former is more common in children and bears a very poor prognosis, whereas the latter is seen in adults, and follows a slower course, but generally recurs after initial therapy. Table 12.1

12.1 Pseudosarcomatous Spindle Cell Proliferations

- Reactive, nonneoplastic fibrous lesions of soft tissue that, because of their clinical presentation, gross appearance, growth pattern, and light microscopic features, may be mistaken for a malignancy, usually a sarcoma, often are referred to as pseudosarcomas. These lesions can be divided into two groups distinguished by differences in etiology and morphological appearance, e.g., postoperative spindle cell nodule and inflammatory myofibroblastic tumor.

12.2 Postoperative Spindle Cell Nodule

- Also called postsurgical inflammatory myofibroblastic tumor, this is a rare benign reparative process occurring within a few months

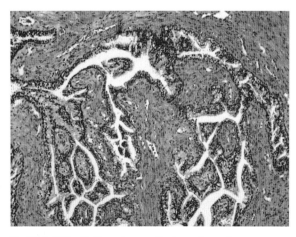

Fig 12.1 BPH with fibroadenoma-like type of growth.

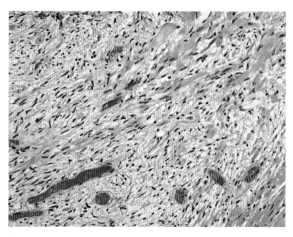

Fig 12.2 BPH nodule of fibromyxoid type.

Table 12.1 Classification of Prostatic Non-epithelial Tumor-like Conditions and Tumors

Tumor-like Proliferations and Inflammatory Pseudotumors
- Postoperative spindle cell nodules
- Inflammatory myofibroblastic tumor
- Blue nevus
- Granulomatous prostatitis

Variants of Prostatic Hyperplasia
- Stromal hyperplasia with atypia
- Fibroadenoma-like foci in benign hyperplasia
- Phyllodes-like hyperplasia

Cystadenoma

Mixed Epithelial-Stromal Tumors (Phyllodes Tumor)
- STUMPs
- Stromal sarcoma

Stromal tumors

Benign
- Leiomyoma, including its variants (atypical leiomyoma, cellular leiomyoma, and leiomyoblastoma)
- Others

Malignant
- Leiomyosarcoma
- Rhabdomyosarcoma
- Others

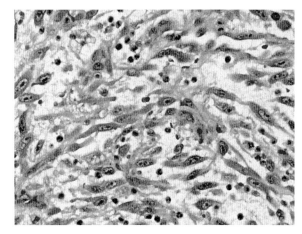

Fig 12.3 Inflammatory myofibroblastic tumor.

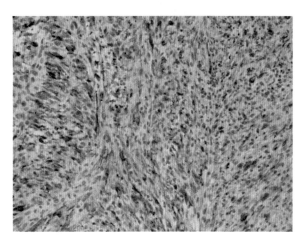

Fig 12.4 ALK positive expression in inflammatory myofibroblastic tumor.

of surgery and consists of nodules of spindle cells arranged in fascicles with a variable number of mitotic figures. The cells have abundant cytoplasm; the nucleus is centrally located and elongated to ovoid in shape; small prominent nucleoli are present.

- The features that can be used to distinguish postoperative spindle cell nodule from a sarcoma are:

  1 lack of significant nuclear pleomorphism and of atypical mitoses
  2 plexiform pattern of blood vessels
  3 presence of chronic inflammation
  4 small size of the nodule
  5 lack of recurrence after conservative excision

12.3 Inflammatory Myofibroblastic Tumor

- Is a rare benign pathological entity of unknown etiology occurring in the prostate, urethra, bladder and other sites without a history of prior surgery.
- Histologically, this lesion resembles granulation tissue with variable cellularity. Cells are more haphazard in their distribution than postoperative spindle cell nodules. Lesions often show a densely cellular spindle cell pattern admixed with a very myxoid component. Cells resemble those seen in nodular fasciitis with a tissue culture appearance.

- Occasionally there may be prominent nucleoli with infrequent, moderately pleomorphic and hyperchromatic cells. These lesions show myofibroblastic differentiation with expression of smooth-muscle markers and focal keratin expression. About 60% of cases may express ALK-1 by immunohistochemistry with gene translocation by FISH. This finding is useful in differential diagnosis with sarcomatoid carcinoma and leiomyosarcoma, which are ALK-1 negative by immunohistochemistry. Figs 12.3–12.5

- The features that can be used to distinguish inflammatory myofibroblastic tumor from a sarcoma are:

Sarcomatoid carcinoma

- Necrosis and atypical mitosis present
- Heterologous differentiation may be present
- ALK1-, CK+, Desmin+/-, EMA+, SMA+/-, Vim+/-, S100-,
- p63+/-, 34βE12+/-, CK5/6+/-

Inflammatory myofibroblastic tumor

- No necrosis. No atypical mitosis
- No heterologous differentiation
- ALK1+, CK+/-, Desmin+/-, EMA+/-, SMA+/-, Vim+, S100-, calponin+/-,
- h-caldesmon+/-, p63-, 34βE12-, CK5/6-

1 areas of the lesion resembling granulation tissue
2 mitotic figures infrequent
3 less pleomorphism
4 prominent myxoid change
5 recurrence rare following incomplete excision

12.4 Atypical Stromal Cells

- Pleomorphic, hyperchromatic nuclei may be seen in the prostatic stroma cells between the epithelial elements in otherwise unremarkable cases of benign prostatic hyperplasia, in circumscribed benign fibromuscular nodules in which smooth muscle typically predominates and in leiomyoma. Fig 12.6
- It is important to be aware that malignant neoplasms of the prostate, such as sarcomas and mixed epithelial-stromal tumors, may contain atypical stromal cells similar to those that can be seen either in nodular hyperplasia or fibromuscular nodules. The distinction of the latter two entities from the former depends on:

1 the absence of a mass
2 the lack of stromal hypercellularity or phyllodes type architecture
3 the degenerative nuclear appearance with smuggled chromatin
4 the lack of mitoses

- Distinction of degenerative stromal atypia from the atypicality seen with neoplasms may be very difficult in a limited sampling, and it has been

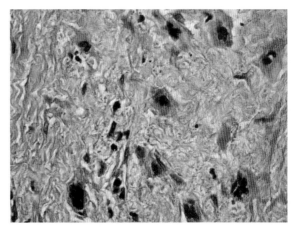

Fig 12.6 Atypical stromal cells (derived from smooth muscle) may be seen in BPH and have no known significance.

suggested the designation "prostatic stromal proliferation of uncertain malignant potential" be used to alert the clinician to this uncertainty.

12.5 Prostatic Stromal Proliferation of Uncertain Malignant Potential (STUMP) and Stromal Sarcomas

- This lesion is also known as atypical stromal hyperplasia, a phyllodes type of atypical stromal hyperplasia, phyllodes tumor or cystic epithelial-stromal tumor.

143

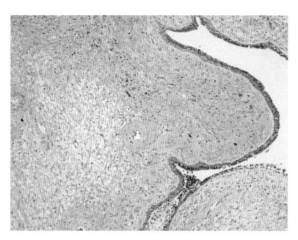

Fig 12.7 Stromal tumor of uncertain malignant potential (STUMP) (low power).

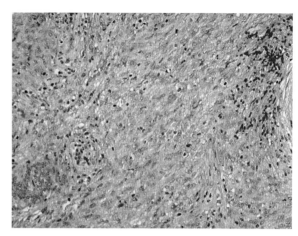

Fig 12.8 Cellular pattern of STUMP.

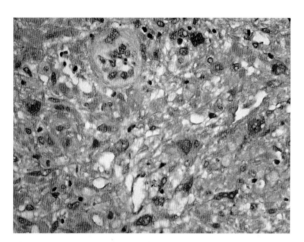

Fig 12.9 Atypical cell pattern of STUMP.

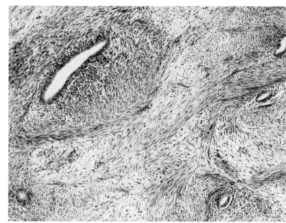

Fig 12.10 STUMP with peri-glandular cellular proliferation and myxoid stroma. This case progressed to stromal sarcoma (depicted in fig 12.14) after several tumor recurrencies.

- Prostatic stromal tumors arising from specialized prostatic stroma are rare and distinct, exhibiting diverse histologic patterns of growth. Currently, the preferred terminology includes prostatic stromal proliferation of uncertain malignant potential (STUMPs) and stromal sarcomas. Figs 12.7–12.14
- Prostatic stromal tumors arising from the specialized prostatic stroma are rare and distinct tumors with diverse histological patterns. In the past, these tumors have been reported under a variety of terms, including atypical stromal (smooth muscle) hyperplasia, phyllodes type of atypical stromal hyperplasia, phyllodes tumor and cystic epithelial-stromal tumors. As the phyllodes 'leaf-like' pattern is only seen in a subset of both

benign and malignant stromal tumors (see below), we prefer to designate stromal tumors of the prostate in more general descriptive terms, such as STUMPs and stromal sarcomas, as has also been recommended by the 2004 World Health Organization Classification of Tumours of the Urinary System and Male Genital Organs. To date, three studies have examined large patient populations in order to address the pathologic and clinical features associated with these lesions.

- Although STUMPs have been generally considered to variably represent either a hyperplastic or benign neoplastic stromal process, a subset of STUMPs has been associated with stromal sarcoma on concurrent biopsy

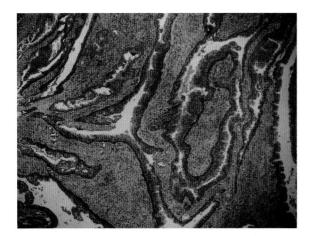

Fig 12.11 Phyllodes type STUMP (low power).

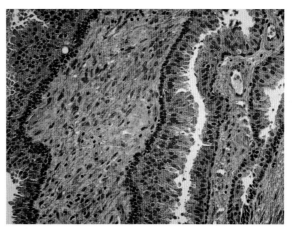

Fig 12.12 Phyllodes type STUMP with cellular stroma. Picture taking from 3rd recurrent lesion after surgery.

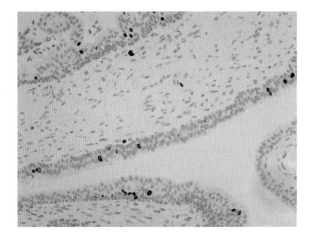

Fig 12.13 Low proliferation index based on Ki67 expression seen in phyllodes type STUMP (same as case fig 12.12).

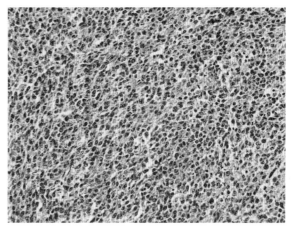

Fig 12.14 Stromal sarcoma of the prostate with monotonous cell proliferation and low mitotic index.

material or has demonstrated stromal sarcoma on repeat biopsy, suggesting a malignant progression in at least some cases. In general, patients with a diagnosis of STUMP have a good prognosis, as most cases are confined to the prostate and rarely progress to sarcoma.

- In contrast, stromal sarcomas can extend out of the prostate and metastasize to distant sites, such as bone, lung, abdomen and retroperitoneum. STUMPs have been reported to occur between the ages of 27 and 83 years, with a median age of 58 years and a peak incidence in the sixth and seventh decades. Patients presented most commonly with urinary obstruction, followed by abnormal rectal examination, hematuria, hematospermia, rectal fullness, palpable rectal mass or elevated serum prostate specific antigen (PSA) levels. On gross

examination, STUMPs appear white-tan and may demonstrate a solid or solid-cystic pattern with smooth-walled cysts filled with bloody, mucinous or clear fluid. These tumors may involve either the transition zone or the peripheral zone and may range in size from microscopic lesions (which are typically incidentally found) to large, cystic lesions up to 15 cm in size.

- Microscopically, four patterns of STUMP have been described and include (1) hypercellular stroma with scattered atypical, but degenerative-appearing cells admixed with benign prostatic glands, (2) hypercellular stroma consisting of bland fusiform stromal cells admixed with benign glands, (3) leaf-like hypocellular fibrous stroma covered by benign-appearing prostatic epithelium

145

similar in morphology to a benign phyllodes tumor of the breast and (4) myxoid stroma containing bland stromal cells and often lacking admixed glands. Cases can exhibit a mixture of the above patterns. Mitotic activity is rare to absent in all of these subtypes and tumor necrosis is not present. Lesions may be present only focally on prostatic biopsies, and care must be taken to detect these lesions when evaluating prostate biopsies for other processes. There appears to be no correlation between the pattern of STUMP and association with stromal sarcoma.

- Approximately half of all reported cases of STUMP demonstrate the first pattern of hypercellular stroma containing atypical cells intermixed with, but not compressing, benign glands (Figure 3). The atypical stromal cells in these cases are pleomorphic and hyperchromatic, with a marked degenerative appearance. Mitotic figures are typically absent and atypical mitoses should not be seen. Although the admixed glands resemble normal benign prostatic glands, the glands within a STUMP may appear more crowded than acini in the surrounding uninvolved prostate. The remaining three patterns of STUMP are seen with varying frequency.

- Cases of STUMP demonstrating hypercellular, elongated bland stromal cells with admixed glands may be occasionally misdiagnosed as a robust stromal proliferation associated with BPH, although the extent of hypercellularity and often more eosinophilic nature of the cytoplasm are unique. The benign phyllodes pattern of STUMP may also contain atypical, degenerative-appearing stromal cells and may be associated with a variety of benign epithelial proliferations, including basal cell hyperplasia, adenosis, and sclerosing adenosis. Finally, the myxoid pattern of STUMP may be confused with stromal nodules of BPH, although the myxoid pattern of STUMP consists of extensive sheets of myxoid stroma without the nodularity identified in BPH, or occasionally myxoid stroma admixed with benign prostate glands.

- In contrast to STUMPs, stromal sarcomas tend to affect a slightly younger population, with a reported age range of 25–86 years. Approximately half of all reported cases of stromal sarcoma occur before the age of 50 years. Stromal sarcomas may arise de novo, or may exist in association with either a pre-existent or concurrent STUMP, thereby suggesting a potential for STUMPs to dedifferentiate to sarcomas in rare cases. Gross examination of stromal sarcomas demonstrates predominantly tan-white, solid, fleshy lesions ranging in size from 2 to 18 cm.

- Occasionally, areas of edema, hemorrhage, or small cysts may be identified. Microscopically, stromal sarcomas demonstrate either a solid growth of neoplastic stromal cells, which may have storiform, epithelioid, fibrosarcomatous, or nonspecific histologic patterns, or may intercalate between benign prostatic glands. Less commonly, stromal sarcomas may demonstrate leaf-like glands with underlying hypercellular stroma, which are also termed malignant phyllodes tumors. Stromal sarcomas have one or more of the following features within the spindle cell component: hypercellularity, cytological atypia, mitotic figures, and necrosis. Stromal sarcomas may additionally be subclassified into low and high grades with high grade tumors defined by moderately marked pleomorphism and hypercellularity, often with increased mitotic activity and occasional necrosis.

- Immunohistochemical findings are similar to those of STUMPs, with strong vimentin reactivity and positivity for CD34 and progesterone receptor. In a subset of cases studied, pancytokeratin and CAM5.2 were negative. One case of stromal sarcoma was reported to demonstrate nuclear reactivity for beta-catenin, although the significance of this finding is unclear. The variability in behavior of STUMPs and stromal sarcomas, and their occasional co-existence, lead to challenges in patient management. Low grade sarcoma can locally invade, despite having at times relatively bland cytology, and high grade sarcoma has the potential to metastasize to distant sites.

- Although many STUMPs may behave in an indolent fashion, their unpredictability in a minority of cases and the lack of correlation between different histological patterns of STUMPs and sarcomatous dedifferentiation warrant close follow-up and consideration of definitive resection in younger individuals. Factors to consider in deciding whether to proceed with definitive resection for STUMPs diagnosed on biopsy include patient age and treatment preference, presence and size of the lesion on rectal exam or imaging studies and extent of the lesion on tissue sampling. Expectant management with close clinical follow-up could be considered in an older individual with a limited lesion on biopsy where there is no lesion identified on digital rectal exam or on imaging studies.

12.6 Histopathology and Immunohistochemistry of STUMPs and Stromal Sarcomas

Four histologic patterns, seen as pure or mixed forms, have been described: i) hypercellular stroma with degenerative-type nuclear atypia admixed with benign prostate glands (most common pattern); ii) hypercellular stroma with bland fusiform eosinophilic admixed with benign glands; iii) leaf-like hypocellular fibrous stroma covered by benign-appearing prostatic epithelium (similar to phyllodes tumor of the breast); iv) myxoid stroma containing bland stromal cells often lacking admixed glands.

- Stromal sarcoma usually shows solid growth of neoplastic stromal cells, which may have fibrosarcomatous, storiform, epithelioid or more rarely leaf-like pattern of growth. Stromal sarcomas may show hypercellularity, cellular atypia, necrosis and mitosis. Stromal sarcomas have been subclassified as low or high grade based on the degree of pleomorphism, hypercellularity, number of mitosis and the presence of tumor necrosis.

- Immunohistochemistry is not useful in differentiating STUMP from stromal sarcoma, which relies on morphologic grounds alone. Both types of lesions are positive for vimentin, SMA, desmin, progesterone receptor and CD34. S100 and CD117 are negative.

- Differential diagnosis may include sarcomatoid carcinoma (cytokeratin and p63 positive), leiomyosarcoma (SMA, desmin and caldesmon positive) or GIST (CD117 positive). Table 12.2

Suggested Reading

Fain JS, Cosnow I, King BF, Zincke H, Bostwick DG. Cystosarcoma Phyllodes of the Seminal Vesicle. Cancer 1993; **71**: 2055–61.

Laurila P, Leivo I, Makisalo H, Ruutu M, Miettinen M. Mullerian Adenosarcoma-like Tumor of the Seminal

Table 12.2 Differential Diagnosis of Adult Prostate Sarcoma vs. Sarcomatoid Prostate Adenocarcinoma by Immunohistochemistry

Marker	Immunoreactivity
Desmin	(+) in LS, may be diffuse Focal (+) in some Sarc. Ca. (−) in SS
Vimentin	Sensitive but not specific for sarcoma
SM Actin	(+) in SS, LS Focal (+) in some Sarc. Ca.
CD34	(+) in most SS 8% of LS (+) (−) in Sarc.Ca.
PANCK	Usually (−) in Sarcomas (+) in up to 27% of prostate LS (+) in 71% Sarc.Ca., yet can be focal No data for SS
HMWCK	Sometimes more sensitive than PANCK (no prostate data available) (−) in bladder LS (no prostate data available) No data for SS
p63	One of most sensitive markers for Sarc. Ca. 0% (+) in LS in general 23% (+) in bladder LS in 1 large study No data on prostatic LS No data for SS
Prostate Markers (PSA, P501S, NKX3.1)	Negative in sarcoma Positive in epithelial component if present Not necessary as H&E presence of carcinoma diagnostic

LS: leiomyosarcoma; Sarc. Ca.: sarcomatoid carcinoma; SS: stromal sarcoma; SM Actin: smooth muscle actin; PANCK: pancytokeratin; HMWCK: high molecular weight cytokeratin; GU: genitourinary

Vesicle. A Case Report with Immunohistochemical and Ultrastructural Observations. Arch Pathol Lab Med. 1992; **116**: 1072–76.

Maheshkumar P, Harper C, Sunderland GT, Conn IG. Cystic Epithelial Stromal Tumour of the Seminal Vesicle. BJU Int. 2000; **85**: 1154.

Mazur MT, Myers JL, Maddox WA. Cystic Epithelial-Stromal Tumor of the Seminal Vesicle. Am J Surg Pathol. 1987; **11**: 210–17.

Reikie BA, Yilmaz A, Medlicott S, Trpkov K. Mixed Epithelial-Stromal Tumor (MEST) of Seminal Vesicle: A Proposal for Unified Nomenclature. Adv Anat Pathol. 2015 Mar; **22**(2): 113–20.

Lamont JS, Hesketh PJ, de las MA, Babayan RK. Primary Angiosarcoma of the Seminal Vesicle. J Urol. 1991; **146**: 165–67.

Fujii T, Shimada K, Tanaka N, Fujimoto K, Konishi N. Phyllodes Tumor of the Prostate. Pathol Int. 2012 Mar; **62**(3): 204–8.

Hossain D, Meiers I, Qian J, MacLennan GT, Bostwick DG. Prostatic Stromal Hyperplasia with Atypia: Follow-up Study of 18 Cases. Arch Pathol Lab Med. 2008 Nov; **132** (11): 1729–33.

Herawi M, Epstein JI. Specialized Stromal Tumors of the Prostate: A Clinicopathologic Study of 50 Cases. Am J Surg Pathol. 2006 Jun; **30**(6): 694–704.

Arya M, Hayne D, Brown RS, O'Donnell PJ, Mundy AR. Hemangiopericytoma of the Seminal Vesicle Presenting with Hypoglycemia. J Urol 2001; **166**: 992.

Gentile AT, Moseley HS, Quinn SF, Franzini D, Pitre TM. Leiomyoma of the Seminal Vesicle. J Urol. 1994; **151**: 1027–29.

Muentener M, Hailemariam S, Dubs M, Hauri D, Sulser T. Primary Leiomyosarcoma of the Seminal Vesicle. J Urol. 2000; **164**: 2027.

Juhasz J, Kiss P. A Hitherto Undescribed Case of 'Collision' Tumour: Liposarcoma of the Seminal Vesicle and Prostatic Carcinoma. Int Urol Nephrol. 1978; **10**: 185–93.

Westra WH, Grenko RT, Epstein J. Solitary Fibrous Tumor of the Lower Urogenital Tract: A Report of Five Cases Involving the Seminal Vesicles, Urinary Bladder, and Prostate. Hum Pathol. 2000; **31**: 63–68.

Montironi R, Lopez-Beltran A, Cheng L, Scarpelli M. Cervical-type Squamous Metaplasia and Myoepithelial Cell Differentiation in Stromal Tumor of the Prostate. Am J Surg Pathol. 2011 Nov; **35**(11): 1752–54.

Wagner DG, Yao JL, di Sant'Agnese PA, Cheng L, Lopez-Beltran A, Montironi R, Huang J. Soft Tissue Tumors of the Prostate: A Review. Anal Quant Cytol Histol. 2007 Dec; **29**(6): 341–50.

Cheng L, Foster SR, MacLennan GT, Lopez-Beltran A, Zhang S, Montironi R. Inflammatory Myofibroblastic Tumors of the Genitourinary Tract–Single Entity or Continuum? J Urol. 2008 Oct; **180**(4): 1235–40.

Mazzucchelli R, Lopez-Beltran A, Cheng L, Scarpelli M, Kirkali Z, Montironi R. Rare and Unusual Histological Variants of Prostatic Carcinoma: Clinical Significance. BJU Int. 2008 Nov; **102**(10): 1369–74.

Galosi AB, Mazzucchelli R, Scarpelli M, Lopez-Beltran A, Cheng L, Muzzonigro G, Montironi R. Solitary Fibrous Tumour of the Prostate Identified on Needle Biopsy. Eur Urol. 2009 Sep; **56**(3): 564–67.

Hodges KB, Abdul-Karim FW, Wang M, Lopez-Beltran A, Montironi R, Easley S, Zhang S, Wang N, MacLennan GT, Cheng L. Evidence for Transformation of Fibroadenoma of the Breast to Malignant Phyllodes Tumor. Appl Immunohistochem Mol Morphol. 2009 Jul; **17**(4): 345–50.

Morichetti D, Mazzucchelli R, Lopez-Beltran A, Cheng L, Scarpelli M, Kirkali Z, Montorsi F, Montironi R. Secondary Neoplasms of the Urinary System and Male Genital Organs. BJU Int. 2009 Sep; **104**(6): 770–76.

Montironi R, Lopez-Beltran A, Cheng L, Scarpelli M. Cervical-type Squamous Metaplasia and Myoepithelial Cell Differentiation in Stromal Tumor of the Prostate. Am J Surg Pathol. 2011 Nov; **35**(11): 1752–54.

Sadimin ET, Epstein JI. Round Cell Pattern of Prostatic Stromal Tumor of Uncertain Malignant Potential: A Subtle Newly Recognized Variant. Hum Pathol. 2016 Jun; **52**: 68–73.

Tang J, He L, Long Z, Wei J. Phyllodes Tumor of the Verumontanum: A Case Report. Diagn Pathol. 2015 Jun 16; **10**: 69.

Löpez-Beltran A, Gaeta JF, Huben R, Croghan GA. Malignant Phyllodes Tumor of Prostate. Urology. 1990 Feb; **35**(2): 164–67.

Kouba E, Simper NB, Chen S, Williamson SR, Grignon DJ, Eble JN, MacLennan GT, Montironi R, Lopez-Beltran A, Osunkoya AO, Zhang S, Wang M, Wang L, Tran T, Emerson RE, Baldrige LA, Monn MF, Linos K, Cheng L. Solitary Fibrous Tumor of the Genitourinary Tract: A Clinicopathologic Study of 11 Cases and Their Association with the NAB2-STAT6 Fusion Gene. J Clin Pathol. 2016; In press.

Chapter 13

Soft Tissue and Miscellaneous Primary Tumors of the Prostate

- A wide variety of soft tissue lesions occur in the prostate, including reactive stromal proliferations, benign neoplasms and sarcomas. Although many of these tumors are distinguished easily, considerable diagnostic difficulty may be encountered with some of the rare and newly identified lesions. Patient age and clinical history are essential in this setting. The serum PSA concentration is usually not significantly elevated. Table 13.1
- The most common sarcomas are rhabdomyosarcoma and leiomyosarcoma. The former is more common in children and bears a very poor prognosis, whereas the latter is seen in adults, and follows a slower course, but generally recurs after initial therapy.

13.1 Leiomyoma

- Unusual prostatic spindle cell lesion. Histologically, the lesion is composed of a well-circumscribed mass of smooth muscle cell proliferation in prostatic or juxtaprostatic tissue that is devoid of epithelial elements and reaches 1 cm or more in diameter. Fig 13.1
- No specific histological criterion exists to differentiate a leiomyoma from a leiomyosarcoma of the prostate as opposed to smooth muscle tumors of the uterus.
- The definition of "atypical leiomyoma" of the prostate is used by some authors to refer to well-circumscribed lesions with a variable amount of nuclear atypia and scattered mitotic activity. Although most atypical leiomyomas have shown no evidence of disease with short follow-up, a few have recurred. Because smooth-muscle tumors of the prostate are rare, the criteria for distinguishing between leiomyosarcoma and leiomyoma in these cases with borderline features have not been elucidated.

13.2 Leiomyosarcoma

- Sarcomas of the prostate are very rare and aggressive tumors, accounting for less than 0.2% of all malignant prostatic tumors. Leiomyosarcoma is the most common sarcoma involving the prostate in adults. Table 13.1
- Microscopically, leiomyosarcoma is hypercellular, composed of intersecting bundles of spindle cells with moderate to severe atypia. Figs 13.3–13.6
- Most reported cases are high grade with high mitotic count and frequent tumor necrosis. Low grade cases are even rarer. Leiomyosarcoma commonly express actin, desmin, caldesmon, and vimentin. Some may focally express cytokeratin and progesterone receptor.

13.3 Rhabdomyosarcoma

- Most frequent in pediatric population, may rarely arise as primary prostatic sarcoma. Histologically, most are of the embryonal subtype. Histologically are similar to those seen in other organs.
- Proliferating cells vary from primitive cells with scant cytoplasm to more well-differentiated tumor cells with more abundant eosinophilic cytoplasm in which cross striations may be seen by conventional H&E staining and light microscopy. Some tumors may have spindle cell appearance or exhibit myxoid growth pattern. Figs 13.7–13.8

13.4 Solitary Fibrous Tumor of the Prostate (SFTs)

- SFTs involving the prostate are uncommon, with only isolated cases reported in the literature. Owing to their relative rarity and lack of long-term follow-up, the clinical behavior of prostatic SFTs is difficult to predict. Complete resection of tumor is currently the single main prognostic factor.
- At low-power magnification, SFTs have a smoothly contoured periphery surrounded

Table 13.1 Differential Diagnosis of Adult Prostate Sarcoma vs. Sarcomatoid Prostate Adenocarcinoma by Immunohistochemistry

Marker	Immunoreactivity
Desmin	(+) in LS, may be diffuse Focal (+) in some Sarc. Ca. (−) in SS
Vimentin	Sensitive but not specific for sarcoma
SM Actin	(+) in SS, LS Focal (+) in some Sarc. Ca.
CD34	(+) in most SS 8% of LS (+) (−) in Sarc. Ca.
PANCK	Usually (−) in Sarcomas (+) in up to 27% of prostate LS (+) in 71% Sarc. Ca., yet can be focal No data for SS
HMWCK	Sometimes more sensitive than PANCK (no prostate data available) (−) in bladder LS (no prostate data available) No data for SS
p63	One of most sensitive markers for Sarc. Ca. 0% (+) in LS in general 23% (+) in bladder LS in 1 large study No data on prostatic LS No data for SS
Prostate Markers (PSA, P501S, NKX3.1)	Negative in sarcoma Positive in epithelial component if present Not necessary as H&E presence of carcinoma diagnostic

LS: leiomyosarcoma; Sarc. Ca.: sarcomatoid carcinoma; SS: stromal sarcoma; SM Actin: smooth muscle actin; PANCK: pancytokeratin; HMWCK: high molecular weight cytokeratin; GU: genitourinary

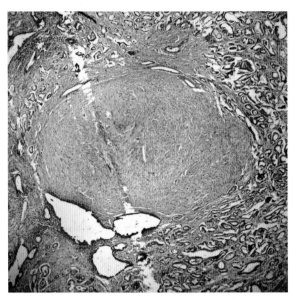

Fig 13.1 Leiomyoma of the prostate incidentally seen in a radical prostatectomy with cancer.

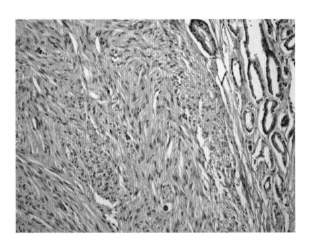

Fig 13.2 High power view of prostatic leiomyoma (same as figure 13.1).

by normal prostatic tissue. Lesional tissue shows a low to moderately cellular process set in a densely sclerotic collagenous matrix interrupted by pockets of edematous stroma. The tumor consists of short spindled cells possessing with eosinophilic cytoplasm and bland nuclei with uniformly distributed chromatin and inconspicuous nucleoli. The mitotic rate is low (2/ 10 HPF). No necrosis is identified. Figs 13.9–13.10

- Separation of the cells from the dense collagen focally imparted a "pseudoangiomatous" appearance. Paucicellular foci with increased sclerotic or edematous stromal matrices are observed. The vascular element consisted of capillary-sized vessels with muscular walls. The vessels had either a rounded configuration or more commonly were ectatic with an irregular contour, resulting in an angiofibromatous appearance.

- The tumor also features scattered cellular zones exhibiting cells arranged in a haphazard pattern. The cells exhibited nuclear atypia in the form of mild hyperchromasia and variation in the nuclear size and shape.

- The tumor cells were immunoreactive to CD34 and bcl-2, and negative for CD117 (c-kit),

ALK-1, smooth muscle actin, and progesterone receptors.

- Some cases of prostate SFT may exhibit NAB2-STAT6 gene fusion and present with nuclear STAT6 expression.

13.5 Gastrointestinal Stromal Tumor (GIST)

- Most cases present with obstructive symptoms and abnormal rectal examination. GISTs are typically large masses arising from the rectum or perirectal space that compress but do not invade the prostate. They can be diagnosed by needle biopsy and are morphologically similar to those found within the gastrointestinal tract. CD117 is uniformly expressed in all cases and CD34 is frequently positive. Figs 13.11–13.12

- Main differential diagnosis includes neural and smooth muscle tumors, SFTs and STUMP.

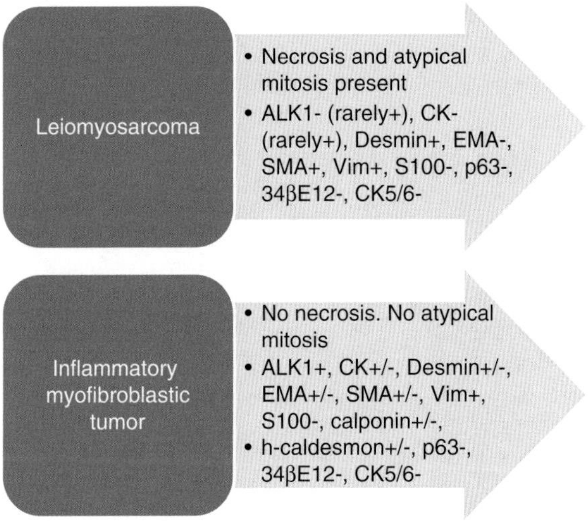

13.6 Prostatic Blue Nevus

- It is a rare spindle cell proliferation containing melanin within prostatic stroma. This histological appearance is reminiscent of the common blue nevus of the skin. Fig 13.13

- It is believed that this lesion does not transform into melanoma, in contrast to the cellular blue nevus, which occasionally undergoes malignant transformation.

- The terms blue nevus and melanosis of the prostate are occasionally used interchangeably, although most authors refer to it as melanosis when melanin is present within both the glandular and stromal melanocytes.

13.7 Miscellaneous Primary Tumors of the Prostate

- This is a very heterogeneous group of tumors which are very rarely observed in the prostate: Wilms'

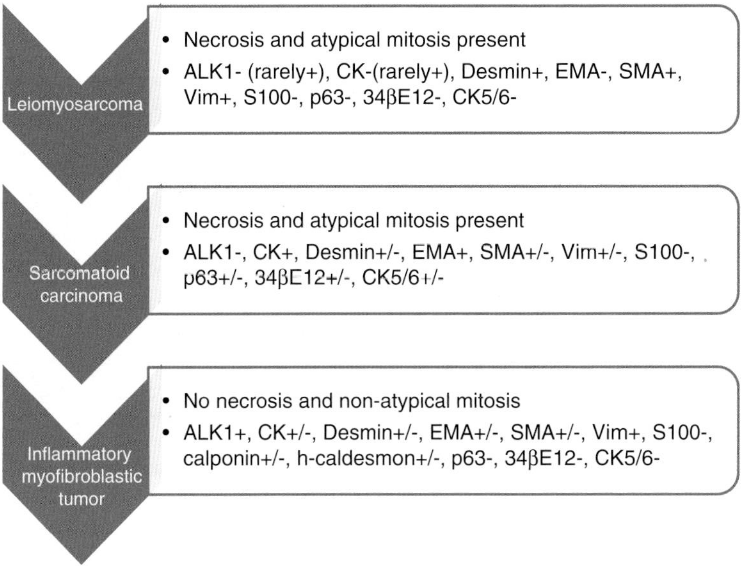

Leiomyosarcoma
- Necrosis and atypical mitosis present
- ALK1- (rarely+), CK- (rarely+), Desmin+, EMA-, SMA+, Vim+, S100-, p63-, 34βE12-, CK5/6-

Inflammatory myofibroblastic tumor
- No necrosis. No atypical mitosis
- ALK1+, CK+/-, Desmin+/-, EMA+/-, SMA+/-, Vim+, S100-, calponin+/-, h-caldesmon+/-, p63-, 34βE12-, CK5/6-

Fig 13.3 Differential diagnosis between leiomyosarcoma and inflammatory myofibroblastic tumor.

Fig 13.4 Differential diagnosis between leiomyosarcoma and sarcomatoid carcinoma.

Leiomyosarcoma
- Necrosis and atypical mitosis present
- ALK1- (rarely+), CK- (rarely+), Desmin+, EMA-, SMA+, Vim+, S100-, p63-, 34βE12-, CK5/6-

Sarcomatoid carcinoma
- Necrosis and atypical mitosis present
- ALK1-, CK+, Desmin+/-, EMA+, SMA+/-, Vim+/-, S100-, p63+/-, 34βE12+/-, CK5/6+/-

Inflammatory myofibroblastic tumor
- No necrosis and non-atypical mitosis
- ALK1+, CK+/-, Desmin+/-, EMA+/-, SMA+/-, Vim+, S100-, calponin+/-, h-caldesmon+/-, p63-, 34βE12-, CK5/6-

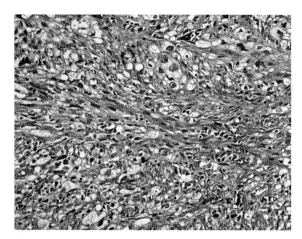

Fig 13.5 Histologic features of leiomyosarcoma of the prostate.

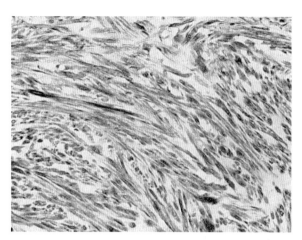

Fig 13.6 Desmin expression in a case of leiomyosarcoma of the prostate (same as figure 13.5).

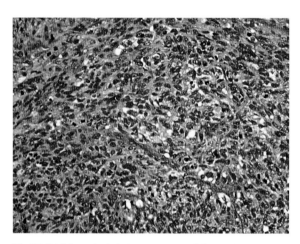

Fig 13.7 High grade rhabdomyosarcoma of the prostate.

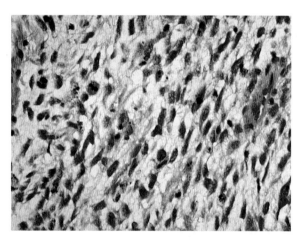

Fig 13.8 Rhabdomyosarcoma of the prostate with myxoid features.

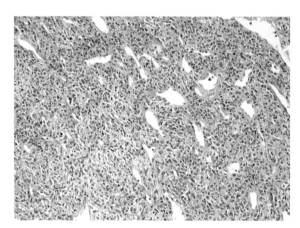

Fig 13.9 Solitary fibrous tumor of the prostate.

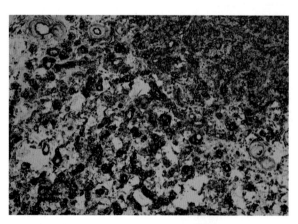

Fig 13.10 CD34 positive expression in solitary fibrous tumor of the prostate.

tumor (nephroblastoma), malignant rhabdoid tumor, tubulo-cystic clear cell adenocarcinoma, melanoma of the prostate, paraganglioma, hemangioma (mostly arising in the prostatic urethra) and neuroblastoma, malignant

perivascular epithelioid cell tumor (pecoma), malignant mixed germ cell tumor, endodermal sinus tumor, renal-type clear cell carcinoma.

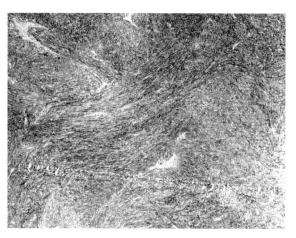

Fig 13.12 CD117 expression in gastrointestinal stromal tumor of the prostate (same as fig 13.11).

Fig 13.11 Gastrointestinal stromal tumor of the prostate.

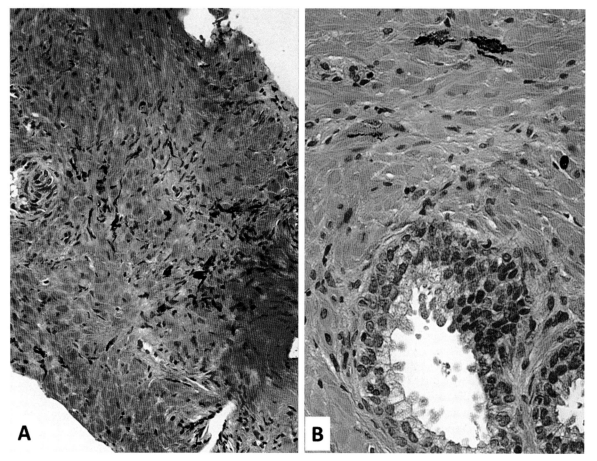

Fig 13.13 Prostatic blue nevus (A) and close up view of proliferating cells (B).

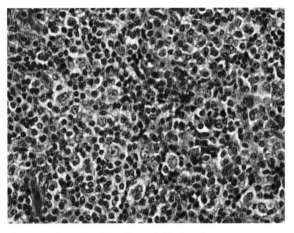

Fig 13.14 Large B cell lymphoma infiltrating the prostate.

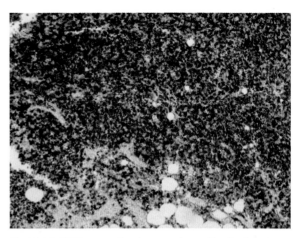

Fig 13.15 CD79a expression decorates the proliferating lymphoma cells.

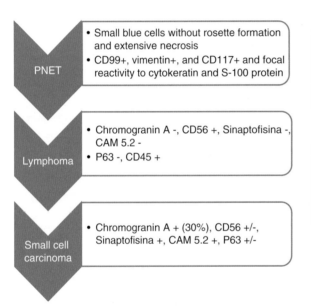

PNET
- Small blue cells without rosette formation and extensive necrosis
- CD99+, vimentin+, and CD117+ and focal reactivity to cytokeratin and S-100 protein

Lymphoma
- Chromogranin A -, CD56 +, Sinaptofisina -, CAM 5.2 -
- P63 -, CD45 +

Small cell carcinoma
- Chromogranin A + (30%), CD56 +/-, Sinaptofisina +, CAM 5.2 +, P63 +/-

Fig 13.16 Differential diagnosis of small blue round cell tumors of the prostate.

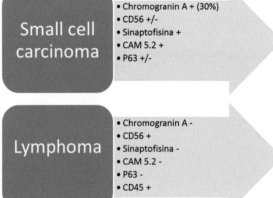

Small cell carcinoma
- Chromogranin A + (30%)
- CD56 +/-
- Sinaptofisina +
- CAM 5.2 +
- P63 +/-

Lymphoma
- Chromogranin A -
- CD56 +
- Sinaptofisina -
- CAM 5.2 -
- P63 -
- CD45 +

Fig 13.17 Differential diagnosis of small cell carcinoma of the prostate vs. lymphoma.

- The most common sarcomas are rhabdomyosarcoma and leiomyosarcoma. Rare cases of malignant fibrous histiocytoma, angiosarcoma, osteosarcoma, chondrosarcoma, malignant peripheral nerve sheath tumors, ectomesenchymoma with rhabdmyosarcoma and ganglioneuroma, PNET, and synovial sarcoma, chondroma, schwannoma, granular cell tumor, neurofibroma or hemagiopericytoma have been reported.

13.8 Lymphoid Tumors of the Prostate

- The prostate is a rare site of extranodal lymphoma which accounts for only 0.1% of all newly diagnosed lymphoma. Typically present in older men. Rarely, Hodgkin's lymphoma and mucosa-associated lymphoid tissue (MALT) lymphoma were reported.
- Most reported non-Hodgkin's lymphomas are diffuse large B-cells followed by small lymphocytic lymphoma. Most frequent symptoms are those related to lower urinary obstruction. Rare cases of myeloma and T-cell lymphoma are on record. The entire spectrum of lymphoma seen in other sites may become manifest in the prostate. Figs 13.14–13.17

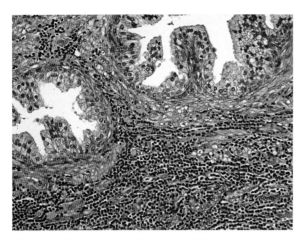

Fig 13.18 Chronic lymphocytic leukemia of the prostate.

- Of patients with chronic lymphocytic leukemia, 20% are reported to have prostate involvement at autopsy. Fig 13.18

Suggested Reading

Raspollini MR, Masieri L, Tosi N, Santucci M. Blue Nevus of the Prostate: Incidental Finding in Radical Prostatectomy Specimen with a Pre-operative Echographic Image of Peripheral Hypoechogenic Nodule. Arch Ital Urol Androl. 2011 Dec; **83**(4): 210–12.

Klock C, Gomes R, João M, Netto G. Prostate Melanosis Associated with Acinar Adenocarcinoma. Int J Surg Pathol. 2010 Oct; **18**(5): 379–80.

Ringoir A, Rappe B, Dhaene K, Schallier D. Prostatic Leiomyoma: A Case Report. Urol Case Rep. 2016 Sep 25; **9**: 45–47.

Venyo AK. A Review of the Literature on Primary Leiomyosarcoma of the Prostate Gland. Adv Urol. 2015; **2015**: 485786.

Ponte R, Ravetti JL, Pacella M, Toncini C. Multifocal Blue Nevus of the Prostate: A Case Report. Anal Quant Cytopathol Histpathol. 2014 Dec; **36**(6): 335–38.

Sbrollini G, Conti A, Galosi AB, Lacetera V, Montironi R, Montesi L, Muzzonigro G. Perivascular Epithelioid Cell Tumor (PEC-ome) of the Prostate: Ultrasound Feature in Case Report. Arch Ital Urol Androl. 2014 Dec 30; **86**(4): 393–94.

Westra WH, Grenko RT, Epstein J. Solitary Fibrous Tumor of the Lower Urogenital Tract: A Report of Five Cases Involving the Seminal Vesicles, Urinary Bladder, and Prostate. Hum Pathol. 2000; **31**: 63–68.

Lamont JS, Hesketh PJ, de las MA, Babayan RK. Primary Angiosarcoma of the Seminal Vesicle. J Urol. 1991; **146**: 165–67.

Laurila P, Leivo I, Makisalo H, Ruutu M, Miettinen M. Mullerian Adenosarcoma-like Tumor of the Seminal

Vesicle. A Case Report with Immunohistochemical and Ultrastructural Observations. Arch Pathol Lab Med. 1992; **116**: 1072–76.

Mazur MT, Myers JL, Maddox WA. Cystic Epithelial-stromal Tumor of the Seminal Vesicle. Am J Surg Pathol. 1987; **11**: 210–17.

Arya M, Hayne D, Brown RS, O'Donnell PJ, Mundy AR. Hemangiopericytoma of the Seminal Vesicle Presenting with Hypoglycemia. J Urol. 2001; **166**: 992.

Huh JS, Park KK, Kim YJ, Kim SD. Diagnosis of a Gastrointestinal Stromal Tumor Presenting as a Prostatic Mass: A Case Report. World J Mens Health. 2014 Dec; **32**(3): 184–88.

Gentile AT, Moseley HS, Quinn SF, Franzini D, Pitre TM. Leiomyoma of the Seminal Vesicle. J Urol. 1994; **151**: 1027–29.

Muentener M, Hailemariam S, Dubs M, Hauri D, Sulser T. Primary Leiomyosarcoma of the Seminal Vesicle. J Urol. 2000; **164**: 2027.

Juhasz J, Kiss P. A Hitherto Undescribed Case of 'Collision' Tumour: Liposarcoma of the Seminal Vesicle and Prostatic Carcinoma. Int Urol Nephrol. 1978; **10**: 185–93.

Montironi R, Lopez-Beltran A, Cheng L, Scarpelli M. Cervical-type Squamous Metaplasia and Myoepithelial Cell Differentiation in Stromal Tumor of the Prostate. Am J Surg Pathol. 2011 Nov; **35**(11): 1752–54. No abstract available.

Wagner DG, Yao JL, di Sant'Agnese PA, Cheng L, Lopez-Beltran A, Montironi R, Huang J. Soft Tissue Tumors of the Prostate: A Review. Anal Quant Cytol Histol. 2007 Dec; **29**(6): 341–50.

Cheng L, Foster SR, MacLennan GT, Lopez-Beltran A, Zhang S, Montironi R. Inflammatory Myofibroblastic Tumors of the Genitourinary Tract–Single Entity or Continuum? J Urol. 2008 Oct; **180**(4): 1235–40.

Mazzucchelli R, Lopez-Beltran A, Cheng L, Scarpelli M, Kirkali Z, Montironi R. Rare and Unusual Histological Variants of Prostatic Carcinoma: Clinical Significance. BJU Int. 2008 Nov; **102**(10): 1369–74.

Galosi AB, Mazzucchelli R, Scarpelli M, Lopez-Beltran A, Cheng L, Muzzonigro G, Montironi R. Solitary Fibrous Tumour of the Prostate Identified on Needle Biopsy. Eur Urol. 2009 Sep; **56**(3): 564–67.

Hodges KB, Abdul-Karim FW, Wang M, Lopez-Beltran A, Montironi R, Easley S, Zhang S, Wang N, MacLennan GT, Cheng L. Evidence for Transformation of Fibroadenoma of the Breast to Malignant Phyllodes Tumor. Appl Immunohistochem Mol Morphol. 2009 Jul; **17**(4): 345–50.

Lopez-Beltran A, Cheng L, Prieto R, Blanca A, Montironi R. Lymphoepithelioma-like Carcinoma of the Prostate. Hum Pathol. 2009 Jul; **40**(7): 982–87.

155

Morichetti D, Mazzucchelli R, Lopez-Beltran A, Cheng L, Scarpelli M, Kirkali Z, Montorsi F, Montironi R. Secondary Neoplasms of the Urinary System and Male Genital Organs. BJU Int. 2009 Sep; **104**(6): 770–76.

Montironi R, Lopez-Beltran A, Cheng L, Scarpelli M. Cervical-type Squamous Metaplasia and Myoepithelial Cell Differentiation in Stromal Tumor of the Prostate. Am J Surg Pathol. 2011 Nov; **35**(11): 1752–54.

Kouba E, Simper NB, Chen S, Williamson SR, Grignon DJ, Eble JN, MacLennan GT, Montironi R, Lopez-Beltran A, Osunkoya AO, Zhang S, Wang M, Wang L, Tran T, Emerson RE, Baldrige LA, Monn MF, Linos K, Cheng L. Solitary Fibrous Tumor of the Genitourinary Tract: A Clinicopathologic Study of 11 Cases and Their Association with the NAB2-STAT6 Fusion Gene. J Clin Pathol. 2016; In press.

Chapter 14

Metastatic and Secondary Tumors of the Prostate

14.1 Secondary Tumors Involving the Prostate

- Prostate involvement by a secondary tumor occurs either as a metastasis or by direct extension. Prostatic metastases from other genitor-urinary primaries, such as kidney and testis, have been rarely cited. Metastases from gastrointestinal tract, lung, skin (melanoma), and endocrine glands are on record. They are reported in 0.1% and 2.9% of all post-mortems and in 0.2% of all surgical prostatic specimens.

Table 14.1 Immunohistochemistry to Identify Tumors of Prostatic Origin

Antibody	Immunoreactivity
PSA	97% sensitive in mets; rare positive cells in GS9-10;
	high specificity; decreased with hormone therapy;
	salivary, bladder adeno, and melanoma may be (+)
PSAP	99% sensitive in mets; less specific than PSA;
	also (+) in NE tumors; decreased with hormone therapy
P501s (prostein)	99% sensitive in mets; limited studies;
	No decrease with hormone therapy
PSMA	88%–100% sensitive in mets; not specific
AMACR	81%–93% sensitive in mets; not specific
NKX3.1	94% sensitive in mets; only lobular breast Ca (+)
ERG	40–50% sensitivity; fairly specific. Also (+) in vascular tumors, meningioma, and some PNETs

mets: metastases; GS9-10: Gleason score 9–10; adeno: adenocarcinoma; PSA: prostate-specific antigen; PSAP: prostate-specific acid phosphatase; AMACR: alpha methylacyl-coaracemase; PSMA: prostate-specific membrane antigen; NE: neuroendocrine; Ca: carcinoma; PNETs: primitive neuroectodermal tumors

- The more common occurrence of secondary involvement of prostate by a bladder urothelial carcinoma can be diagnostically challenging in needle biopsy specimens.
- Immunohistochemistry is a relevant tool in establishing prostate primary. Table 14.1; Figs 14.1–14.7

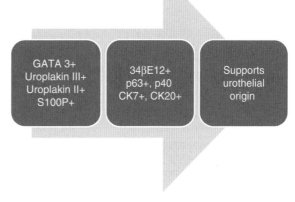

Fig 14.1 Immunohistochemical markers used to establish urothelial origin.

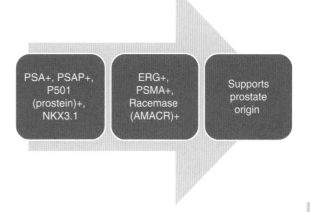

Fig 14.2 Immunohistochemical markers used to establish prostate origin.

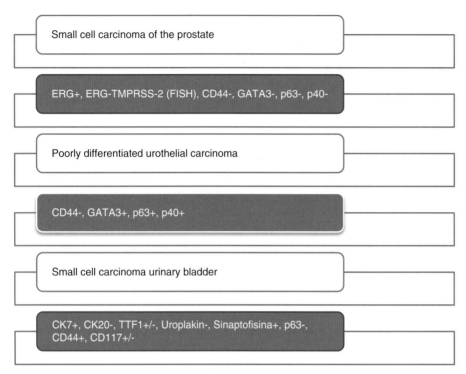

Fig 14.3 Immunohistochemical markers used to establish differential diagnosis between small cell carcinoma and poorly differentiated urothelial carcinoma.

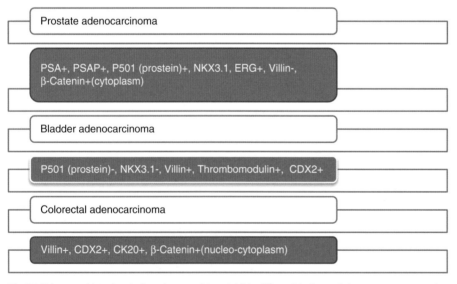

Fig 14.4 Immunohistochemical markers used to establish differential diagnosis between prostate adenocarcinoma, bladder adenocarcinoma, and colorectal adenocarcinoma.

14.2 Prostate Involvement from Bladder Urothelial Carcinoma

- Attention to subtle histological features such as papillary or solid growth, the relatively higher degree of nuclear pleomorphism, brisk mitotic activity or the occasional squamoid cytoplasm should raise the possibility of urothelial carcinoma (UC).

- Another helpful feature is the identification of pre-existing prostatic duct/acini distended by the

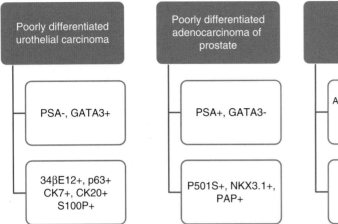

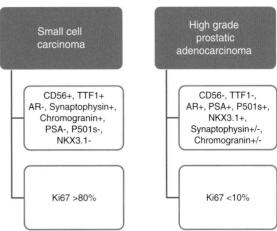

Fig 14.5 Immunohistochemical markers used to assess poorly differentiated adenocarcinoma of prostate vs. poorly differentiated urothelial carcinoma.

Fig 14.6 Immunohistochemical markers used to assess poorly differentiated adenocarcinoma of prostate vs. small cell carcinoma.

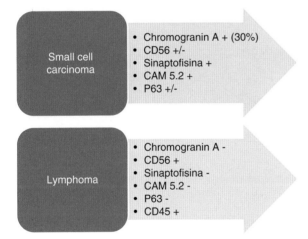

Fig 14.7 Immunohistochemical markers used to assess prostatic small cell carcinoma vs. lymphoma.

Fig 14.8 Poorly differentiated prostate adenocarcinoma infiltrating the urinary bladder.

malignant urothelial cells with occasional pagetoid or undermining pattern of spread. Some of the latter structures can be surrounded by concentric fibrosis even in the absence of stromal prostatic invasion. Figs 14.8–14.13

- The differential diagnosis for the intraductal spread of UC into the prostate should include high grade prostatic intraepithelial neoplasia, prostatic ductal adenocarcinoma and "intraductal" prostatic adenocarcinoma. Unlike UC, the latter lesions demonstrate positive reactivity for prostate-specific markers, i.e., PSA, prostate-specific membrane antigen (PSMA) and P504S,

and are negative for high molecular weight cytokeratins (34betaE12). Furthermore, intraductal UC spread into prostate is positive for uroplakin, thrombomodulin and/or p63. Table 14.2

- Intraductal UC spread into prostate could be extensive and can involve the peripheral prostate zone and rarely the seminal vesicle through the ejaculatory duct. The latter should be distinguished from invasion into prostatic stroma, which usually has a more infiltrative pattern, displaying irregular rather than smooth bordered urothelial nests and is associated with desmoplastic response.

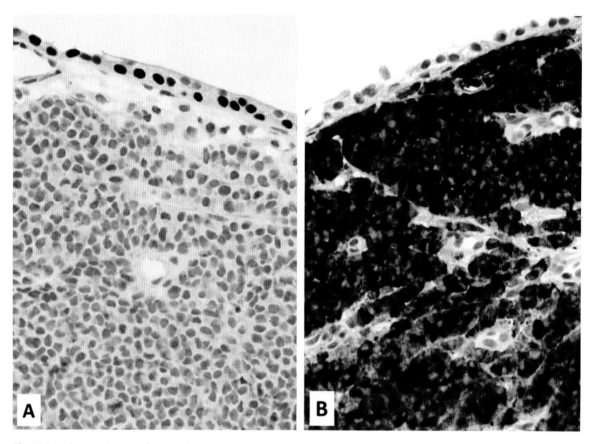

Fig 14.9 In this case (same as fig 14.8), the negative expression of p63 (A) and the positive expression of PSMA (B) may support prostate primary.

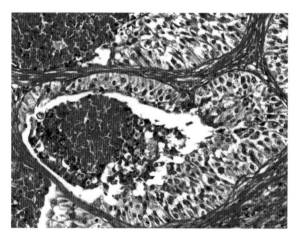

Fig 14.10 High grade urothelial carcinoma infiltrating the prostate.

- In cases of advanced urinary bladder UC, direct extension into the prostate through transmural bladder wall penetration may be seen. Given the significant difference in management of the two diseases, their distinction is crucial.
- Even in poorly differentiated Pca, there is relatively little pleomorphism or mitotic activity compared to poorly differentiated UC. A subtler finding is that the cytoplasm of prostatic adenocarcinoma is often foamy and pale, imparting a "soft" appearance. The findings of infiltrating cords of cells or focal cribriform glandular differentiation are other features more typical of prostatic adenocarcinoma than transitional cell carcinoma.

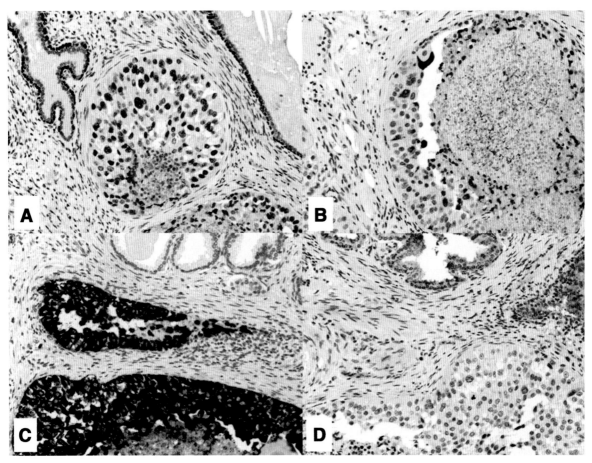

Fig 14.11 In this case (same as fig 14.10), the immunohistochemical profile p63 positive (A), Ck20 focally positive (B), CK7 positive (C) and PSA negative (D) supports bladder primary.

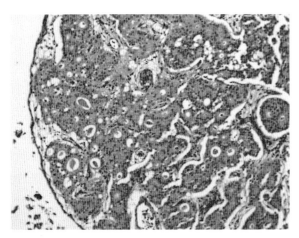

Fig 14.12 Poorly differentiated prostate adenocarcinoma infiltrating the urinary bladder.

- In the differential diagnosis of high grade Pca vs. urothelial carcinoma (UC), the primary option is to use PSA as a first test to identify Pca and GATA3 to identify UC. If GATA3 is not available, then HMWCK and p63. If the tumor is PSA positive with intense staining and HMWCK and p63 negative, the findings are diagnostic of Pca. If the tumor is equivocal/weak/negative for PSA and negative/focal for p63 and HMWCK, then one needs to do P501S, NKX3.1 and GATA3. Some experts also include PAP in this second round of staining. If the tumor is negative for PSA and diffusely strongly positive for p63 and HMWCK, the findings are diagnostic of UC. If the tumor is negative for PSA and moderate-strong positive for GATA3, it is diagnostic of UC.

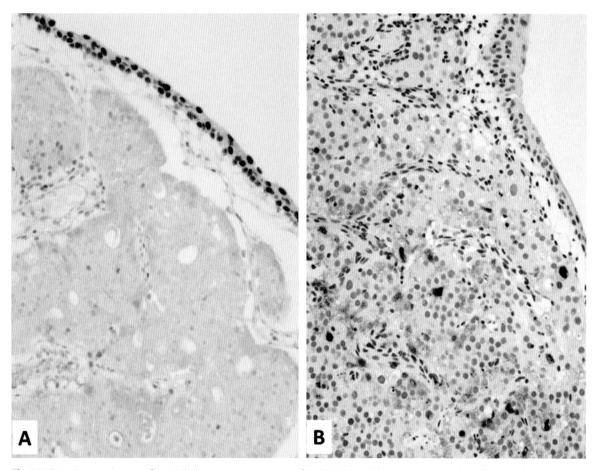

Fig 14.13 In this case (same as fig 14.12), the negative expression of GATA 3 (A) and the positive expression of PSA (B) support prostate primary.

14.3 Prostate Involvement from Colorectal Carcinoma

- A source of secondary tumor extension into the prostate is the topographically adjacent colorectal tract. Attention to some characteristic morphologic features should raise the possibility of a secondary spread on prostate needle biopsy specimens. The presence of goblet/columnar cell differentiation, pseudo-stratified nuclei and characteristic "dirty necrosis" are more likely encountered in colorectal carcinoma.
Figs 14.14–14.16
- One should be cautioned that single infiltrating glands of prostatic duct adenocarcinoma can resemble infiltrating colonic adenocarcinoma.

The differentiation between prostatic duct adenocarcinoma and secondary involvement of the prostate by colorectal carcinoma can be facilitated by finding more typical prostatic duct adenocarcinoma elsewhere within the biopsy.

- An immunohistochemical profile of positive nuclear CDX2 staining, positive nuclear (cytoplasmic staining can occur in Pca), β-catenin and villin, and positive staining for CK20 in the face of negative reactivity for prostate-specific antigen (PSA) and prostatic acid phosphatase (PAP), prostate-specific membrane (PSMA), can be used to confirm the diagnosis of colorectal carcinoma spread.
Table 14.3

Table 14.2 Differential Diagnosis of Prostate Adenocarcinoma vs. Urothelial Carcinoma Based on Immunohistochemistry

Antibody	Immunoreactivity
	PSA ~85%–90% (+) in GS10; negative in a subset of high grade Pca; weak non-specific cytoplasmic (+) lead to false (+); negative in UC.
PSAP	Polyclonal (+) in ~85%–90% GS10; monoclonal used in many kits lower sensitivity; negative in UC
P501S (Prostein)	(+) in many PSA (–) Pca; negative in UC; coarse cytoplasmic granules reduce false (+)
NKX3.1	(+) in many PSA (–) Pca; negative in UC nuclear stain reduce false (+)
AR	High sensitivity for Pca; positive in some UC
AMACR	High sensitivity for Pca; positive in some UC
PSMA	High sensitivity for Pca; positive in 14% of UC
CK7/CK20	Negative CK7 favors Pca; not specific, as both can be positive in Pca
HMWCK	Diffuse positive rules out Pca; only positive in ~70% of UC; occasionally false positive cells in Pca
p63	Less false positive in Pca; only positive in ~70% of UC Diffuse positive rules out Pca; occasionally false positive in Pca
Thrombomodulin	Positive in only 63% of high grade UC; focal positive in 5% Pca
Uroplakin	Negative in Pca; positive in only 60% of high grade UC
GATA3	Almost always negative in Pca; positive in 80% of high grade UC

GS10: Gleason score 5+5=10 adenocarcinoma; Pca: prostate adenocarcinoma; UC: urothelial carcinoma; PSA: prostate-specific antigen; PSAP: prostate-specific acid phosphatase; AR: androgen receptor; AMACR: alpha methylacyl-coaracemase; PSMA: prostate-specific membrane antigen; HMWCK: high molecular weight cytokeratin; UC: Urothelial carcinoma

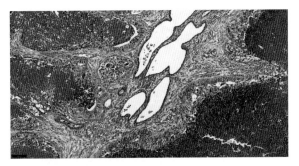

Fig 14.14 Colorectal adenocarcinoma infiltrating prostatic tissues.

histological patterns of adenocarcinoma arising in the gastrointestinal tract that can assist in differential diagnosis. Prostatic extension from bladder adenocarcinoma may occur either by metastasis or direct invasion. Immunohistochemical stains can be utilized in the differential diagnosis with prostatic adenocarcinoma.

- Monoclonal PSA antibodies do not label bladder adenocarcinoma, although polyclonal PSA and PSAP are positive in a significant percentage of bladder adenocarcinomas.
- Of the more recently discovered prostatic markers, PSMA lacks specificity, but NKX3.1 and P501S do not react with bladder adenocarcinomas. Table 14.4

14.5   Other Metastatic Deposits

- Prostate cancer may extend to other sites, such as the lymph nodes, liver or lung. Assessing prostate origin in patients with second or even third primary cancers is becoming more relevant in clinical practice.
- Seminal vesicle extension by prostate cancer is usually solved by H&E, but may occasionally require immunohistochemistry. Clinical information and immunohistochemistry are critical in achieving the correct diagnosis. Figs 14.17–14.22

14.4   High Grade Prostatic Adenocarcinoma vs. Bladder Adenocarcinoma

- Morphologically, there are differences in that bladder adenocarcinoma shares all of the various

Suggested Reading

Rao Q, Williamson SR, Lopez-Beltran A, Montironi R, Huang W, Eble JN, Grignon DJ, Koch MO, Idrees MT, Emerson RE, Zhou XJ, Zhang S, Baldridge LA, Cheng L. Distinguishing Primary Adenocarcinoma of the Urinary Bladder from Secondary Involvement by Colorectal Adenocarcinoma: Extended

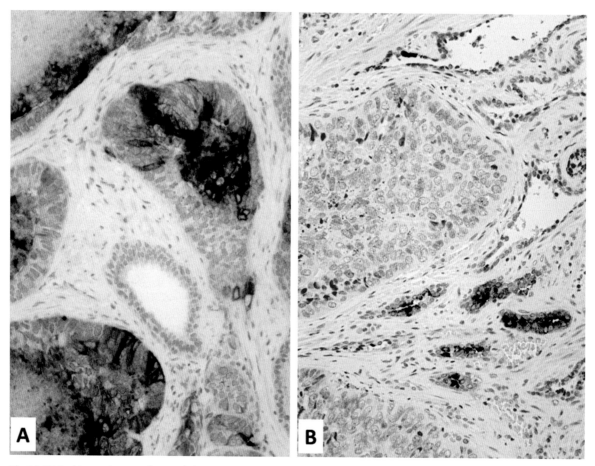

Fig 14.15 In this case (same as fig 14.14), the positive expression of monoclonal CEA (A) and the negative expression of PSA (B) support colorectal primary. Notice PSA positive benign glands in (B).

Immunohistochemical Profiles Emphasizing Novel Markers. Mod Pathol. 2013 May; 26(5): 725–32. doi: 10.1038/modpathol.2012.229.

Liu H, Shi J, Wilkerson ML, Lin F. Immunohistochemical Evaluation of GATA3 Expression in Tumors and Normal Tissues: A Useful Immunomarker for Breast and Urothelial Carcinomas. Am J Clin Pathol. 2012; 138: 57–64.

Miettinen M, McCue PA, Sarlomo-Rikala M, et al. GATA3: A Multispecific but Potentially Useful Marker in Surgical Pathology: A Systematic Analysis of 2500 Epithelial and Nonepithelial Tumors. Am J Surg Pathol. 2013.

Chang A, Amin A, Gabrielson E, et al. Utility of GATA3 Immunohistochemistry in Differentiating Urothelial Carcinoma from Prostate Adenocarcinoma and Squamous Cell Carcinomas of the Uterine Cervix, Anus, and Lung. Am J Surg Pathol. 2012; 36: 1472–76.

Genega EM, Hutchinson B, Reuter VE, Gaudin PB. Immunophenotype of High-grade Prostatic

Adenocarcinoma and Urothelial Carcinoma. Mod Pathol. 2000; 13: 1186–91.

Mhawech P, Uchida T, Pelte MF. Immunohistochemical Profile of High-grade Urothelial Bladder Carcinoma and Prostate Adenocarcinoma. Hum Pathol. 2002; 33: 1136–40.

Epstein JI, Kuhajda FP, Lieberman PH. Prostate-specific Acid Phosphatase Immunoreactivity in Adenocarcinomas of the Urinary Bladder. Hum Pathol. 1986; 17: 939–42.

Wang W, Epstein JI. Small Cell Carcinoma of the Prostate. A Morphologic and Immunohistochemical Study of 95 Cases. Am J Surg Pathol. 2008; 32: 65–71.

Yao JL, Madeb R, Bourne P, et al. Small Cell Carcinoma of the Prostate: An Immunohistochemical Study. Am J Surg Pathol. 2006; 30: 705–12.

Agoff SN, Lamps LW, Philip AT, et al. Thyroid Transcription Factor-1 Is Expressed in Extrapulmonary

Table 14.3 Differential Diagnosis of Colorectal Adenocarcinoma vs. High Grade Prostate Adenocarcinoma by Immunohistochemistry

Antibody	Immunoreactivity
Villin	(+) in most CRC; (−) in Pca
CDX2	(+) in most CRC; rare (+) in Pca
CK20	(+) in most CRC; (+) in 20% Pca
Prostate markers	(−) in CRC; (+) in >90% Pca; rare (−) Pca cases
Polyclonal CEA MUC1, MUC2	(+) in CRC; overlap with Pca
Beta-catenin	(+) in CRC, diffuse nuclear staining diagnostic
	Typically (+) cytoplasmic
	Nuclear (+) in some studies of Pca

CRC: colorectal adenocarcinoma; Pca: prostate adenocarcinoma

Small Cell Carcinomas but Not in Other Extrapulmonary Neuroendocrine Tumors. Mod Pathol. 2000; **13**: 238–42.

Ordonez NG. Value of Thyroid Transcription Factor-1 Immunostaining in Distinguishing Small Cell Lung Carcinomas from Other Small Cell Carcinomas. Am J Surg Pathol. 2000; **24**: 1217–23.

Lotan TL, Gupta NS, Wang W, et al. ERG Gene Rearrangements Are Common in Prostatic Small Cell Carcinomas. Mod Pathol. 2011; **24**: 820–28.

Han B, Mehra R, Lonigro RJ, et al. Fluorescence in Situ Hybridization Study Shows Association of PTEN Deletion with ERG Rearrangement During Prostate Cancer Progression. Mod Pathol. 2009; **22**: 1083–93.

Williamson SR, Zhang S, Yao JL, et al. ERG-TMPRSS2 Rearrangement Is Shared by Concurrent Prostatic Adenocarcinoma and Prostatic Small Cell Carcinoma

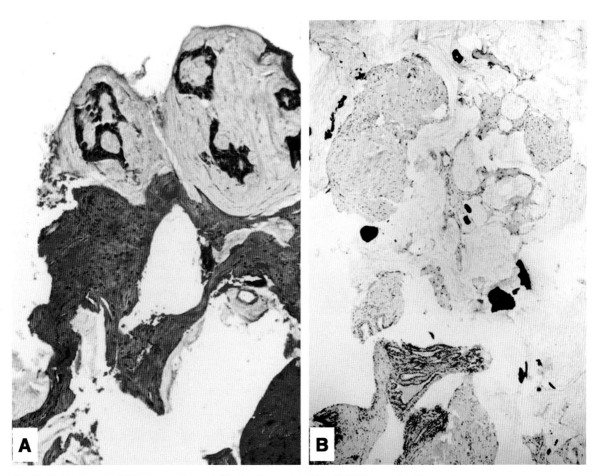

Fig 14.16 Mucinous (colloid) adenocarcinoma infiltrating the prostate (A) with CK 7 expression (B).

Table 14.4 Differential Diagnosis of High Grade Prostatic Adenocarcinoma vs. Primary Bladder Adenocarcinoma

Antibody	Immunoreactivity
PSA	High sensitivity; 7–13% high grade Pca (–); 13% bladder adeno (+) polyclonal
PAP	High sensitivity; 5% GS8-10 (–); 33% bladder adeno (+) polyclonal
p501S (prostein)	High sensitivity (83%–100%) and high specificity
NKX3.1	High sensitivity (95%); high specificity in general; not investigated in bladder adenocarcinoma
PSMA	High sensitivity (88%–92%); 11% bladder adenocarcinoma cytoplasmic staining; 8% bladder adenocarcinoma membrane staining
Villin	High specificity for bladder; sensitivity 65% for bladder adeno
Thrombomodulin	95% negative in Pca; sensitivity 60% for bladder adeno
CDX2	94% negative in Pca; sensitivity 47% for bladder adeno
Monoclonal CEA	>95% negative in Pca; sensitivity 52% for bladder adeno
CA125	>95% negative in Pca; sensitivity 28% for bladder adeno
HMWCK	92% negative in high grade Pca; sensitivity 40% for bladder adeno
CK7/CK20	77% (CK7) & 64% (CK20) sensitivity for bladder adeno; not specific: CK7 in 57% of high grade Pca and CK20 in 20%

GS10: Pca: prostate adenocarcinoma; adeno: adenocarcinoma; GS8-10: Gleason score 8–10 adenocarcinoma; PSA: prostate-specific antigen; PSAP: prostate-specific acid phosphatase; PSMA: prostate-specific membrane antigen; CEA: carcinoembryonic antigen; CA125: cancer antigen 125

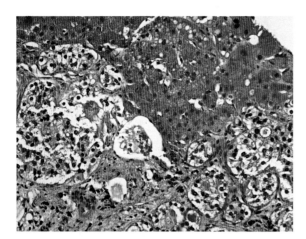

Fig 14.17 Liver metastasis of high grade prostate adenocarcinoma.

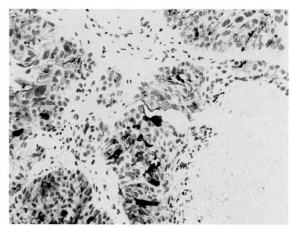

Fig 14.18 In this case (same as fig 14.17), the expression of PSA favors prostate primary.

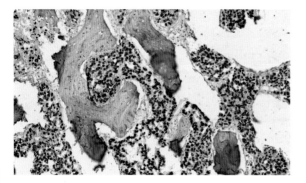

Fig 14.19 In this case, the expression of P501S (prostein) favors prostate primary.

and Absent in Small Cell Carcinoma of the Urinary Bladder: Evidence Supporting Monoclonal Origin. Mod Pathol. 2011; **24**: 1120–27.

Scheble VJ, Braun M, Wilbertz T, et al. ERG Rearrangement in Small Cell Prostatic and Lung Cancer. Histopathology. 2010; **56**: 937–43.

Schelling LA, Williamson SR, Zhang S, et al. Frequent TMPRSS2-ERG Rearrangement in Prostatic Small Cell Carcinoma Detected by Fluorescence in Situ Hybridization: The Superiority of Fluorescence in Situ Hybridization over ERG Immunohistochemistry. Hum Pathol. 2013.

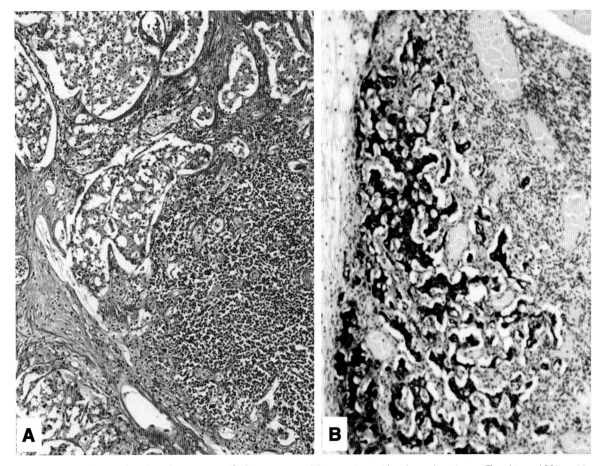

Fig 14.20 Peri colorectal lymph node metastasis of adenocarcinoma (A) in a patient with colorectal carcinoma. The observed PSA positive expression (B) supports prostate primary.

Slater D. Carcinoid Tumour of the Prostate Associated with Inappropriate ACTH Secretion. Br J Urol. 1985; **57**: 591–92.

Bodey B, Bodey B, Jr, Kaiser HE. Immunocytochemical Detection of Prostate Specific Antigen Expression in Human Primary and Metastatic Melanomas. Anticancer Res. 1997; **17**: 2343–46.

Varinot J, Drouin S, Rouprêt M, Montironi R, Lopez-Beltran A, Compérat E. Prostate Cancer with Clear Cell Features and an Unusual Nested-like Pattern of Growth: A Case Report. Anal Quant Cytol Histol. 2012 Oct; **34**(5): 289–92.

Cheng L, MacLennan GT, Lopez-Beltran A, Montironi R. Anatomic, Morphologic and Genetic Heterogeneity of Prostate Cancer: Implications for Clinical Practice. Expert Rev Anticancer Ther. 2012 Nov; **12**(11): 1371–74. doi: 10.1586/era.12.127. No.

Morichetti D, Mazzucchelli R, Lopez-Beltran A, Cheng L, Scarpelli M, Kirkali Z, Montorsi F, Montironi R.

Secondary Neoplasms of the Urinary System and Male Genital Organs. BJU Int. 2009 Sep; **104**(6): 770–76.

Quick Charles M. MDa, Gokden Neriman MDa, Sangoi Ankur R. MDb, Brooks James D. MDc, McKenney Jesse K. MDa. The Distribution of PAX-2 Immunoreactivity in the Prostate Gland, Seminal Vesicle, and Ejaculatory Duct: Comparison with Prostatic Adenocarcinoma and Discussion of Prostatic Zonal Embryogenesis. Human Pathology. 2010; **41**: 1145–49.

Harvey Aaron M. MD, Grice Beverly HTL, Hamilton Candice HTL, Truong Luan D. MD, Ro Jae Y. MD, Ayala Alberto G. MD, Zhai Qihui "Jim". MD Diagnostic Utility of P504S/p63 Cocktail Prostate-specific Antigen, and Prostatic Acid Phosphatase in Scarpelli M, Mazzucchelli R, Barbisan F, Santinelli A, Lopez-Beltran A, Cheng L, Montironi R. Is There a Role for Prostate Tumour Overexpressed-1 in the Diagnosis of HGPIN and of Prostatic

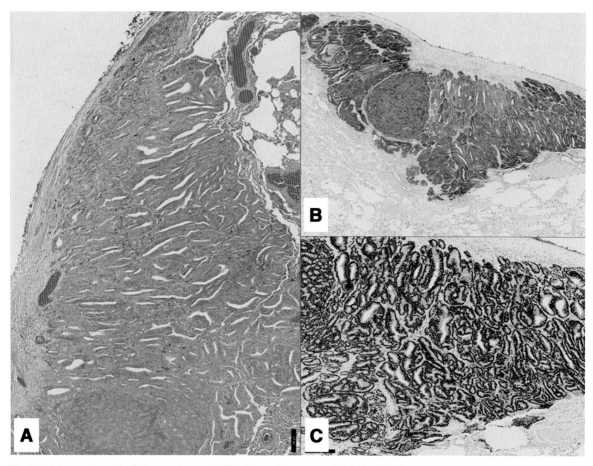

Fig 14.21 Lung metastasis of adenocarcinoma (A). The observed expression of PSA (B) and androgen receptor (C) supports prostate primary.

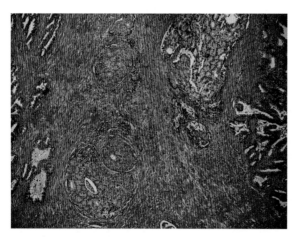

Fig 14.22 Seminal vesicle infiltration by prostate adenocarcinoma. Prostate origin can be suggested by morphology alone.

Adenocarcinoma? A Comparison with Alpha-Methylacyl CoA Racemase. Int J Immunopathol Pharmacol. 2012 Jan–Mar; **25**(1): 67–74.

Williamson SR, Zhang S, Yao JL, Huang J, Lopez-Beltran A, Shen S, Osunkoya AO, MacLennan GT, Montironi R, Cheng L. ERG-TMPRSS2 Rearrangement Is Shared by Concurrent Prostatic Adenocarcinoma and Prostatic Small Cell Carcinoma and Absent in Small Cell Carcinoma of the Urinary Bladder: Evidence Supporting Monoclonal Origin. Mod Pathol. 2011 Aug; **24**(8): 1120–27. doi: 10.1038/modpathol.2011.56.

Lopez-Beltran A, Eble John N, Bostwick David G. Pleomorphic Giant Cell Carcinoma of the Prostate. Archives of Pathology and Laboratory Medicine. 2005; **129**: 683–85.

Montironi R, Scattoni V, Mazzucchelli R, Lopez-Beltran A, Bostwick DG, Montorsi F. Atypical Foci Suspicious but Not Diagnostic of Malignancy in Prostate Needle Biopsies (Also Referred to as "Atypical Small Acinar Proliferation Suspicious for but Not Diagnostic of Malignancy"). Eur Urol. 2006 Oct; **50**(4): 666–74.

Chapter 15

The Seminal Vesicles and Ejaculatory Ducts

15.1 The Seminal Vesicles and Ejaculatory Ducts: Basic Anatomy and Histology

- Seminal vesicles lie posterolateral to the base of the urinary bladder and anterior to Denonvilliers fascia. The seminal vesicle wall consists of a thick circumferential coat of smooth muscle and the ejaculatory ducts are surrounded by a collagenous stroma. Uncommonly, one may see small hyaline globules in the SV's wall. Figs 15.1–15.5
- Seminal vesicle and ejaculatory ducts share histogenesis from the wolffian system with the prostatic central zone.
- The SV's epithelium is composed of ducts and acini with a two-cell lining layer of secretory cells and basal cells. Lipofuscin (yellow-brown pigment) can be found in the cytoplasm of secretory cells in SVs and ejaculatory duct epithelium, and rarely in stromal cells. It is characteristic to see scattered nuclei exhibiting enlargement and degenerative-type

hyperchromasia. This is a helpful feature to separate SV/ejaculatory duct epithelium from prostate epithelium.
- The immunoprofile of secretory cells of SVs/ejaculatory ducts is CKAE1/AE3 +, CAM5.2+, PAX-2+, MUC 6+, PSA-, PAP- and P504S- (racemase). Basal cells are p63+. Fig 15.6

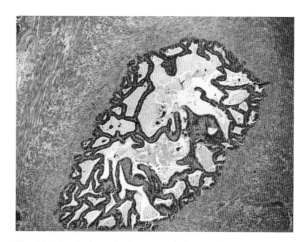

Fig 15.1 Seminal vesicle showing a thick smooth muscle layer.

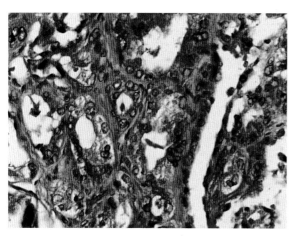

Fig 15.2 Lipochrome pigment in SV epithelium.

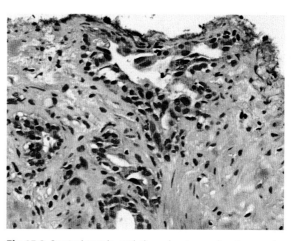

Fig 15.3 Seminal vesicle epithelium showing no lipochrome pigment may be seen in limited prostate biopsies and should not be misdiagnosed as malignancy.

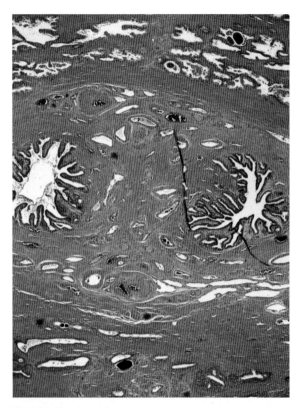

Fig 15.4 Ejaculatory ducts seen at low power.

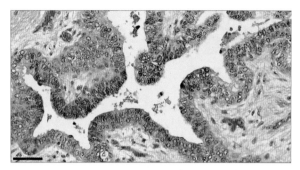

Fig 15.5 Ejaculatory ducts may occasionally show no pigment and should not be misdiagnosed as malignancy.

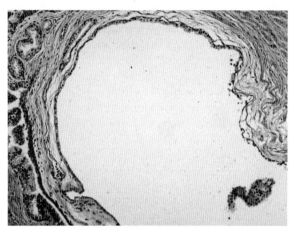

Fig 15.7 Cystically dilated ejaculatory duct.

Secretory/basal cells of SVs/ejaculatory ducts	Prostate adenocarcinoma
CKAE1/AE3 +, CAM5.2+, PAX-2 +, MUC 6+, CEA+, CK7+	CKAE1/AE3+, CAM5.2+, PAX-2-, MUC 6-,
PSA-, PAP- and P504S (racemase) -	PSA+, PAP+, P504S (racemase)+
Basal cells: p63+, p40+	No basal cells: P63-, p40-

Fig 15.6 Differential diagnosis between SV/ejaculatory epithelium vs. prostate adenocarcinoma.

- Cysts seen in the seminal vesicle, ejaculatory ducts or vas deferens are rare and most frequently diagnosed during work up of infertility. A case of cystic dilatation of the ejaculatory duct at the opening into an enlarged prostatic utricle was recently described.

- The opening of the ejaculatory ducts is seen lateral to the prostatic utricle and may occasionally be cystic of size enough to be detected by ultrasound. Fig 15.7 The epithelial lining includes a basal cell layer and a luminal cell layer. The former are morphologically and immunohistochemically similar to those of the prostate. The luminal cells show acidophilic abundant cytoplasm with a variable amount of yellow pigment, whereas the nuclei show condensed chromatin and size variation.

- Occasionally, large epithelial cells with hyperchromatic nuclei can be seen. This

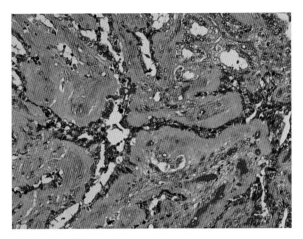

Fig 15.8 Amyloidosis of the seminal vesicle.

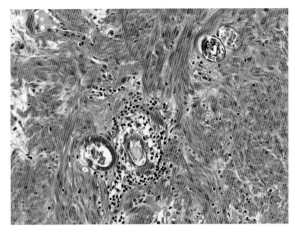

Fig 15.9 Schistosoma hematobium in seminal vesicle muscle wall.

epithelium is similar to that of the seminal vesicles. There is no morphological equivalent.

15.2 The Seminal Vesicles and Ejaculatory Ducts

15.2.1 Inflammatory and Tumor-like Conditions

- Rare infections, ectopic tissues, age-related changes and cysts may occasionally present as tumor-like lesions.
- With age, the columnar epithelium is replaced by flattened cuboidal cells and the muscular stroma becomes hyalinized and fibrotic. Lipochrome pigment is frequently present in SV epithelium. Occasionally, stromal hyaline bodies may be present. The epithelium shows highly atypical cells with large, hyperchromatic nuclei with prominent nucleoli. Multinucleated cells may be present. Mitotic figures are absent. When present in needle biopsies, this should not be mistaken as prostate cancer.
- Ectopic prostate tissue may be seen in the SVs, frequently in the wall of a vesicle cyst. Urothelial or squamous metaplasia has been reported rarely arising in the SVs.
- SV amyloidosis (localized amyloidosis), which is Congo Red + with apple-green polarization birefringence. Fig 15.8
- Fibrosis associated with retroperitoneal and mediastinal fibrosis.

- Chronic or acute seminal vesiculitis, including SV abscess, tuberculosis, BCG therapy-related granuloma, seminal schistosomiasis (usually secondary to schistosoma haematobium infection from urinary bladder), malakoplakia, viral lesions and SV wall calcification or calculi. Fig 15.9
- Androgen deprivation therapy in patients with prostate cancer may result in shrinkage of the SVs, and radiation therapy causes atrophy and fibrosis of the SVs.
- Muscular/fibromuscular hyperplasia is rare in the SV wall and rarely may present seminal vesicle glands entrapped within smooth muscle hyperplasia (adenomiosis).
- Primary tumors arising in the seminal vesicles (SVs) are extremely rare with anecdotal cases reported. Pelvic pain and urinary or rectal obstructive symptoms are frequently the onset of disease.
- Some may be asymptomatic, and detected by digital rectal examination and imaging, but final diagnosis frequently requires biopsy. It may be difficult to ascertain the site of origin of a given tumor when adjacent pelvic organs are involved.

15.2.2 Cysts

- Seminal vesicle cysts are rare and may be congenital or acquired. Most are asymptomatic, unilateral, and < 5 cm. Cysts >12 cm are known as giant cysts. The contents may include blood cells and sperm.

171

- Histologic analysis of the SV shows a unilocular cyst with flattened epithelium (PSA+, PSAP+). A malignancy may develop in an otherwise benign SV cyst, typically squamous cell carcinoma or adenocarcinoma.
- Hydatidic cyst has been described in retro vesicular space.
- Cystic ejaculatory ducts have also been described at the opening in the urethra.

15.2.3 Cystadenoma

- Cystadenoma is a rare benign tumor of the seminal vesicles. Patients range in age from 37 to 66 years. They may be asymptomatic or have symptoms of bladder outlet obstruction. Imaging reveals a complex, solid-cystic pelvic mass. Tumors may recur when incompletely removed.
- Microscopically, cystadenoma is a well-circumscribed tumor containing variable-sized glandular spaces with branching contours and cysts separated by spindle cell stroma. The glands are grouped in a lobular pattern, contain pale intraluminal secretions, and are lined by one or two layers of cuboidal to columnar cells. Table 15.1
- No significant cytologic atypia, mitotic activity or necrosis is present. Figs 15.10–15.11

15.2.4 Adenocarcinoma

- Primary adenocarcinoma is rare, with less than 100 acceptable cases reported.
- Presenting symptoms usually include obstructive uropathy due to a non-tender perirectal mass and, less commonly, hematuria or hematospermia. Serum carcinoembryonic antigen may be elevated. Most are in older men (mean 62 years), but may occur under the age 40 years.
- Strict criteria for the diagnosis of this lesion require the exclusion of a concomitant prostatic, bladder or rectal carcinoma. Suggested criteria include: i) Tumor located primarily in the SVs; ii) no evidence of carcinoma in the prostate, bladder or rectum; iii) histology of adenocarcinoma with papillary, sheet-like growth or mucinous differentiation; iv) in situ adenocarcinoma in the adjacent seminal epithelium (criteria yet undefined); v) cytoplasmic inmunorreactivity for CEA; and vi) absence of staining for PSA and PAP.

Table 15.1 Tumors of the Seminal Vesicles

Epithelial Tumors
- Cystadenoma
- Adenocarcinoma (primary)

Mesenchymal Tumors (Benign and Malignant)
- Angiosarcoma
- Hemangiopericytoma
- Leiomyoma
- Leiomyosarcoma
- Liposarcoma
- Malignant fibrous histiocytoma
- Solitary fibrous tumor

Mixed Epithelial-Stromal Tumors (Benign and Malignant)
- Fibroadenoma
- Adenomyoma
- Malignant epithelial-stromal tumors
  - low grade
  - high grade

Other
- Germ cell tumors

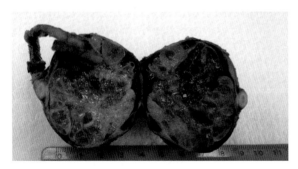

Fig 15.10 Gross aspect of SV cystadenoma.

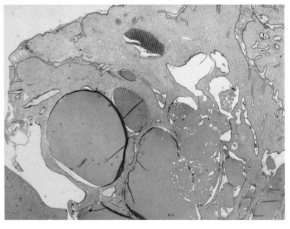

Fig 15.11 Microscopic features of SV cystadenoma.

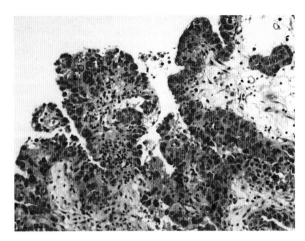

Fig 15.12 Adenocarcinoma of the seminal vesicle with papillary configuration.

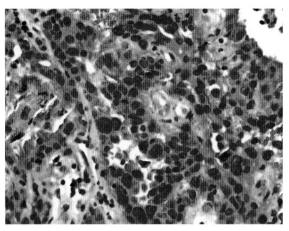

Fig 15.13 Close up view of the cells in adenocarcinoma of the seminal vesicle.

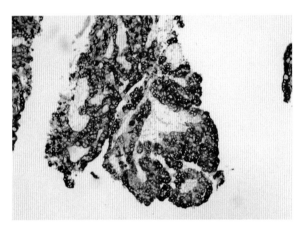

Fig 15.14 Adenocarcinoma of the seminal vesicle positive for CK7 (anti-CK7 immunohistochemistry).

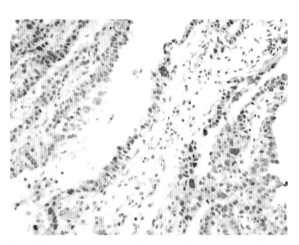

Fig 15.15 Adenocarcinoma of the seminal vesicle negative for PSA (anti-PSA immunohistochemistry).

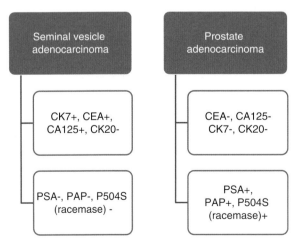

Seminal vesicle adenocarcinoma	Prostate adenocarcinoma
CK7+, CEA+, CA125+, CK20-	CEA-, CA125- CK7-, CK20-
PSA-, PAP-, P504S (racemase) -	PSA+, PAP+, P504S (racemase)+

Fig 15.16 Differential diagnosis of adenocarcinoma of the seminal vesicle vs. prostate adenocarcinoma.

- The tumors are usually large (3–5 cm) and often invade the bladder, ureter or rectum. Tumors can show a mixture of glandular, papillary and trabecular features with varying degrees of differentiation. Tumors with a colloid pattern have been described.
- The tumor cells' cytoplasm may show clear cell or hobnail morphology. It is important to exclude a prostatic adenocarcinoma.
- Carcinoembryonic antigens (CEA) and CK7 are detectable in normal seminal vesicle. Tumor of the SVs should be positive for CK 7 (unlike many prostatic adenocarcinomas), CEA, and for CA125 (unlike carcinoma arising in a mullerian duct cyst) and negative for CK 20 (unlike bladder and colonic carcinoma), PSA and PAP. Figs 15.12–15.16

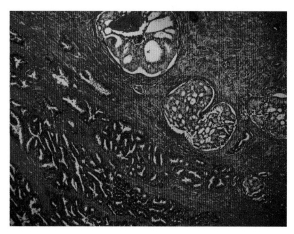

Fig 15.17 Prostate adenocarcinoma infiltrating the wall of seminal vesicle.

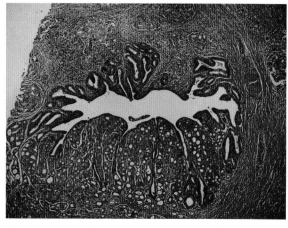

Fig 15.18 Prostate adenocarcinoma infiltrating the wall of the ejaculatory ducts.

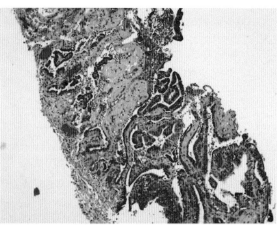

Fig 15.19 Ductal carcinoma of prostate extending through seminal vesicle.

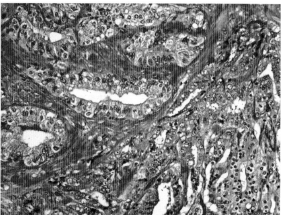

Fig 15.20 Lipochrome pigment may assist in differentiating prostate adenocarcinoma vs. epithelium of the seminal vesicle.

- The prognosis of primary seminal vesicle adenocarcinoma is poor. Since most patients present with metastases at diagnosis, overall survival in 95% of patients is less than three years. Table 15.1

15.2.5 Secondary Carcinoma

- The seminal vesicle is involved by secondary tumors much more frequently than it contains primary adenocarcinoma. Most frequent secondary involvement is from prostate acinar adenocarcinoma or adenocarcinomas with variant histology (ductal or intraductal carcinoma), but urothelial carcinoma may also invade the SVs by direct extension (stage T4) or mucosal spread from the urethra, in this case as pagetoid spread or mucosal replacement from in situ urothelial carcinoma. Figs 15.17–15.20

- Rectal adenocarcinoma occasionally invades SVs. Other metastases to SVs and/or retrovesical space may originate in renal cell carcinoma, hepatocellular carcinoma, thymoma and seminoma.

15.2.6 Differentiating Prostate Gland, Seminal Vesicle and Ejaculatory Duct Tissues

- Occasionally, uropathologists face a differential diagnosis between prostate tissue, seminal vesicle or ejaculatory duct in the setting of needle biopsies.

- Seminal vesicle wall consists of a thick circumferential coat of smooth muscle and the ejaculatory ducts are surrounded by a collagenous stroma. SVs are CKAE1/AE3+, p63+, PAX-2 +, PSA-, PAP- and P504S-(racemase).
- The use of a panel based on the P504S/p63 one-color cocktail is a practical and cost-effective stain to differentiate prostatic carcinoma that involves the seminal vesicle from seminal vesicle epithelium. It is superior to PSA and PAP, since these cannot distinguish benign from malignant glands.
- More recently, the use of nuclear PAX-2 immunoreactivity has been suggested as a robust marker in this setting. PAX-2 is typically positive in epithelium of the seminal vesicle and ejaculatory duct, but the intensity of staining is less in the ejaculatory duct. No reactivity for PAX-2 is seen in prostatic adenocarcinoma or prostatic intraepithelial neoplasia.

15.2.7 Angiosarcoma

- Reported patients present with pelvic pain and died of distant metastasis within four months after the diagnosis.

15.2.8 Hemangiopericytoma

- Anecdotal cases of malignant hemangiopericytoma of the seminal vesicle have been reported with patients who died of disseminated disease after surgery.

15.2.9 Leiomyosarcoma

- Imaging methods show a large pelvic mass in the region of the SVs. Most reported patients with seminal vesicle leiomyosarcoma presented with pelvic pain and obstructive symptoms.
- Resection of the tumor mass by radical prostatectomy and vesiculectomy is the therapy of choice. This approach may result as curative in some cases, although others may develop metastasis. Morphologically, it is identical to leiomyosarcoma of other locations.

15.2.10 Liposarcoma

- Only rare cases of liposarcoma of the SVs have been described. One case had associated prostatic carcinoma.

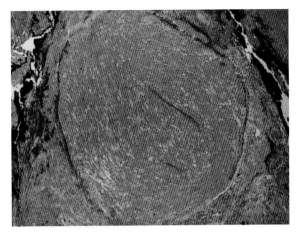

Fig 15.21 Leiomyoma of the seminal vesicle.

15.2.11 Malignant Fibrous Histiocytoma (Undifferentiated Sarcoma)

- This tumor is exceedingly rare in the seminal vesicle. The therapy should be the complete surgical resection if possible.

15.2.12 Leiomyoma

- It is usually asymptomatic with smaller tumors seen incidentally at time of prostatectomy. Larger tumors may be detected on digital rectal examination or imaging. Fig 15.21
- Leiomyoma ranges 0.5 to 5 cm, and local excision yields no recurrence.

15.2.13 Solitary Fibrous Tumor

- Anecdotal cases have been reported in the seminal vesicle, most frequently in the right organ. The origin of the tumor was established by imaging methods. The clinical presentation includes pelvic pain and/or hematuria. Complete local excision appears to be curative.

15.2.14 Other

- Rare examples of fibroma, schwannoma, paraganglioma, mammary-type myofibroblastoma, fibrosarcoma, osteosarcoma, rhabdomyosarcoma, pleomorphic sarcoma, malignant myoblastoma, PNET, carcinoid and GIST are on record.

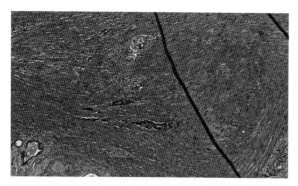

Fig 15.22 Mesonephric remnant in seminal vesicle wall.

- Rare primary germ cell (choriocarcinoma, seminoma) tumors have been reported in the SVs.
- A case of primary squamous cell carcinoma arising in a patient with seminal cyst and few lymphoma cases are on record.
- Recently, a unique case of an intraepithelial abnormality in pre-existing ducts and acini in the left SV of a 73-year-old patient with prostatic adenocarcinoma has been reported. The case shows morphological and immunohistochemical features similar to those of basal cell hyperplasia of the prostate.
- The epithelial lining was thicker than the surrounding normal ducts with obliteration of the acinar lumen, and there was some degree of cell stratification.
- PSA, PSAP, PSMA, Prostein (P501S) and AMACR, as well as GATA3, were negative. CK5/6, p63, 34betaE12 and p53 were positive in cells in a basal and suprabasal position, whereas CA-125 was expressed in the luminal cells. The clinical significance of this lesion is not known.
- Mesonephric remnants may also be seen in the SVs. Fig 15.22

15.2.15 Benign and Malignant Mixed Epithelial-Stromal Tumors

- There have been about 35 acceptable cases reported on this category.
- The criteria for the diagnosis of mixed epithelial-stromal tumors are:
  i They arise from the seminal vesicle.
  ii There is no normal seminal vesicle within the tumor.
  iii They do not invade the prostate (with rare exceptions).
  iv They have a less conspicuous and less cellular stromal component than cystadenoma.
  v They are not immunoreactive for prostatic markers.

15.2.15.1 Fibroadenoma and Adenomyoma

- These tumors have been reported in men aged 39–66 years, and presented with pain and voiding symptoms. These lesions are grossly solid and cystic, ranging from 3.5 to 16 cm.
- The distinction from epithelial-stromal tumor of low grade (below) is based on stromal characteristic (bland cytology) and inconspicuous to absent mitotic activity.
- Some cases referred to as low grade phyllodes tumor or benign mesenchymoma.

15.2.15.2 Malignant Epithelial-Stromal Tumors

- Seminal vesicles are male sex accessory glands derived from the mesonephric ducts. The SVs are located posterolaterally, at the base of the bladder. These accessory glands show four major components, the lumen, mucosa, smooth muscle wall and surrounding adipose tissue. The most common malignant neoplasm of the seminal vesicle is adenocarcinoma, followed by primary sarcomas and rare neoplasms with epithelial and stromal components.
- The cysts and the glands are mostly round-to-oval, but may also be irregular or slit-like. The epithelial lining of the cysts may exhibit polypoid or papillary luminal infoldings. Epithelial cells lining the cysts vary from cuboidal to columnar and flat, and may show focal hobnailing or tufting. The basal cell layer is typically preserved, but may be inconspicuous on microscopy. The stromal component between the glands shows variable cellularity, with pleomorphism and nuclear atypia, which range from benign to malignant in their histologic appearance and behavior, but most of the reported cases in the benign (or low grade) category demonstrated absent or very low mitotic activity. Fibrous or muscular differentiation and condensation around the cysts has also been reported.
- These neoplasms have been described in the literature under various names, including "epithelial-stromal tumor," "cystic epithelial-stromal tumor," "cystadenoma," "cystomyoma,"

"mesenchymoma," "Mullerian adenosarcoma-like tumor," "phyllodes tumor" and "cystosarcoma phyllodes." "Cystadenoma" is the most commonly used term, but has often been used to describe tumors with a distinct stromal component. In these cases, the term "cystadenoma" failed to account for the tumoral stromal component.

- We propose that term seminal vesicle "mixed epithelial-stromal tumor" be used to designate the tumors of the seminal vesicle containing epithelial and stromal components, with a distinction of grade based on the histologic features and the biological behavior. Histologic features to be evaluated for grade separation include stromal atypia, mitotic activity, nuclear pleomorphism and tumor necrosis.

- The histologic spectrum of benign-to-malignant MEST is primarily determined by the degree of atypia of the stromal component. Some authors have recently proposed reclassifying the previously described "cystadenomas" to MEST, based on the reported descriptions of the "non-neoplastic" versus neoplastic stroma, although they have acknowledged that the majority of reports had not provided sufficient detail to differentiate reliably between the two. The term "cystadenoma" should therefore be restricted only to those rare benign tumors that demonstrate hypocellular (normal or almost normal) seminal vesicle stroma and can be considered part of the spectrum of the low grade MEST, rather than a separate category.

- Designations "low grade MEST," "intermediate grade MEST (uncertain malignant potential)," and "high grade MEST" of seminal vesicles can be applied to these tumors to better characterize and study them in the future.

- Low grade MEST. Absence of stromal atypia and any mitotic activity; nuclear pleomorphism absent or focal and mild (at most); tumor necrosis absent.

- Intermediate grade MEST-UMP. Increased stromal cellularity with low mitotic activity; nuclear atypia and pleomorphism present; tumor necrosis absent.

- High grade MEST. Increased stromal cellularity and significant mitotic activity; marked nuclear atypia and pleomorphism; usually extensive tumor necrosis.

- Important considerations in the differential diagnosis include the stromal tumor of uncertain malignant potential of the prostate (STUMP) and its malignant variant, the prostatic stromal sarcoma (PSS). In contrast to the tumors arising in the prostate, the seminal vesicle MEST are centered on and recapitulate the morphology and the immunoprofile of the seminal vesicle. Unlike STUMP and PSS, MEST of the seminal vesicle are negative for PSA and PSAP and the epithelium of the cysts are reactive for cytokeratin 7 (as demonstrated in our index cases). The stromal expression of vimentin, actin, desmin and CD34 cannot reliably differentiate between STUMP/PSS and MEST. Both index tumors, presented herein, showed strong stromal reactivity for estrogen and progesterone receptors, which has not always been the case with the STUMP/PSS. Both STUMP and PSS are also rare tumors, and similar to MEST, defining a tumor as high grade PSS is dependent on the morphologic features of the stroma. PSS are distinguished from the lower grade STUMP based on a higher degree of cellularity, stromal overgrowth, mitoses, and necrosis.

- Documented surgical approaches used to treat MEST have varied and included isolated complete tumor resection (if technically feasible), vesiculectomy, vesiculoprostatectomy and cystoprostatectomy. Postsurgical clinical outcome is paramount to ultimately classify the neoplasm, but unfortunately, of all reported MEST cases of the seminal vesicle, only nine had follow-up of three years (five of which were in the low grade category). As the collected data so far is incomplete to confidently define the malignant potential of these tumors, surgical resection still remains an appropriate course of action, even for low grade tumors.

Suggested Reading

López JI, Angulo JC. The Ejaculatory Ducts and Their Implications in Prostate Adenocarcinoma. Anal Quant Cytopathol Histpathol. 2013 Aug; **35**(4): 205–09.

Montironi R, Lopez-Beltran A, Cheng L, Galosi AB, Montorsi F, Scarpelli M. Seminal Vesicle Intraepithelial Neoplasia versus Basal Cell Hyperplasia in a Seminal Vesicle. Eur Urol. 2014 Mar 4; **pii**: S0302–2838 (14) 00183–83.

Santos LD, Wong CS, Killingsworth M. Cystadenoma of the Seminal Vesicle: Report of a Case with Ultrastructural Findings. Pathology. 2001; **33**: 399–402.

Ormsby AH, Haskell R, Ruthven SE, Mylne GE. Bilateral Primary Seminal Vesicle Carcinoma. Pathology. 1996; **28**: 196–200.

Ormsby AH, Haskell R, Jones D, Goldblum JR. Primary Seminal Vesicle Carcinoma: An Immunohistochemical Analysis of Four Cases. Mod Pathol. 2000; **13**: 46–51.

Fain JS, Cosnow I, King BF, Zincke H, Bostwick DG. Cystosarcoma Phyllodes of the Seminal Vesicle. Cancer. 1993; **71**: 2055–61.

Laurila P, Leivo I, Makisalo H, Ruutu M, Miettinen M. Mullerian Adenosarcoma-like Tumor of the Seminal Vesicle. A Case Report with Immunohistochemical and Ultrastructural Observations. Arch Pathol Lab Med. 1992; **116**: 1072–76.

Maheshkumar P, Harper C, Sunderland GT, Conn IG. Cystic Epithelial Stromal Tumour of the Seminal Vesicle. BJU Int. 2000; **85**: 1154.

Mazur MT, Myers JL, Maddox WA. Cystic Epithelial-Stromal Tumor of the Seminal Vesicle. Am J Surg Pathol. 1987; **11**: 210–17.

Lamont JS, Hesketh PJ, de las MA, Babayan RK. Primary Angiosarcoma of the Seminal Vesicle. J Urol. 1991; **146**: 165–67.

Arya M, Hayne D, Brown RS, O'Donnell PJ, Mundy AR. Hemangiopericytoma of the Seminal Vesicle Presenting with Hypoglycemia. J Urol. 2001; **166**: 992.

Gentile AT, Moseley HS, Quinn SF, Franzini D, Pitre TM. Leiomyoma of the Seminal Vesicle. J Urol. 1994; **151**: 1027–29.

Muentener M, Hailemariam S, Dubs M, Hauri D, Sulser T. Primary Leiomyosarcoma of the Seminal Vesicle. J Urol. 2000; **164**: 2027.

Juhasz J, Kiss P. A Hitherto Undescribed Case of 'Collision' Tumour: Liposarcoma of the Seminal Vesicle and Prostatic Carcinoma. Int Urol Nephrol. 1978; **10**: 185–93.

Westra WH, Grenko RT, Epstein J. Solitary Fibrous Tumor of the Lower Urogenital Tract: A Report of Five Cases Involving the Seminal Vesicles, Urinary Bladder, and Prostate. Hum Pathol. 2000; **31**: 63–68.

Quick Charles M. MDa, Neriman Gokden MDa, Sangoi Ankur R. MDb, Brooks James D. MDc, McKenney Jesse K. MDa. The Distribution of PAX-2 Immunoreactivity in the Prostate Gland, Seminal Vesicle, and Ejaculatory Duct: Comparison with Prostatic Adenocarcinoma and Discussion of Prostatic Zonal Embryogenesis. Human Pathology. 2010; **41**: 1145–49.

Harvey Aaron M. MD, Grice Beverly HTL, Hamilton Candice HTL, Truong Luan D. MD, Ro Jae Y. MD, Ayala Alberto G. MD, Zhai Qihui "Jim" MD. Diagnostic Utility of P504S/p63 Cocktail Prostate-specific Antigen, and Prostatic Acid Phosphatase in Verifying Prostatic Carcinoma Involvement in Seminal Vesicles: A Study of 57 Cases of Radical Prostatectomy Specimens of Pathologic Stage pT3b. Arch Pathol Lab Med. 2010; **134**: 983–88.

Chapter 16

Pathology of the Prostatic Urethra

16.1 The Prostatic Urethra: Basic Anatomy and Histology

- In males, the epithelium is derived from the urogenital sinus except in the fossa navicularis, where it is derived from ectodermal cells migrating from the glans penis. The connective tissue and smooth muscle surrounding the male urethra is derived from splanchnic mesenchyme. The epithelium of the urethra is derived from the urogenital sinus. Figs 16.1–16.3
- The urothelium has a characteristic immunophenotype. It expresses cytokeratins of both low and high molecular weights, including keratins 7, 8, 13 and 19.

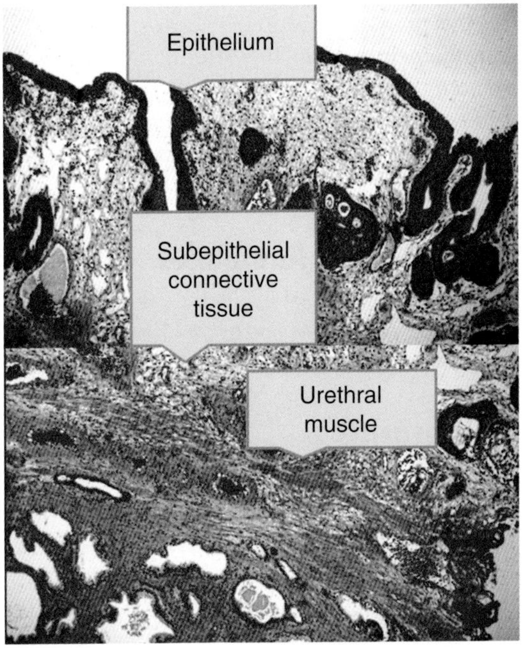

- Cytokeratin 18 and 20 are present in the superficial (umbrella cells) cells. This pattern of expression differs from that of normal stratified squamous epithelium that show predominantly high molecular weight keratin immunoreactivity, and from colorectum, endometrium, endocervix and prostate, which demonstrate a preponderance of low molecular weight keratin.
- High molecular weight keratin immunoreactivity is restricted to the basal cell layer of the urothelium.
- The verumontanum bulges from the posterior wall at the bend of the urethra and distally forms the *crista urethralis*. Just proximal to the verumontanum is the prostatic utricle. The utriculus is generally regarded as an embryonal relic when seen in the adult.
- The utricle forms as an ingrowth of specialized cells from the dorsal wall of the urogenital sinus as the entire caudal ends of the Müllerian ducts undergo complete regression. Histologically, utricle cysts are lined by epithelium indistinguishable from adult prostate in younger

Epithelium

Subepithelial connective tissue

Urethral muscle

Fig 16.1 Prostatic urethra including epithelium, subepithelial connective tissue and urethral muscle that mark the limit between urethra and prostate.

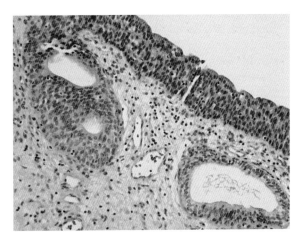

Fig 16.2 Close up view of the urothelium covering prostatic urethra.

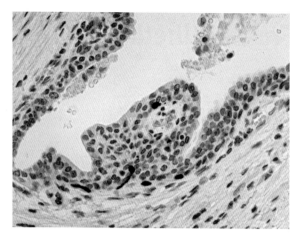

Fig 16.3 Neuroendocrine cells may be seen within the urothelium (anti-chromogranin immunohistochemistry).

patients. The covering is usually squamous epithelium.

- The prostatic urethra is formed at the bladder neck and exits the prostate at the apex; anteriorly, it turns 35 degrees to form the urethral angle.
- Most prostatic ducts, as well as the ejaculatory ducts, empty into the urethra in the area of the verumontanum.
- Orifices of the prostatic ducts are located in the area of the verumontanum, separately from the utricle and ejaculatory ducts. The ducts are lined by a bilayer prostatic epithelium histologically identical to that seen in the ducts and acini away from the urethra.
- Intraductal and invasive neoplasms originating from the periurethral ducts can grow within the urethral lumen or infiltrate the prostatic utricle. In particular, intraductal carcinoma of the prostate and prostatic ductal adenocarcinomas can be seen in the periurethral prostatic ducts. The former is similar morphologically to the counterpart duct carcinoma in situ in the female breast and the latter shows similarities with the endometrioid carcinoma of the female genital tract.
- Pre-prostatic, prostatic, and membranous urethra regions are covered by urothelium similar to what is seen in the bladder with stratified layers of urothelium and a superficial (umbrella) cell layer. Focal secretory urethral cells may be admixed with urethral lining.
- The lamina propria consists of loose connective tissue and small thin-walled blood vessels. A rim

of smooth muscle fibers (urethral muscle) marks the limit with prostatic tissue.

- The male urethra is 15 to 20 cm long and is divided in three anatomical segments. The prostatic urethra begins at the internal urethral orifice at the bladder neck and extends through the prostate to the prostatic apex. In the central part of the urethral crest is an eminence called the verumontanum.
- The verumontanum contains a slit-like opening that leads to an epithelium-lined sac called the prostatic utricle, a Mullerian vestige.
  The ejaculatory ducts empty into the urethra on either side of the prostatic utricle.
  The membranous urethra extends from the prostatic apex to the bulb of the penis.
- Cowper's glands are located on the left and right sides of the membranous urethra and their ducts empty into it. Bulbourethral glands are located in the proximal (bulbous) portion of the penile urethra. In addition, scattered mucus-secreting periurethral glands (Littré glands) are present at the periphery of the penile urethra except anteriorly. The female urethra is approximately 4 cm long, and, at its periphery, contains paraurethral Skene's glands.
- The type of epithelium lining the urethra varies along its length. In general, urothelium line the prostatic urethra, pseudostratified columnar epithelium line the membranous segment and most of the penile urethra, and nonkeratinized stratified squamous epithelium line the fossa navicularis and external urethral orifice.

16.2 Congenital Anomalies

- The most common lesions include duplication, diverticula, congenital urethral polyps (usually in the prostatic urethra) and urethral valves.

16.3 Urethritis

- Urethritis is a descriptive and often nonspecific term that refers to a variety of benign, acute or chronic inflammatory lesions that can be seen along the urinary tract, though they are more common in the bladder, and may occasionally be polypoid. Histologically, they are similar to those seen in the urinary bladder.

16.4 Urethral Polyp

- Urethral inflammatory polyps show inflamed and vascular stroma lined by normal or hyperplastic urothelium with inflammatory cells extending to the urothelium. Similar to other locations in the urinary tract, fibroepithelial polyps may also occur in the urethra. Table 16.1; Figs 16.4–16.7

16.5 Urethral Diverticulum

- Histologically, is lined by urothelium, but squamous and glandular metaplasia can be seen. Nephrogenic adenoma or carcinoma may develop in diverticula.

16.6 Ectopic Prostatic Tissue

- Occurs in adolescents or young adults and presents with hematuria or irritative symptoms that may shed atypical cells into the urine. It is often located in the posterior portion of the prostatic urethra. These lesions may be better classified as benign prostatic-type polyps composed of benign prostatic glands with overlying, frequently intact urothelium. Glands are PSA+, high molecular weight cytokeratin+, and p63+. Fig 16.8

16.7 Epithelial Tumors of the Urethra

- This includes epithelial neoplasms of the prostatic urethra and tumors arising in the accessory glands (Cowper and Littré glands in

Table 16.1 Inflammatory Conditions of the Prostatic Urethra

Non-specific Acute and Chronic Urethritis
Specific Urethritis
  Follicular
  Interstitial
  Eosinophilic
  Encrusted
  Emphysematous
  Gangrenous
  Hemorrhagic
  Viral
  Urethritis with atypical giant cells
  Denuding (CIS)
Granulomatous Lesions
  Postsurgical
  Suture granuloma
  BCG-Induced
  Schistosomiasis
  Malacoplakia
  Tuberculosis
  Xanthoma
  Other
Other Infection Cystitides
  Fungal
  Actinomycosis
  Other

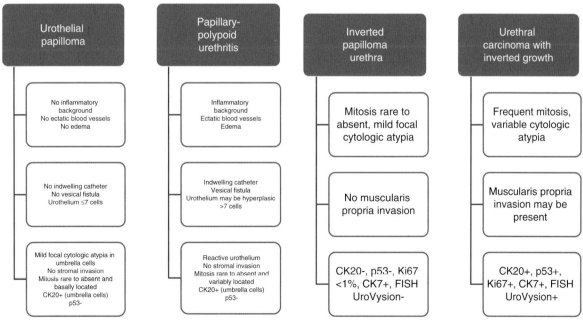

Fig 16.4 Differential diagnosis between urothelial papilloma and papillary-polypoid urethritis.

Fig 16.5 Differential diagnosis between inverted papilloma and urothelial carcinoma with inverted growth.

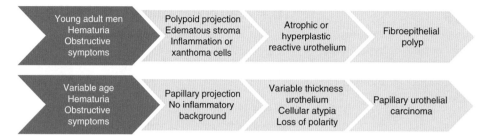

Fig 16.6 Differential diagnosis between fibroepithelial polyp and papillary urothelial carcinoma.

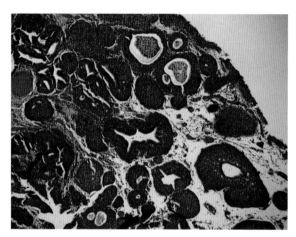

Fig 16.7 Urethritis glandularis should not be mistaken as carcinoma.

the male, as well as Skene glands in the female). Table 16.2

16.7.1 Benign Epithelial Tumors of the Urethra

- Benign epithelial tumors are rare. A variety of lesions have been reported, including squamous papilloma, villous adenoma, condyloma acuminatum, nephrogenic adenoma, inverted papilloma and urothelial papilloma.
  The histological features are identical to tumors described in the urinary bladder.

16.7.2 Carcinoma of the Urethra

- These are uncommon but aggressive tumors most frequently involving the distal urethra and meatus, with an overall poor prognosis. Tumor stage and location are important predictive factors. High tumor stage and the presence of lymph node metastasis are adverse prognostic parameters.

These tumors may occur within urethral diverticula.

- Proximal tumors have better overall survival than distal tumors, and five-year survival is 50% for proximal tumors vs. 20% for distal tumors in males.
- Most tumors present as frequent ulcerated exophytic nodular, infiltrative, papillary or ill-defined lesion masses.
- Urothelial tumors involving the proximal urethra exhibit macroscopic diversity with cases showing papillary growth, erythematous or white plaque-like areas (carcinoma in situ) and nodular/infiltrative growth in invasive carcinoma. Fig 16.9
- Adenocarcinomas are often large, infiltrative or expansile neoplasms which may have an exophytic surface, and appear mucinous, gelatinous or cystic.
- Other tumors may occur in the penile urethra, bulbomembranous urethra or the prostatic urethra, which often determines the gross and histological appearance.
- Microscopically, most tumors of the proximal urethra are urothelial carcinomas or adenocarcinomas with rare examples of squamous cell carcinoma.

16.7.2.1 Urothelial Carcinoma

- Tumors are classified as outlined in the urinary bladder and include noninvasive, papillary urothelial carcinomas, carcinoma in situ or invasive urothelial carcinoma, and may be synchronous or metachronous to bladder neoplasia. Fig 16.10
- Deeply invasive urothelial carcinomas are high grade, with or without papillary components, and characterized by irregular nests, sheets and cords

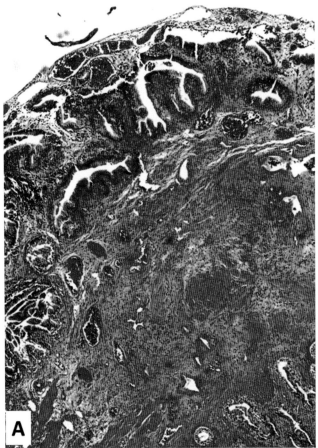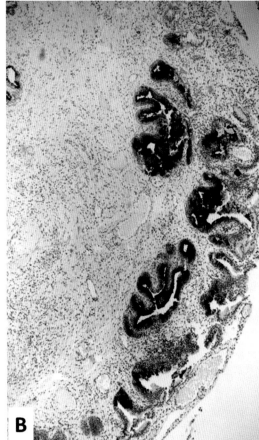

Fig 16.8 Ectopic prostate tissue (A) with PSA expression (B).

of cells accompanied by desmoplasia and/or inflammatory response.

- Tumors may exhibit squamous or glandular differentiation or unusual morphologic variations (nested microcystic, micropapillary, glycogenic-type clear cell, plasmacytoid). Coexisting small cell or sarcomatoid carcinoma components are rarely seen.

- Tumors should be graded using the low vs. high grade scheme as outlined in 2004/2016 WHO grading system. Carcinoma in situ may involve periurethral glands, focally or extensively, and should not be mistaken as invasion.

  The association of urothelial carcinoma with HPV, in both the urethra and the urinary bladder, remains controversial.

- Urothelial carcinoma may involve the prostatic urethra, exhibiting the same grade and histological spectrum of histologic subtypes seen in the bladder. Features unique to prostatic urethral urothelial cancers are the frequent proclivity of high grade tumors to extend into the prostatic ducts and acini in a pagetoid fashion.

- In females, differentiation from Paget disease of the vulva extending through the urethra is mandatory, as is the exclusion of melanoma extending to the urethra (HMB45+, Melan A+). Urothelial carcinomas are often CK7+/CK20+; Paget disease of the vulva is typically CK7+/CK20−. Fig 16.11

- Direct extension of prostatic adenocarcinoma into the urethra must be considered in male patients. These tumors are often categorized as prostatic ductal adenocarcinoma and are PSA, PSMA and PAP positive, and p63 negative. Figs 16.12–16.14

- Occasionally, prostate adenocarcinoma extending to the urethra shows a streaking papillary pattern, a finding that should not be misdiagnosed as primary urothelial carcinoma.

183

Table 16.2 Histological Classification of the Tumors of the Urethra

Epithelial Tumors
Benign
    Villous adenoma
    Squamous papilloma
    Urothelial papilloma, including inverted papilloma
Malignant
Primary
    Squamous cell carcinoma
    Urothelial carcinoma
    Adenocarcinoma

        Clear cell carcinoma
        Non-clear cell carcinoma

            Enteric
            Colloid (mucinous) carcinoma
            Signet-ring cell carcinoma
            Adenocarcinoma, not otherwise specified (NOS)

    Adenosquamous carcinoma
    Neuroendocrine carcinoma
    Undifferentiated carcinoma
Secondary
Non-epithelial Tumors
Benign
    Leiomyoma
    Hemangioma
    Glomangiomyoma
Malignant
    Malignant melanoma
    Non-Hodgkin lymphoma
    Plasmocytoma
Tumor-like Lesions
    Fibroepithelial polyp
    Prostatic polyp
    Caruncle
    Condyloma accuminatum
    Nephrogenic adenoma (metaplasia)
Tumors of Accessory Glands
Malignant
    Carcinoma of Skene, Littré and Cowper glands

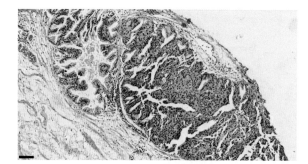

Fig 16.9 Urothelial CIS of the prostatic urethra.

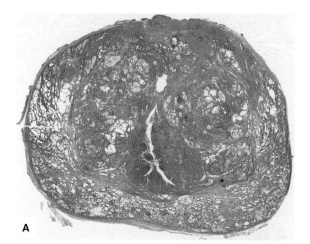

A

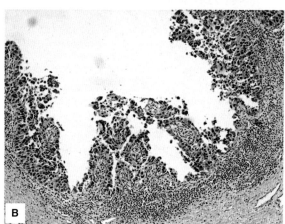

B

Fig 16.10 Macro-section of urothelial carcinoma of the prostatic urethra (A). Microscopic feature of urothelial carcinoma of the urethra (B).

- A number of tumor-like conditions enter the differential diagnosis, including nephrogenic adenoma (metaplasia), fibroepithelial and prostatic polyps and condyloma acuminatum. Low-risk HPV infection plays a crucial role in the etiology of condyloma acuminatum of the urethra. Figs 16.15–16.16

16.7.2.2 Squamous Cell Carcinoma

- About 75% of carcinomas of the male urethra and 70% of carcinomas in women are squamous cell carcinoma, and are associated with a very poor outcome. Squamous cell carcinoma of the urethra is associated with HPV infection in both sexes.

- High-risk human papillomavirus (HPV) 16 or 18 may be detected in up to 60% of cases in women, and about 30% of squamous cell carcinomas tested positive for HPV16 in men. Some HPV16 positive

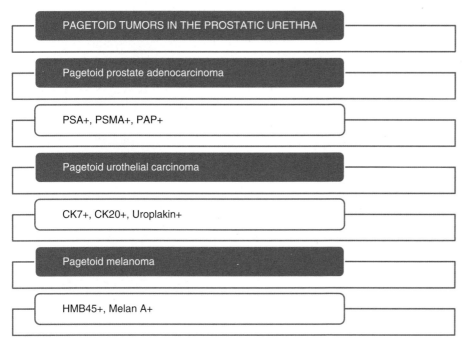

```
PAGETOID TUMORS IN THE PROSTATIC URETHRA

Pagetoid prostate adenocarcinoma

    PSA+, PSMA+, PAP+

Pagetoid urothelial carcinoma

    CK7+, CK20+, Uroplakin+

Pagetoid melanoma

    HMB45+, Melan A+
```

Fig 16.11 Differential diagnosis of pagetoid tumors of the prostatic urethra.

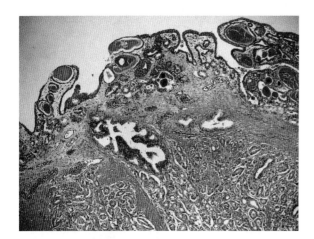

Fig 16.12 Prostate adenocarcinoma infiltrating the verumontanum, but not the urethra.

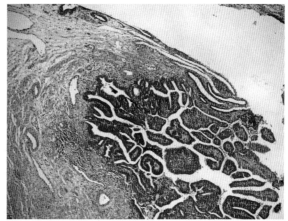

Fig 16.13 Papillary cystadenocarcinoma of the periurethral duct.

tumors might have a more favorable prognosis. Tumors in the bulbar urethra are usually negative for HPV.

- Squamous cell carcinomas of the urethra span the range from well differentiated (including the rare verrucous carcinoma) to moderately differentiated (most common) to poorly differentiated. Squamous cell carcinomas are similar in histology to those of other sites and may be of keratinizing and non-keratinizing type, with rare cases showing basaloid or clear cell features.

- Squamous cell carcinomas are graded based on the degree of differentiation as well, moderately or poorly differentiated. Fig 16.17

16.7.2.3 Adenocarcinoma of the Prostatic Urethra

- Adenocarcinoma of the female and male urethra may be seen in two forms: clear cell adenocarcinoma (approximately 40%) and non-clear cell adenocarcinoma (approximately 60%), the latter frequently exhibiting similar patterns to those of the bladder (enteric, mucinous, signet-ring cell or adenocarcinoma not otherwise specified). Rare cases may resemble prostate adenocarcinoma on histology, but they are CEA+/PSA-. Fig 16.18

- Clear cell adenocarcinomas are rare in men. Clear cell adenocarcinoma is usually characterized by histologic heterogeneity within the neoplasm, including solid, tubular, tubule-cystic or papillary histologic patterns. Figs 16.19–16.20

- The cytologic features vary from low grade (resembling nephrogenic adenoma focally) to high grade (more frequently). Hobnail cells are frequent findings in clear cell adenocarcinoma. Necrosis, mitotic activity and extensive infiltrative growth are commonly observed. Clear cell adenocarcinoma express CK 7, CK 20, PAX-2 and PAX-8, although some cases may be negative.

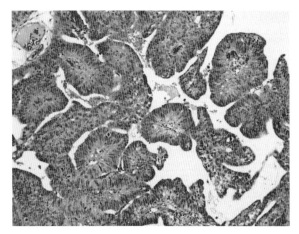

Fig 16.14 Rarely, this papillary configuration of prostate carcinoma may be mistaken as papillary urothelial carcinoma of the urethra.

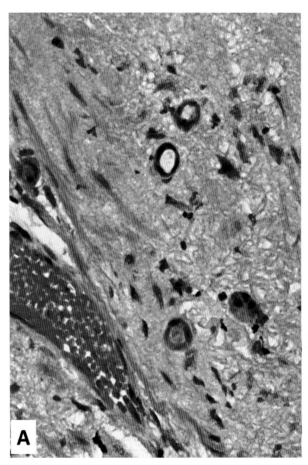

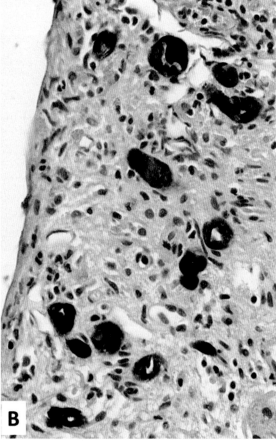

A

B

Fig 16.15 Nephrogenic adenoma (A) positive with cytokeratin (B).

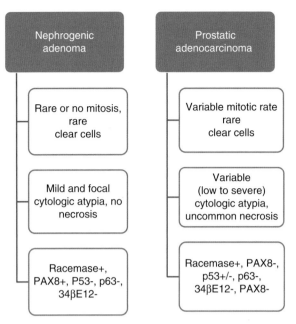

Fig 16.16 Differential diagnosis between nephrogenic adenoma and prostate carcinoma.

Nephrogenic adenoma
- Rare or no mitosis, rare clear cells
- Mild and focal cytologic atypia, no necrosis
- Racemase+, PAX8+, P53-, p63-, 34βE12-

Prostatic adenocarcinoma
- Variable mitotic rate rare clear cells
- Variable (low to severe) cytologic atypia, uncommon necrosis
- Racemase+, PAX8-, p53+/-, p63-, 34βE12-, PAX8-

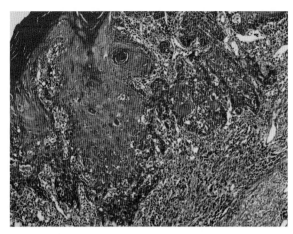

Fig 16.17 Primary squamous cell carcinoma of the urethra.

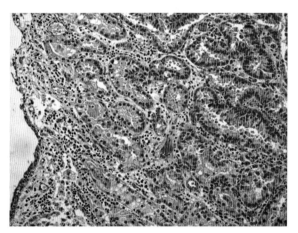

Fig 16.19 Clear cell adenocarcinoma of the urethra.

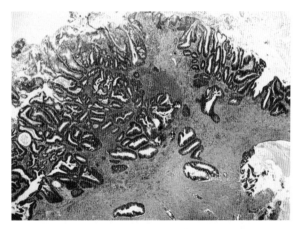

Fig 16.18 Primary adenocarcinoma of the urethra.

- Adenocarcinomas are graded based on the degree of differentiation (well differentiated, moderately differentiated and poorly differentiated)
- As primary adenocarcinoma is rare, the possibility of urothelial carcinoma with glandular differentiation, extension from a bladder primary or metastases (colon mainly) should be ruled out. The immunoprofile CK7+/CK20+/CDX2-, β-catenin-, may be helpful since it supports the diagnosis of primary adenocarcinoma.

- Even rarer are cases of in situ and infiltrating mucinous adenocarcinoma arising from the prostatic urethra with invasion into the prostate. The histological growth patterns found in these tumors were identical to mucinous adenocarcinoma of the bladder consisting of lakes of mucin lined by tall columnar epithelium with goblet cells showing varying degrees of nuclear atypia and, in some of these cases, mucin-containing signet cells. These tumors have been negative immunohistochemically for PSA, PAP and other markers of prostatic origin. TNM classification seems to be relevant to prognosis. Table 16.3

187

Table 16.3 TNM Classification of Tumors of the Urethra

T – Primary Tumor

TX Primary tumor cannot be assessed

T0 No evidence of primary tumor

Urethra (male and female)

Ta Noninvasive papillary, polypoid or verrucous carcinoma

Tis Carcinoma in situ

T1 Tumor invades subepithelial connective tissue

T2 Tumor invades any of the following: corpus spongiosum, prostate, periurethral muscle

T3 Tumor invades any of the following: corpus cavernosum, beyond prostatic capsule, anterior vagina, bladder neck

T4 Tumor invades other adjacent organs

Urothelial (transitional cell) carcinoma of prostate (prostatic urethra)

Tis pu Carcinoma in situ, involvement of prostatic urethra

Tis pd Carcinoma in situ, involvement of prostatic ducts

T1 Tumor invades subepithelial connective tissue

T2 Tumor invades any of the following: prostatic stroma, corpus spongiosum, periurethral muscle

T3 Tumor invades any of the following: corpus cavernosum, beyond prostatic capsule, bladder neck (extra-prostatic extension)

T4 Tumor invades other adjacent organs (invasion of bladder)

N – Regional Lymph Nodes

NX Regional lymph nodes cannot be assessed

N0 No regional lymph node metastasis

N1 Metastasis in a single lymph node 2 cm or less in greatest dimension

N2 Metastasis in a single lymph node more than 2 cm in greatest dimension, or multiple lymph nodes

M – Distant Metastasis

MX Distant metastasis cannot be assessed

M0 No distant metastasis

M1 Distant metastasis

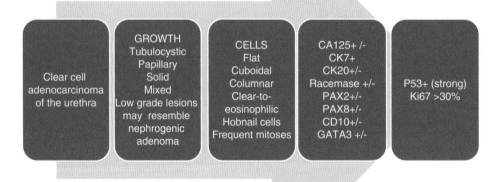

| Clear cell adenocarcinoma of the urethra | GROWTH Tubulocystic Papillary Solid Mixed Low grade lesions may resemble nephrogenic adenoma | CELLS Flat Cuboidal Columnar Clear-to-eosinophilic Hobnail cells Frequent mitoses | CA125+ /- CK7+ CK20+/- Racemase +/- PAX2+/- PAX8+/- CD10+/- GATA3 +/- | P53+ (strong) Ki67 >30% |

Fig 16.20 Differential diagnosis of clear cell adenocarcinoma of the urethra.

16.7.2.4 Adenocarcinoma of Accessory Glands (Synonyms: Urethral, Periurethral or Paraurethral Accessory Glands)

- Exceedingly rare adenocarcinomas arising from Cowper and Littré glands in the male and Skene glands in the female, presenting with hematuria, dysuria and urinary obstruction. The typical case is a large exophytic or nodular ulcerated tumor with infiltrative or expansile margins that appear gelatinous or cystic.
- In males, adenocarcinoma arising from Littré glands is seen centered in the penile urethra, while Cowper (bulbourethral) gland adenocarcinoma occurs in the bulbomembranous (proximal) urethra. These tumors share histologic features with adenocarcinoma arising from urethral mucosa. Growth patterns include papillary/micropapillary, acinar, tubular or admixture thereof. Tumor cells are cuboidal or columnar with eosinophilic or clear cytoplasm and large hyperchromatic nuclei. Intracytoplasmic mucin or frank mucinous component is rare.
- In females, Skene gland adenocarcinoma is more common distally, and shows papillary/micropapillary or glandular architecture with tumor cells either columnar or cuboidal with eosinophilic or clear cytoplasm frequently showing intraluminal mucin. The nuclei are large and hyperchromatic with prominent nucleoli. Some cases may have a similar histology to that seen in prostatic adenocarcinoma, including PSA expression. A reported case was positive for CK7, CK20 and PAX-8 and negative for CDX-2, GATA3 and S100P. Adenoid cystic carcinoma showing perineural invasion has been reported to occur from Skene gland. A Bartholin gland origin should be excluded before definitive diagnosis. A rare case of adenomyomatous hyperplasia of the Skene gland has been reported.
- The diagnosis of accessory glands adenocarcinoma is difficult because the tumor has usually destroyed the anatomic landmarks at time of diagnosis. Partial involvement of recognizable periurethral gland remains as the best indicator of origin.
- Pathologic stage at time of presentation is the best predictor. PSA is a reliable marker for therapeutic response in Skene gland adenocarcinoma.

16.8 Soft Tissue Tumors

- There are rare examples of soft tissue tumors arising in the urethra. Benign tumors include leiomyoma, which shows a similar morphology and immunoprofile to other organs. In female patients, leiomyoma may show expression of estrogen receptors. Leiomyoma may occur as a part of diffuse leiomyomatosis syndrome (esophageal and rectal leiomyoma).
- Paraurethral cystic lesions may also be rarely seen in practice.
- Hemangioma and neurofibroma, paraganglioma, granular cell tumors, papillary endothelial hyperplasia (Masson tumor), rhabdomyosarcoma and Kaposi's sarcoma are on record.

16.9 Other Rare Tumors and Tumor-like Conditions

- Teflon-related foreign body reactions may produce tumor-like lesions. Fig 16.21
- Melanoma may primarily occur in the urethra, is more common in females, polypoid and often diagnosed in distal urethra. The histologic spectrum, including nested, fascicular or diffuse as seen in other locations, and tumor cells may be pleomorphic or epithelioid with rhabdoid phenotype, and may be amelanotic.
- Extramammary Paget disease extending from the vulva (CEA+, EMA+, CK7+, CK20–) and poorly differentiated urothelial carcinoma (CK7+, CK20+, uroplakin+) enters differential diagnosis.

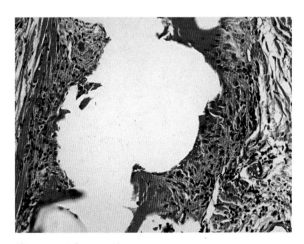

Fig 16.21 Teflon granuloma.

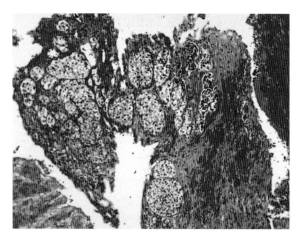

Fig 16.22 Von Brunn hyperplasia following therapy.

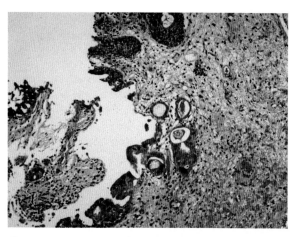

Fig 16.23 Reactive atypia after radiotherapy for prostate cancer.

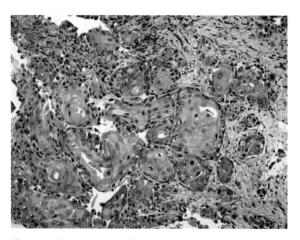

Fig 16.24 Reactive atypia after brachytherapy for prostate cancer.

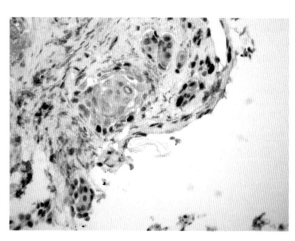

Fig 16.25 Weak p53 staining supports diagnosis of reactive atypia.

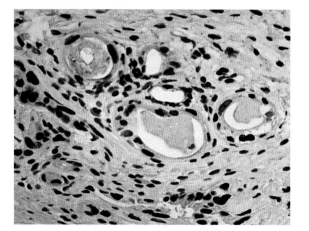

Fig 16.26 The presence of basal cells highlighted by p63 immunohistochemistry also supports the reactive nature of the lesion.

- Primary non-Hodgkin lymphoma and plasmacytoma has also been described to occur in the urethra.
- Secondary tumor deposits from neighboring organs are always an important consideration when dealing with urethral tumors.

Suggested Reading

Badhiwala N, Chan R, Zhou HJ, Shen S, Coburn M. Sarcomatoid Carcinoma of Male Urethra with Bone and Lung Metastases Presenting as Urethral Stricture. Case Rep Urol. 2013; **2013**: 931893.

Grivas PD, Davenport M, Montie JE, Kunju LP, Feng F, Weizer AZ. Urethral Cancer. Hematol Oncol Clin North Am. 2012; **26**: 1291–314.

Kanagarajah P, Ayyathurai R, Saleem U, Manoharan M. Small Cell Carcinoma Arising from the Bulbar Urethra:

A Case Report and Literature Review. Urol Int. 2012; **88**: 477–79.

Rabbani F. Prognostic Factors in Male Urethral Cancer. Cancer. 2011; **117**: 2426–34.

Reis LO, Ferreira F, Almeida M, Ferreira U. Urethral Carcinoma: Critical View on Contemporary Consecutive Series. Med Oncol. 2011; **28**: 1405–10.

Rudloff U, Amukele SA, Moldwin R, Qiao X, Morgenstern N. Small Cell Carcinoma Arising from the Proximal Urethra. Int J Urol. 2004; **11**: 674–77.

Swartz MA, Porter MP, Lin DW, Weiss NS. Incidence of Primary Urethral Carcinoma in the United States. Urology. 2006; **68**: 1164–68.

Thyavihally YB, Tongaonkar HB, Srivastava SK, Mahantshetty U, Kumar P, Raibhattanavar SG. Clinical Outcome of 36 Male Patients with Primary Urethral Carcinoma: A Single Center Experience. Int J Urol. 2006; **13**: 716–20.

Visser O, Adolfsson J, Rossi S, Verne J, Gatta G, Maffezzini M, Franks KN. Group Rw. Incidence and Survival of Rare Urogenital Cancers in Europe. Eur J Cancer. 2012; **48**: 456–64.

Yoo KH, Kim GY, Kim TG, Min GE, Lee HL. Primary Small Cell Neuroendocrine Carcinoma of the Female Urethra. Pathol Int. 2009; **59**: 601–03.

Adley BP, Maxwell K, Dalton DP, et al. Urothelial-type Adenocarcinoma of the Prostate Mimicking Metastatic Colorectal Adenocarcinoma. Int Braz J Urol. 2006; **32**: 681–88.

Amin MB, Young RH. Primary Carcinomas of the Urethra. Seminars in Diagnostic Pathology. 1997; **14**: 147–60.

Curtis MW, Evans AJ, Srigley JR. Mucin-producing Urothelial-type Adenocarcinoma of Prostate: Report of Two Cases of a Rare and Diagnostically Challenging Entity. Mod Pathol. 2005; **18**: 585–90.

Dimitroulis D, Patsouras D, Katsargyris A, et al. Primary Enteric-type Mucinous Adenocarcinoma of the Urethra in a Patient with Ulcerative Colitis. Int Surg. 2014; **99**: 669–72.

Dodson MK, Cliby WA, Keeney GL, et al. Case Report: Skene's Glands Adenocarcinoma with Increased Serum Level of Prostate-specific Antigen. Gynecol Oncol. 1994; **55**: 304–07.

Yvgenia R, Meir DB, Sibi J, et al. Mucinous Adenocarcinoma of the Posterior Urethra. Report of a Case. Pathol Res & Pract. 2005; **201**: 137–40.

Lightbourn GA, Abrams M, Seymour L. Primary Mucoid Adenocarcinoma of the Prostate Gland with Bladder Invasion. J Urol. 1969; **101**: 78–80.

Loo KT, Chan JKC. Colloid Adenocarcinoma of the Urethra Associated with Mucosal in Situ Carcinoma. Arch Path Lab Med. 1992; **116**: 976–77.

Osunkoya AO, Epstein JI. Primary Mucin-producing Urothelial-type Adenocarcinoma of Prostate: Report of 15 Cases. Am J Surg Pathol. 2007; **31**: 1323–29.

Massari F, Ciccarese C, Modena A, et al. Adenocarcinoma of the Paraurethral Glands: A Case Report. Histol Histopathol. 2014; **29**: 1295–303.

Sebesta EM, Mirheydar HS, Parsons JK, et al. Primary Mucin-producing Urothelial-type Adenocarcinoma of the Prostatic Urethra Diagnosed on TURP: A Case Report and Review of the Literature. BMC Urol. 2014; **14**: 39–43.

Sakamoto N, Ohtsubo S, Iguchi A, et al. Intestinal-type Mucinous Adenocarcinoma Arising from the Prostatic Duct. Int J Urol. 2005; **12**: 509–12.

Tran KP, Epstein JI. Mucinous Adenocarcinoma of the Urinary Bladder Type Arising in the Prostatic Urethra. Distinction from Mucinous Adenocarcinoma of the Prostate. Am Surg J Pathol. 1996; **20**: 1346–50.

Williamson SR, Scarpelli M, Lopez-Beltran A, Montironi R, Conces MR, Cheng L. Urethral Caruncle: A Lesion Related to IgG4-associated Sclerosing Disease? J Clin Pathol. 2013; **66**: 559–62.

Borislav A, Tavora A, Tavora F. Histology and Immunohistochemistry of Clear Cell Adenocarcinoma of the Urethra: Histogenesis and Diagnostic Problems. Virchows Arch. 2013; **462**: 193–201.

Raspollini MR, Carini M, Montironi R, Cheng L, Lopez-Beltran A. Mucinous Adenocarcinoma of the Male Urethra. Two Cases' Report and Literature Review. Anal Quant Cytopathol Histopathol. 2015; (In press).

Keen MR, Golden RL, Richardson JF, Melicow MM. Carcinoma of Cowper's Gland Treated with Chemotherapy. J Urol. 1970 Dec; **104**(6): 854–59.

Korytko TP, Lowe GJ, Jimenez RE, Pohar KS, Martin DD. Prostate-specific Antigen Response after Definitive Radiotherapy for Skene's Gland Adenocarcinoma Resembling Prostate Adenocarcinoma. Urol Oncol. 2012 Sep; **30**(5): 602–06. doi: 10.1016/j.urolonc.2010.06.015. Epub 2010 Sep 25.

Aronson P, Ronan SG, Briele HA, Bardawil WA, Manaligod JR. Adenoid Cystic Carcinoma of Female Periurethral Area. Light and Electron Microscopic Study. Urology. 1982 Sep; **20**(3): 312–15.

Halat S, Eble JN, Grignon DJ, Lacy S, Montironi R, MacLennan GT, Lopez-Beltran A, Tan PH, Baldridge LA, Cheng L. Ectopic Prostatic Tissue: Histogenesis and Histopathological Characteristics. Histopathology. 2011 Apr; **58**(5): 750–58. doi: 10.1111/j.1365-2559.2011.03799.x. Epub 2011 Mar 25.

Velazquez EF, Soskin A, Bock A, Codas R, Cai G, Barreto JE. Cubilla AL Epithelial Abnormalities and Precancerous Lesions of Anterior Urethra in Patients with Penile Carcinoma: A Report of 89 Cases. Mod Pathol. 2005; **18**(7): 917–23.

Fine SW, Chan TY, Epstein JI. Inverted Papillomas of the Prostatic Urethra. Am J Surg Pathol. 2006; **30**(8): 975–79.

Noel JC, Fayt I, Aguilar SF. Adenosquamous Carcinoma Arising in Villous Adenoma from Female Vulvar Urethra. Acta Obstet Gynecol Scand. 2006; **85**(3): 373–76.

Kuroda N, Shiotsu T, Ohara M, Hirouchi T, Mizuno K, Miyazaki E. Female Urethral Adenocarcinoma with a Heterogeneous Phenotype. APMIS. 2006; **114**(4): 314–18.

Achiche MA, Bouhaoula MH, Madani M, Azaiez M, Chebil M, Ayed M. Primary Transitional Cell Carcinoma of the Bulbar Urethra. Prog Urol. 2005; **15**(6): 1145–48.

Shalev M, Mistry S, Kernen K, Miles BJ. Squamous Cell Carcinoma in a Female Urethral Diverticulum. Urology. 2002; **59**(5): 773.

Hruby G, Choo R, Lehman M, Herschorn S, Kapusta L. Female Clear Cell Adenocarcinoma Arising within a Urethral Diverticulum. Can J Urol. 2000; **7**(6): 1160–63.

Practical Immunohistochemistry of Prostate Cancer and Related Lesions

- This chapter incorporates consensus data reported from the International Society of Urological Pathology recommendations for the use of immunohistochemistry in prostate specimens.
- General recommendations are relevant to approach Pca diagnosis and will be reviewed in this chapter. Box 17.1 summarizes main current recommendations as bullet points.

17.1 The Diagnosis of Limited Prostate Adenocarcinoma on Needle Biopsy

- The most common use of immunohistochemistry in the evaluation of prostate samples is for the identification of basal cells, which are absent with rare exceptions in adenocarcinoma of the prostate.
- Typically, benign glands are positive for basal cells with immunohistochemistry, but adenosis, partial atrophy and high grade prostatic intraepithelial neoplasia can have very patchy or near complete absence of basal cells in a given focus. This is of particular relevance on needle biopsies. Figs 17.1–17.6
- The most commonly used basal cell antibodies are high molecular weight cytokeratin (34ßE12, cytokeratin 5/6) and p63 or p40, which are cytoplasmic and nuclear antibodies, respectively; p63 and p40 show comparable results.

BOX 17.1 ISUP Recommendations for the Use of Immunohistochemistry in Prostate Specimens

- In the setting of obvious carcinoma or benign glands, there is no justification to do immunohistochemistry.
- If there is Gleason score 3+4=7 or higher grade cancer in at least one part, the work-up of other parts with an atypical focus suspicious for Gleason score 3+3–6 cancer is not recommended.
- In the setting of Gleason score 4+3 or 4+4=8 cancer on at least one part, the extent of high grade cancer could affect clinical treatment such that work-up of other atypical possible high grade cancer foci is justified.
- In the setting of Gleason score 4+3 or higher grade cancer on at least one part, given that intraductal carcinoma in the vast majority of cases is considered extension of high grade cancer into prostatic ducts and acini, it is not recommended in the setting of definitive invasive high grade cancer that work-up of additional cribriform lesions be pursued.
- In the setting of Gleason score 3+3 on at least one part, the number of positive cores and/or their location could possibly affect subsequent therapy in terms of suitability for active surveillance or focal therapy, such that unless one knows with certainty that it would not affect therapy, it is justified to perform an immunohistochemical work-up of additional atypical foci.
- In the differential diagnosis of high grade Pca vs. urothelial carcinoma (UC), the primary option is to use PSA as a first test to identify Pca and GATA3 to identify UC. If GATA3 is not available, then HMWCK and p63 may be used. If the tumor is PSA positive with intense staining and HMWCK and p63 negative, the findings are diagnostic of Pca. If the tumor is equivocal/weak/negative for PSA and negative/focal for p63 and HMWCK, then one needs to do P501S, NKX3.1 and GATA3.
- Some experts also include PAP in this second round of staining. If the tumor is negative for PSA and diffusely strongly positive for p63 and HMWCK, the findings are diagnostic of UC. If the tumor is negative for PSA and moderate-strong positive for GATA3, it is diagnostic of UC.
- Laboratories should be encouraged to use GATA3 for UC and add P501S and NKX3.1 as prostate markers in addition to PSA, p63 and HMWCK. If GATA3, p501s and NKX3.1 are not available in equivocal cases, the case should be sent out for consultation to laboratories with these antibodies.

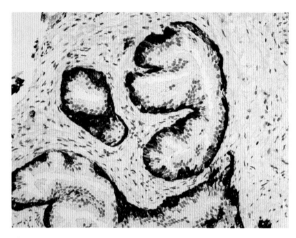

Fig 17.1 Prostatic gland with focal loss of basal cells (anti-34βE12 immunohistochemistry).

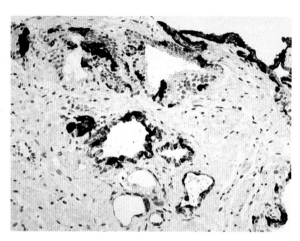

Fig 17.2 Prostatic atrophy with focal loss of basal cells (anti-34βE12 immunohistochemistry).

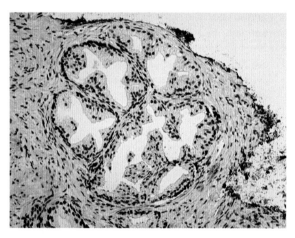

Fig 17.3 Prostatic gland with focal loss of basal cells (anti-p63 immunohistochemistry).

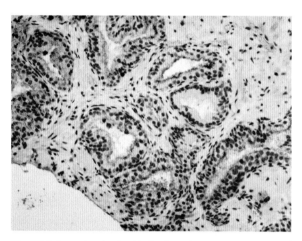

Fig 17.4 Prostatic gland with focal weak positive expression of racemase.

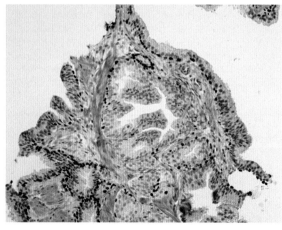

Fig 17.5 PIN with focal loss of basal cells (anti-p63 immunohistochemistry).

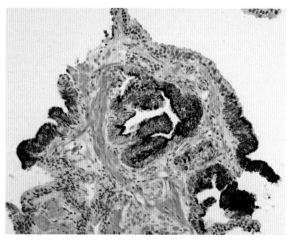

Fig 17.6 PIN with positive expression of racemase.

Table 17.1 Immunohistochemistry in The Diagnosis of Limited Adenocarcinoma of the Prostate on Needle Biopsy

Antibody	Immunoreactivity
p63	Less non-specific staining, p63 aberrant Pca false (−) in mimics
p40	Less non-specific staining; no aberrant Pca expression, false (−) in mimics
HMWCK	No diffuse aberrant; increased non-specificity HMWCK Pca; false (−) in mimics
HMWCK/p63	Conserves tissue; may not recognize p63; aberrant Pca
AMACR	Positive in 80% of Pca; false (+) in mimics
AMACR/p63	See AMACR and p63 in same tissue; hard to see rare p63 basal cells if both same chromogen
Triple (p63/AMACR/CK)	AMACR and basal cell; dual color technically more labeling in same cells difficult to evaluate
ERG	More specific; only ~40% Pca positive; HGPIN (+); limited experience with mimickers

- P40 which is an isoform of p63 shows less aberrant p63 immunoreactivity in adenocarcinoma of the prostate. Table 17.1; Figs 17.7–17.13
- Studies comparing high molecular weight cytokeratin and p63 have showed p63 to be slightly superior, and ck5/6 seems to be superior to 34ßE12.
- Diffuse expression of p63 (aberrant expression) in acinar adenocarcinoma is a recently recognized phenomenon in which the staining for p63 is strong and diffuse within the malignant glands. Other basal cell markers such as cytokeratin 5/6 and 34βE12 are negative. Figs 17.14–17.16
- The use of a double cocktail combining HMWCK and p63 can increase the sensitivity of basal cell detection with a decrease in staining variability.
- Alpha-methylacyl-CoA-racemase (AMACR; P504S) is significantly up-regulated in prostate cancer. By immunohistochemistry, the majority of prostate cancers are positive for AMACR. The observed sensitivity varies amongst studies

(82%–100%). There are no differences between polyclonal and monoclonal P504s in the sensitivity for diagnosis of prostate cancer.
- Different cocktails have been investigated combining antibodies for AMACR and basal cell specific markers. One combination is with antibodies to p63 and AMACR, both labeled with a brown chromogen. A limitation is that in some cases, focal nuclear staining for p63 can be difficult to detect if the cytoplasmic staining for AMACR is intensely positive. The main application is the case with small foci of atypical glands and the lesion may not survive sectioning to do separate stains for basal cell markers and AMACR on different slides.
- There is also a triple stain cocktail using a brown chromogen for both high molecular weight cytokeratin and p63 and a red chromogen for AMACR that optimizes the preservation of tissue for immunohistochemistry.
- Fusions between the androgen-regulated transmembrane protease serine 2 gene (TMPRSS2) and the ERG gene is present in approximately 40%–50% of prostate adenocarcinomas. ERG has been proposed as an aid to the diagnosis of limited adenocarcinoma of the prostate. This gene fusion is highly specific for prostate cancer, with the exception that about 20% of high grade PINs also show the gene fusion.
- Monoclonal anti-ERG antibodies correlate well with TMPRSS2-ERG gene fusions in fusion-positive cancer. ERG antibodies have been shown to be negative in post-atrophic hyperplasia, partial atrophy and adenosis, but rarely some benign glands may express ERG, as an ERG labels endothelium (internal control). Fig 17.17 The heterogeneous and weak ERG expression (20–30% of cases) further contributes to potentially false negative staining on biopsy. The major limitation of ERG as a diagnostic test is its low sensitivity, such that a negative stain does not exclude prostate carcinoma. There are conflicting studies on the diagnostic utility of ERG.
- It is therefore recommended to use either HMWCK (34BE12 or CK5/6 or others) or p63 or a combination of the two with AMACR either in a double or triple cocktail for the work-up of small foci of atypical glands suspicious for

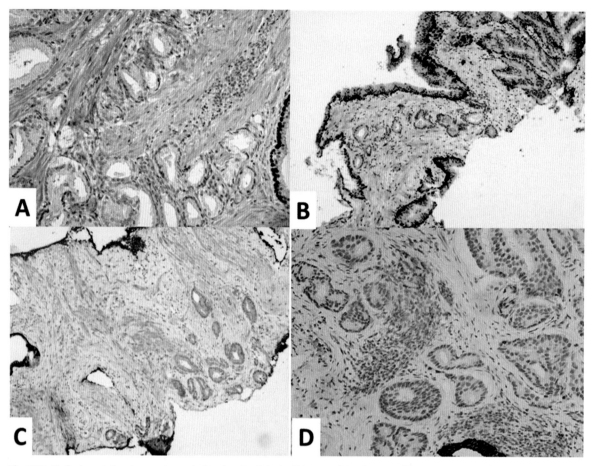

Fig 17.7 Limited prostatic adenocarcinoma lacking basal cell. Anti-p63 immunohistochemistry (A), anti-p40 immunohistochemistry (B), anti-CK5/6 immunohistochemistry (C), anti-34βE12 immunohistochemistry (D).

adenocarcinoma of the prostate. Currently, ERG remains as an option.

- In the setting of obvious carcinoma or obviously benign glands, there is no justification to do immunohistochemistry.
- Distorted rectal glands included in the biopsy represent a potential immunohistochemical pitfall, since they are racemase positive and negative for 34βE12/p63. Fig 17.18

17.2 Poorly Differentiated Prostate Adenocarcinoma vs. Urothelial Carcinoma

- Although the distinction between urothelial carcinoma and prostatic adenocarcinoma can usually be made on routine stained sections, there may be overlap in cases where prostate

adenocarcinoma has marked pleomorphism and pseudo-papillary structures mimicking urothelial carcinoma.

- Therefore, the distinction between poorly differentiated urothelial carcinoma and poorly differentiated adenocarcinoma of the prostate, even in a metastatic site, is critical, as both are treated differently. Consequently, in a poorly differentiated tumor involving the bladder and prostate without any glandular differentiation typical of prostate adenocarcinoma, the case should be worked up immunohistochemically. Table 17.2; Figs 17.19–17.20
- Situations that can cause diagnostic difficulty include PSA and PSAP within periurethral glands, as well as cystitis cystica and cystitis glandularis in both men and women. Periurethral gland carcinomas in women and

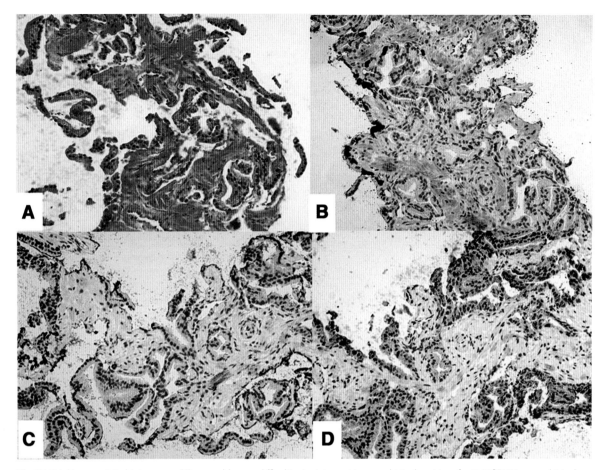

Fig 17.8 Inking prostate biopsy cores (A) may add some difficulties to interpret immunohistochemistry of anti-34βE12 immunohistochemistry (B), anti-p63 immunohistochemistry (C), anti-racemase immunohistochemistry (D).

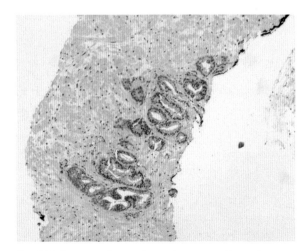

Fig 17.9 Prostate adenocarcinoma in prostate biopsy (same as Fig 17.10).

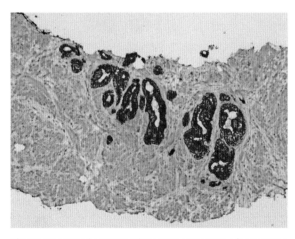

Fig 17.10 Limited prostatic adenocarcinoma positive for racemase and lacking basal cells (cocktail 34βE12/racemase).

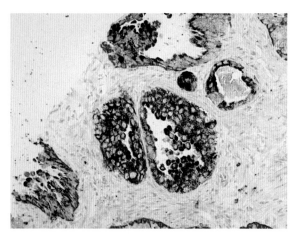

Fig 17.11 PIN ATYP as seen with cocktail 34βE12 (red)/racemase (brown) immunohistochemistry.

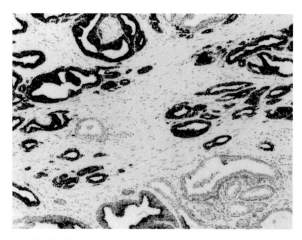

Fig 17.12 Racemase expression in prostate adenocarcinoma with perineural invasion and negative staining in non-neoplastic glands.

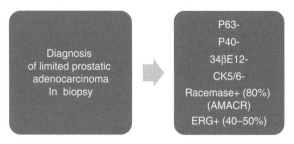

Fig 17.13 Basic criteria for the diagnosis of limited prostatic adenocarcinoma using immunohistochemistry.

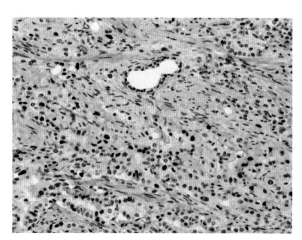

Fig 17.14 Prostate adenocarcinoma with aberrant p63 expression (anti-p63 immunohistochemistry).

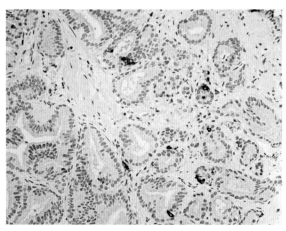

Fig 17.15 Prostate adenocarcinoma with aberrant 34βE12 expression (anti-34βE12 immunohistochemistry).

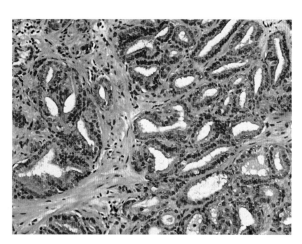

Fig 17.16 Prostate adenocarcinoma (same case as Fig 17.15).

Table 17.2 Differential Diagnosis of Prostate Adenocarcinoma vs. Urothelial Carcinoma Based on Prostate Related Markers

Antibody	Immunoreactivity
	PSA~85%–90% (+) in GS10; negative in a subset of high grade Pca; weak non-specific cytoplasmic (+) lead to false (+); negative in UC
PSAP	Polyclonal (+) in ~85%–90% GS10;
	monoclonal used in many kits lower sensitivity;
	negative in UC
P501S (Prostein)	(+) in many PSA; (−) Pca; negative in UC;
	Coarse cytoplasmic granules reduce false (+)
NKX3.1	(+) in many PSA (−) Pca; negative in UC
	Nuclear stain reduce false (+)
AR	High sensitivity for Pca; positive in some UC
AMACR	High sensitivity for Pca; positive in some UC
PSMA	High sensitivity for Pca; positive in 14% of UC
CK7/CK20	Negative CK7 favors Pca; not specific as both can be positive in Pca
HMWCK	Diffuse positive rules out Pca; only positive in ~70% of UC; occasionally false positive cells in Pca
p63	Less false positive in Pca; only positive in ~70% of UC
	Diffuse positive rules out Pca; occasionally
	false positive in Pca

GS10: Gleason score 5+5=10 adenocarcinoma; Pca: prostate adenocarcinoma; UC: urothelial carcinoma; PSA: prostate-specific antigen; PSAP: prostate-specific acid phosphatase; AR: androgen receptor; AMACR: alpha methylacyl-coaracemase; PSMA: prostate-specific membrane antigen; HMWCK: high molecular weight cytokeratin

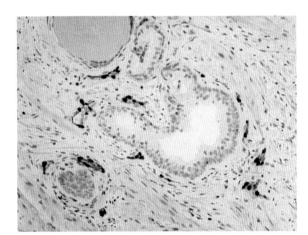

Fig 17.17 ERG expression in endothelial cells but negative expression in non-neoplastic prostate.

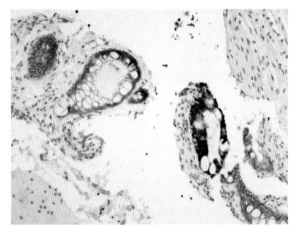

Fig 17.18 Racemase expression in distorted rectal glands should not be misdiagnosed as malignancy.

various salivary gland tumors may also be PSA and PSAP positive.

- Other examples of cross-reactive staining include anal glands in men (PSA, PSAP) and urachal remnants (PSA). Some intestinal carcinoids and pancreatic islet cell tumors are strongly reactive with antibodies to PSAP, yet are negative with antibodies to PSA. Weak false-positive staining for PSAP has been reported in several breast and renal cell carcinomas. Therefore, weak focal positive staining

for either antigen should be interpreted with caution.

- With only a few exceptions, immunohistochemical staining for PSA and PSAP is very specific for prostatic tissue.
- Although PSA and PSAP have proven to be useful in identifying prostate lineage, their sensitivity decreases in poorly differentiated prostate adenocarcinoma with cases showing focal positive staining in <25% of the tumor cells staining with

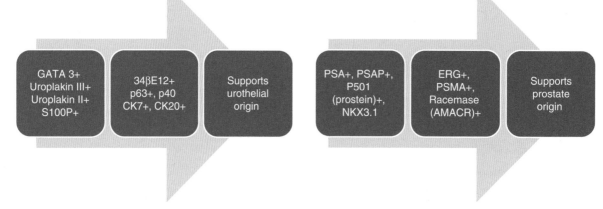

Fig 17.19 Basic immunohistochemistry to establish urothelial origin.

Fig 17.20 Basic immunohistochemistry to establish prostatic origin.

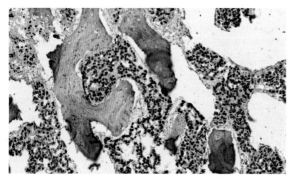

Fig 17.21 Prostein (p501S) expression in metastatic prostate cancer.

PSAP and PSA, respectively. 5–13% of cases may be completely negative to PSAP or PSA.

- Newer prostate lineage markers such as prostein (P501S), prostate-specific membrane antigen (PSMA), NKX3.1 and androgen receptor could be of added utility. Of these markers, PSMA has lower specificity and androgen receptor can be positive in some urothelial carcinoma cases. Fig 17.21

- Combining some of the above markers with urothelial lineage markers will further facilitate resolving urothelial vs. prostatic carcinoma differential diagnoses. HMWCK positivity has been shown in over 90% of urothelial carcinoma. HMWCK may be seen rarely in prostate cancer, but focal (8%).

- p63 has a greater specificity albeit lower sensitivity for urothelial carcinoma compared to high molecular weight cytokeratin (100% specificity

and 83% sensitivity). A cautionary note is warranted, given that HMWCK labels areas of squamous differentiation in post therapy prostate carcinoma lesions.

- Uroplakins are urothelium-specific transmembrane proteins expressed by the majority of non-invasive and up to two-thirds of advanced invasive and metastatic urothelial carcinomas as assessed by UPIII. Although highly specific for urothelial differentiation, UPIII is only of low degree of sensitivity (40%) in high grade urothelial carcinoma. Thrombomodulin is an endothelial cell associated co-factor for thrombin-mediated activator of protein C. Its expression, predominantly as membranous staining, has been found in 69%–100% of urothelial carcinoma. Thrombomodulin is only rarely positive in prostate adenocarcinoma. Compared to uroplakin III, thrombomodulin has a higher degree of sensitivity, but lower specificity as a marker for urothelial carcinoma. Likewise, p63 seems to be superior to thrombomodulin as a urothelial marker in high grade tumors.

- GATA3 (GATA binding protein 3 to DNA sequence [A/T]GATA[A/G]) is a member of a zinc finger transcription factor family. It is an excellent marker for urothelial carcinoma with >90% of urothelial carcinomas positive for GATA3. The nuclear staining is usually diffuse in more than 50% of cells. Very uncommonly, prostatic adenocarcinomas can be focally positive for GATA3.

Table 17.3 Urothelial Antibodies Used in the Differential Diagnosis of Prostate Adenocarcinoma vs. Urothelial Carcinoma

Antibody	Immunoreactivity
Thrombomodulin	Positive in only 63% of high grade UC; focal positive in 5% Pca
Uroplakin	Negative in Pca; positive in only 60% of high grade UC
GATA3	Almost always negative in Pca; positive in 80% of high grade UC

Pca: prostate adenocarcinoma; UC: urothelial carcinoma

- CK7 and CK20 are of limited utility in this differential, given that they may be both positive in a subset of adenocarcinoma of the prostate.
- It is recommended to use PSA as a first test to identify Pca and GATA3 to identify UC. If GATA3 not available, then HMWCK and p63 may be used. If the tumor is PSA positive with intense staining and HMWCK and p63 negative, the findings are diagnostic of Pca. Table 17.3
- If the tumor is negative for PSA and diffusely strongly positive for p63 and HMWCK, the findings are diagnostic of UC. If the tumor is negative for PSA and moderate-strong positive for GATA3, then it is diagnostic of UC.
- If the tumor is equivocal/weak/negative for PSA and negative/focal for p63 and HMWCK, then it must be tested for 501S, NKX3.1 and GATA3. PAP may be included in this second round of immunostaining.

17.3 High Grade Prostatic Adenocarcinoma vs. Bladder Adenocarcinoma

- In the differential diagnosis of bladder adenocarcinoma, one must first consider the possibility of secondary adenocarcinoma involving the bladder either by metastasis or direct invasion, such as from the prostate. Morphologically, there are differences in that bladder adenocarcinoma shares all of the various histological patterns of adenocarcinoma arising in the gastrointestinal tract. However, if necessary, certain immunohistochemical stains can be utilized in the differential diagnosis with prostatic

Table 17.4 Differential Diagnosis of High Grade Prostatic Adenocarcinoma vs. Bladder Adenocarcinoma

Antibody	Immunoreactivity
PSA	High sensitivity; 7–13% high grade Pca (–); 13% bladder adeno (+) polyclonal
PAP	High sensitivity; 5% GS8-10 (–); 33% bladder adeno (+) polyclonal
p501S (prostein)	High sensitivity (83%–100%) and high specificity
NKX3.1	High sensitivity (95%); high specificity in general; not investigated in bladder adenocarcinoma
PSMA	High sensitivity (88%–92%); 11% bladder adenocarcinoma cytoplasmic staining; 8% bladder adenocarcinoma membrane staining
Villin	High specificity for bladder; sensitivity 65% for bladder adeno
Thrombomodulin	95% negative in Pca; sensitivity 60% for bladder adeno
CDX2	94% negative in Pca; sensitivity 47% for bladder adeno
Monoclonal CEA	>95% negative in Pca; sensitivity 52% for bladder adeno
CA125	>95% negative in Pca; sensitivity 28% for bladder adeno
HMWCK	92% negative in high grade Pca; sensitivity 40% for bladder adeno
CK7/CK20	77% (CK7) and 64% (CK20) sensitivity for bladder adeno; not specific: CK7 in 57% of high grade Pca and CK20 in 20%

GS10: Gleason score 5+5=10 adenocarcinoma; Pca: prostate adenocarcinoma; adeno: adenocarcinoma; GS8-10: Gleason score 8–10 adenocarcinoma; PSA: prostate-specific antigen; PSAP: prostate-specific acid phosphatase; PSMA: prostate-specific membrane antigen; CEA: carcinoembryonic antigen; CA125: cancer antigen 125

adenocarcinoma. Monoclonal PSA antibodies do not label bladder adenocarcinoma, although polyclonal PSA and PSAP are positive in a significant percentage of bladder adenocarcinomas.

- Of the more recently discovered prostatic markers, PSMA lacks specificity, but NKX3.1 and P501S do not react with bladder adenocarcinomas. Table 17.4

17.4 Prostatic Small Cell Carcinoma vs. High Grade Prostatic Adenocarcinoma

- It is critical to identify a small cell component, as prostatic small cell carcinomas are treated with the same chemotherapy as is used in pulmonary small cell carcinomas, whereas advanced high grade prostatic adenocarcinoma is initially treated with hormonal therapy.
- The diagnosis of small cell carcinoma of the prostate is reached based on morphologic features (H&E) similar to those found in small cell carcinomas of the lung. Morphological variations of small cell carcinoma include the intermediate cell type with slightly more open chromatin and visible small nucleoli where it can be difficult to distinguish from high grade adenocarcinoma of the prostate. About 50% of the tumors are mixed small cell carcinoma and adenocarcinoma of the prostate.
- In some cases, the transition between the small cell and acinar components is abrupt and in other cases, the two components merge together.
- Using immunohistochemical techniques, the small cell component is positive for one or more neuroendocrine markers (synaptophysin, chromogranin, CD56) in almost 90% of cases. PSA and other prostatic markers such as P501s are positive in about 17%–25% of cases, although often very focally. In 24% and 35% of cases respectively, positivity is noted for p63 and high molecular weight cytokeratin, markers typically negative in prostatic carcinoma. Table 17.5
- Studies have demonstrated TTF-1 expression in over 50% of small cell carcinomas of the prostate, limiting its utility in distinguishing primary small cell carcinoma of the prostate from a metastasis from the lung.
- A technique that can distinguish small cell carcinoma of the prostate from other small cell carcinomas is documentation by FISH or RT-PCR of a gene fusion between members of the ETS family of genes, in particular ERG (ETS-related gene) and TMPRSS2, found in approximately one-half of usual prostatic adenocarcinoma.
- In a similar percent of cases, small cell carcinoma of the prostate is positive for

Table 17.5 Differential Diagnosis of Prostatic Small Cell Carcinoma vs. High Grade Prostatic Adenocarcinoma

Antibody	Immunoreactivity
CD56	Sensitivity 83%–92% for SCC; limited studies; specific; Pca (–)
TTF-1	Specific; Pca positive in 1%; sensitivity 52% SCC
Ki67	83% rate in SCC; ~10% rate in high grade Pca
NE stains	Syn (85%) and Chromo (75%) in SCC; strong staining in 10% Pca
Prostate markers	95%–100% in Pca; 25% SCC(+); usually rare (+) (PSA, P501s, NKX3.1)
AR	90% high grade Pca; 17% SCC

SCC: small cell carcinoma; Pca: prostate adenocarcinoma; Syn: synaptophysin; Chromo: chromogranin; AR: androgen receptor

TMPRSS2-ERG gene fusion by FISH. Importantly, it should be noted that compared to usual acinar carcinoma harboring TMPRSS2-ERG rearrangements, small cell carcinoma with TMPRSS2-ERG rearrangement is not reliably positive for ERG protein by immunohistochemistry, presumably due to lack of androgen receptor expression in small cell carcinoma. Additionally, in the setting of standard treatment for castrate-resistant prostate cancer, ERG protein expression may not be present by immunohistochemistry requiring the use of membrane staining for CD44 in all prostatic NE small cell carcinomas, whereas in usual prostatic adenocarcinomas, only rare positive scattered tumor cells are CD44 positive.

- In cases where the routinely stained sections are equivocal, a combination of prostate markers, neuroendocrine markers, TTF-1 and ki67 can be used. CD44 has in one study claimed to be positive in prostatic small cell carcinoma and negative in usual Pca. However, the results need to be verified.
- It should be recognized that not all small cell carcinomas express neuroendocrine markers. CD56 is the most sensitive, yet least specific. Synaptophysin has the best combination of sensitivity and specificity. Chromogranin is the most specific, but is often negative or only shows rare positive cells.

Table 17.6 Immunohistochemistry to Identify Tumors of Prostatic Origin

Antibody	Immunoreactivity
PSA	97% sensitive in mets; rare positive cells in GS 9–10;
	High specificity; Decreased with hormone therapy;
	Salivary, bladder adeno and melanoma may be (+)
PSAP	99% sensitive in mets; less specific than PSA;
	also (+) in NE tumors; decreased with hormone therapy
P501s (prostein)	99% sensitive in mets; limited studies
	No decrease with hormone therapy
PSMA	88%–100% sensitive in mets; not specific
AMACR	81%–93% sensitive in mets; not specific
NKX3.1	94% sensitive in mets; only lobular breast Ca (+)
ERG	40–50% sensitivity; fairly specific; also (+) in vascular tumors, meningioma, and some PNETs

mets: metastases; GS 9–10: Gleason score 9–10 adenocarcinoma; adeno: adenocarcinoma; PSA: prostate-specific antigen; PSAP: prostate-specific acid phosphatase; AMACR: alpha methylacyl-coaracemase; PSMA: prostate-specific membrane antigen; NE: neuroendocrine; Ca: carcinoma; PNETs; primitive neuroectodermal tumors

Table 17.7 Differential Diagnosis of Nonspecific Granulomatous Prostatitis/Xanthoma vs. High Grade Prostate Adenocarcinoma

Antibody	Immunoreactivity
CD68	Sensitive and specific for histiocytes
Keratins	Sensitive and specific for reactive epithelial cells; positive in associated benign glands
PSA	6.7% positive in histiocytes; may be negative in high grade Pca
PAP	11.8% positive in histiocytes; may be negative in high grade Pca
AMACR	8.3% positive in histiocytes 20% negative in limited Pca

Pca: prostate adenocarcinoma; AMACR: alpha methylacyl-coaracemase

17.5 Prostate Origin in Metastatic Carcinoma of Unknown Primary

- Given that there is a treatment for metastatic adenocarcinoma of the prostate which can provide symptomatic relief and in some cases increased survival, it is critical to determine whether a metastatic carcinoma is of prostatic origin. There are several antibodies that can be used for this purpose. One must also be aware that immunoreactivity for PSA and PSAP decreases after androgen deprivation therapy. Table 17.6

17.6 Nonspecific Granulomatous Prostatitis/Xanthoma Vs. High Grade Prostate Adenocarcinoma

- One of the principal entities that can be confused with high grade prostate cancer is nonspecific granulomatous prostatitis (NSGP). Although most cases of NSGP seen on needle biopsy do not

histologically resemble prostate cancer, 4% of cases can closely resemble cancer. Xanthomas of the prostate can similarly mimic high grade adenocarcinoma of the prostate. Table 17.7

17.7 Adult Prostate Sarcoma Vs. Sarcomatoid Prostate Adenocarcinoma

- The differential diagnosis of a malignant spindle cell tumor in the prostate is sarcomatoid prostate adenocarcinoma (carcinosarcoma) versus a sarcoma. The most common sarcomas in the prostate of an adult are stromal sarcoma and leiomyosarcoma. Morphologically, leiomyosarcoma has a distinctive fascicular growth pattern that can be distinguished from a sarcomatoid carcinoma. A pitfall is the expression of keratin in some prostate leiomyosarcomas with conflicting studies on the presence of p63 in these tumors. Table 17.8

17.8 Colorectal Adenocarcinoma vs. High Grade Prostate Adenocarcinoma

- Colorectal adenocarcinomas may directly invade the prostate where they may resemble one of the patterns of prostatic duct adenocarcinomas. Usually, colorectal adenocarcinomas that invade the prostate are not occult, although occasionally they may present in the prostate.
- Histological features favoring colorectal adenocarcinoma are prominent desmoplasia,

Table 17.8 Differential Diagnosis of Adult Prostate Sarcoma vs. Sarcomatoid Prostate Adenocarcinoma by Immunohistochemistry

Marker	Immunoreactivity
Desmin	(+) in LS, may be diffuse
	Focal (+) in some Sarc Ca
	(−) in SS
Vimentin	Sensitive, but not specific for sarcoma
SM Actin	(+) in SS, LS
	Focal (+) in some Sarc Ca
CD34	(+) in most SS
	8% of LS (+)
	(−) in Sarc Ca
PANCK	Usually (−) in Sarcomas
	(+) in up to 27% of prostate LS
	(+) in 71% Sarc Ca, yet can be focal
	No data for SS
HMWCK	Sometimes more sensitive than PANCK (no prostate data available)
	(−) in bladder LS (no prostate data available)
	No data for SS
p63	One of most sensitive markers for Sarc Ca
	0% (+) in LS in general
	23% (+) in bladder LS in one large study
	No data on prostatic LS
No data for SS	
Prostate Markers	Negative in sarcoma
(PSA, P501S, NKX3.1)	Positive in epithelial component if present
	Not necessary as H&E presence of carcinoma diagnostic

LS: leiomyosarcoma; Sarc Ca: sarcomatoid carcinoma; SS: stromal sarcoma; SM Actin; smooth muscle actin; PANCK; pancytokeratin; HMWCK: high molecular weight cytokeratin; GU: genitourinary

Table 17.9 Differential Diagnosis of Colorectal Adenocarcinoma vs. High Grade Prostate Adenocarcinoma by Immunohistochemistry

Antibody	Immunoreactivity
Villin	(+) in most CRC; (−) in Pca
CDX2	(+) in most CRC; rare (+) in Pca
CK20	(+) in most CRC; (+) in 20% Pca
Prostate markers	(−) in CRC; (+) in >90% Pca; rare (−) Pca cases
Polyclonal CEA MUC1, MUC2	(+) in CRC; overlap with Pca
Beta-catenin	(+) in CRC, diffuse nuclear staining diagnostic
	Typically (+) cytoplasmic
	Nuclear (+) in some studies of Pca

CRC: colorectal adenocarcinoma; Pca; prostate adenocarcinoma

- There have been, however, multiple immunohistochemical markers that have been proposed for prognostic purposes. The more promising ones that have been studied to a greater extent are PTEN loss, increased ki67 proliferation index, abnormal expression of p53 protein, abnormal expression of ERG, loss of NKX3.1 and abnormal expression of MYC protein.
- A limitation of all of them is they have not been validated in prospective studies.

Suggested Reading

Hedrick L, Epstein JI. Use of Keratin 903 as an Adjunct in the Diagnosis of Prostate Carcinoma. Am J Surg Pathol. 1989; **13**: 389–96.

Goldstein NS, Underhill J, Roszka J, Neill JS. Cytokeratin 34 Beta E-12 Immunoreactivity in Benign Prostatic Acini. Quantitation, Pattern Assessment, and Electron Microscopic Study. Am J Clin Pathol. 1999; **112**: 69–74.

Wojno KJ, Epstein JI. The Utility of Basal Cell-specific Anti-cytokeratin Antibody (34 Beta E12) in the Diagnosis of Prostate Cancer. A Review of 228 Cases. Am J Surg Pathol. 1995; **19**: 251–60.

Shah RB, Zhou M, LeBlanc M, Snyder M, Rubin MA. Comparison of the Basal Cell-specific Markers, 34betaE12 and p63, in the Diagnosis of Prostate Cancer. Am J Surg Pathol. 2002; **26**: 1161–68.

Weinstein MH, Signoretti S, Loda M. Diagnostic Utility of Immunohistochemical Staining for p63, a Sensitive Marker of Prostatic Basal Cells. Mod Pathol. 2002; **15**: 1302–08.

"dirty necrosis," chronic inflammatory response, tall columnar epithelium with mucin or mucin-positive signet-ring cells that may be seen occasionally. Table 17.9

17.9 Prognostic Immunohistochemical Markers

- Currently, there are no prognostic immunohistochemical markers that are recommended to be routinely performed on biopsy or resection specimens.

Parsons JK, Gage WR, Nelson WG, De Marzo AM. p63 Protein Expression Is Rare in Prostate Adenocarcinoma: Implications for Cancer Diagnosis and Carcinogenesis. Urology. 2001; **58**: 619–24.

Sailer V, Stephan C, Wernert N, et al. Comparison of p40 (DeltaNp63) and p63 Expression in Prostate Tissues–Which One Is the Superior Diagnostic Marker for Basal Cells? Histopathology. 2013; **63**: 50–56.

Abrahams NA, Ormsby AH, Brainard J. Validation of Cytokeratin 5/6 as an Effective Substitute for Keratin 903 in the Differentiation of Benign from Malignant Glands in Prostate Needle Biopsies. Histopathology. 2002; **41**: 35–41.

Rubin MA, Zhou M, Dhanasekaran SM, et al. Alpha-Methylacyl Coenzyme A Racemase as a Tissue Biomarker for Prostate Cancer. JAMA. 2002; **287**: 1662–70.

Zhou M, Shah R, Shen R, Rubin MA. Basal Cell Cocktail (34betaE12 + p63) Improves the Detection of Prostate Basal Cells. Am J Surg Pathol. 2003; **27**: 365–71.

Brimo F, Epstein JI. Immunohistochemical Pitfalls in Prostate Pathology. Hum Pathol. 2012; **43**: 313–24.

Giannico GA, Ross HM, Lotan T, Epstein JI. Aberrant Expression of p63 in Adenocarcinoma of the Prostate: A Radical Prostatectomy Study. Am J Surg Pathol. 2013; **37**: 1401–06.

Zhou M, Chinnaiyan AM, Kleer CG, Lucas PC, Rubin MA. Alpha-Methylacyl-CoA Racemase: A Novel Tumor Marker Over-expressed in Several Human Cancers and Their Precursor Lesions. Am J Surg Pathol. 2002; **26**: 926–31.

Jiang Z, Wu CL, Woda BA, et al. Alpha-Methylacyl-CoA Racemase: A Multi-institutional Study of a New Prostate Cancer Marker. Histopathology. 2004; **45**: 218–25.

Magi-Galluzzi C, Luo J, Isaacs WB, Hicks JL, de Marzo AM, Epstein JI. Alpha-Methylacyl-CoA Racemase: A Variably Sensitive Immunohistochemical Marker for the Diagnosis of Small Prostate Cancer Foci on Needle Biopsy. Am J Surg Pathol. 2003; **27**: 1128–33.

Zhou M, Jiang Z, Epstein JI. Expression and Diagnostic Utility of Alpha-Methylacyl-CoA-Racemase (P504S) in Foamy Gland and Pseudohyperplastic Prostate Cancer. Am J Surg Pathol. 2003; **27**: 772–78.

Kunju LP, Rubin MA, Chinnaiyan AM, Shah RB. Diagnostic Usefulness of Monoclonal Antibody P504S in the Workup of Atypical Prostatic Glandular Proliferations. Am J Clin Pathol. 2003; **120**: 737–45.

Jiang Z, Iczkowski KA, Woda BA, Tretiakova M, Yang XJ. P504S Immunostaining Boosts Diagnostic Resolution of "Suspicious" Foci in Prostatic Needle Biopsy Specimens. Am J Clin Pathol. 2004; **121**: 99–107.

Kunju LP, Chinnaiyan AM, Shah RB. Comparison of Monoclonal Antibody (P504S) and Polyclonal Antibody to Alpha Methylacyl-CoA Racemase (AMACR) in the Work-up of Prostate Cancer. Histopathology. 2005; **47**: 587–96.

Hameed O, Sublett J, Humphrey PA. Immunohistochemical Stains for p63 and Alpha-Methylacyl-CoA Racemase, versus a Cocktail Comprising both, in the Diagnosis of Prostatic Carcinoma: A Comparison of the Immunohistochemical Staining of 430 Foci in Radical Prostatectomy and Needle Biopsy Tissues. Am J Surg Pathol. 2005; **29**: 579–87.

Sanderson SO, Sebo TJ, Murphy LM, Neumann R, Slezak J, Cheville JC. An Analysis of the p63/Alpha-Methylacyl Coenzyme A Racemase Immunohistochemical Cocktail Stain in Prostate Needle Biopsy Specimens and Tissue Microarrays. Am J Clin Pathol. 2004; **121**: 220–25.

Jiang Z, Li C, Fischer A, Dresser K, Woda BA. Using an AMACR (P504S)/34betaE12/p63 Cocktail for the Detection of Small Focal Prostate Carcinoma in Needle Biopsy Specimens. Am J Clin Pathol. 2005; **123**: 231–36.

He H, Magi-Galluzzi C, Li J, et al. The Diagnostic Utility of Novel Immunohistochemical Marker ERG in the Workup of Prostate Biopsies with "Atypical Glands Suspicious for Cancer." Am J Surg Pathol. 2011; **35**: 608–14.

Green WM, Hicks JL, De Marzo A, Illei PP, Epstein JI. Immunohistochemical Evaluation of TMPRSS2-ERG Gene Fusion in Adenosis of the Prostate. Hum Pathol. 2013; **44**: 1895–901.

Cheng L, Davidson DD, Maclennan GT, et al. Atypical Adenomatous Hyperplasia of Prostate Lacks TMPRSS2-ERG Gene Fusion. Am J Surg Pathol. 2013; **37**: 1550–54.

Yaskiv O, Zhang X, Simmerman K, et al. The Utility of ERG/p63 Double Immunohistochemical Staining in the Diagnosis of Limited Cancer in Prostate Needle Biopsies. Am J Surg Pathol. 2011; **35**: 1062–68.

Minner S, Gartner M, Freudenthaler F, et al. Marked Heterogeneity of ERG Expression in Large Primary Prostate Cancers. Mod Pathol. 2013; **26**: 106–16.

Mosquera JM, Mehra R, Regan MM, et al. Prevalence of TMPRSS2-ERG Fusion Prostate Cancer among Men Undergoing Prostate Biopsy in the United States. Clin Cancer Res. 2009; **15**: 4706–11.

Shah RB, Tadros Y, Brummell B, Zhou M. The Diagnostic Use of ERG in Resolving an "Atypical Glands Suspicious for Cancer" Diagnosis in Prostate Biopsies beyond That Provided by Basal Cell and Alpha-Methylacyl-CoA-Racemase Markers. Hum Pathol. 2013; **44**: 786–94.

Pollen JJ, Dreilinger A. Immunohistochemical Identification of Prostatic Acid Phosphatase and Prostate Specific Antigen in Female Periurethral Glands. Urology. 1984; **23**: 303–04.

Nowels K, Kent E, Rinsho K, Oyasu R. Prostate Specific Antigen and Acid Phosphatase-reactive Cells in Cystitis

Cystica and Glandularis. Arch Pathol Lab Med. 1988; **112**: 734–37.

Golz R, Schubert GE. Prostatic Specific Antigen: Immunoreactivity in Urachal Remnants. J Urol. 1989; **141**: 1480–82.

Kamoshida S, Tsutsumi Y. Extraprostatic Localization of Prostatic Acid Phosphatase and Prostate-specific Antigen: Distribution in Cloacogenic Glandular Epithelium and Sex-dependent Expression in Human Anal Gland. Hum Pathol. 1990; **21**: 1108–11.

Sobin LH, Hjermstad BM, Sesterhenn IA, Helwig EB. Prostatic Acid Phosphatase Activity in Carcinoid Tumors. Cancer. 1986; **58**: 136–38.

Spencer JR, Brodin AG, Ignatoff JM. Clear Cell Adenocarcinoma of the Urethra: Evidence for Origin within Paraurethral Ducts. J Urol. 1990; **143**: 122–25.

van Krieken JH. Prostate Marker Immunoreactivity in Salivary Gland Neoplasms. A Rare Pitfall in Immunohistochemistry. Am J Surg Pathol. 1993; **17**: 410–14.

Downes MR, Torlakovic EE, Aldaoud N, Zlotta AR, Evans AJ, van der Kwast TH. Diagnostic Utility of Androgen Receptor Expression in Discriminating Poorly Differentiated Urothelial and Prostate Carcinoma. J Clin Pathol. 2013; **66**: 779–86.

Chuang AY, DeMarzo AM, Veltri RW, Sharma RB, Bieberich CJ, Epstein JI. Immunohistochemical Differentiation of High-grade Prostate Carcinoma from Urothelial Carcinoma. Am J Surg Pathol. 2007; **31**: 1246–55.

Miyamoto H, Yao JL, Chaux A, et al. Expression of Androgen and Oestrogen Receptors and Its Prognostic Significance in Urothelial Neoplasm of the Urinary Bladder. BJU Int. 2012; **109**: 1716–26.

Varma M, Morgan M, Amin MB, Wozniak S, Jasani B. High Molecular Weight Cytokeratin Antibody (clone 34betaE12): A Sensitive Marker for Differentiation of High-grade Invasive Urothelial Carcinoma from Prostate Cancer. Histopathology. 2003; **42**: 167–72.

Huang HY, Shariat SF, Sun TT, et al. Persistent Uroplakin Expression in Advanced Urothelial Carcinomas: Implications in Urothelial Tumor Progression and Clinical Outcome. Hum Pathol. 2007; **38**: 1703–13.

Parker DC, Folpe AL, Bell J, et al. Potential Utility of Uroplakin III, Thrombomodulin, High Molecular Weight Cytokeratin, and Cytokeratin 20 in Noninvasive, Invasive, and Metastatic Urothelial (Transitional Cell) Carcinomas. Am J Surg Pathol. 2003; **27**: 1–10.

Ordonez NG. Thrombomodulin Expression in Transitional Cell Carcinoma. Am J Clin Pathol. 1998; **110**: 385–90.

Esheba GE, Longacre TA, Atkins KA, Higgins JP. Expression of the Urothelial Differentiation Markers GATA3 and Placental S100 (S100P) in Female Genital Tract Transitional Cell Proliferations. Am J Surg Pathol. 2009; **33**: 347–53.

Liu H, Shi J, Wilkerson ML, Lin F. Immunohistochemical Evaluation of GATA3 Expression in Tumors and Normal Tissues: A Useful Immunomarker for Breast and Urothelial Carcinomas. Am J Clin Pathol. 2012; **138**: 57–64.

Miettinen M, McCue PA, Sarlomo-Rikala M, et al. GATA3: A Multispecific but Potentially Useful Marker in Surgical Pathology: A Systematic Analysis of 2500 Epithelial and Nonepithelial Tumors. Am J Surg Pathol. 2013.

Chang A, Amin A, Gabrielson E, et al. Utility of GATA3 Immunohistochemistry in Differentiating Urothelial Carcinoma from Prostate Adenocarcinoma and Squamous Cell Carcinomas of the Uterine Cervix, Anus, and Lung. Am J Surg Pathol. 2012; **36**: 1472–76.

Genega EM, Hutchinson B, Reuter VE, Gaudin PB. Immunophenotype of High-grade Prostatic Adenocarcinoma and Urothelial Carcinoma. Mod Pathol. 2000; **13**: 1186–91.

Mhawech P, Uchida T, Pelte MF. Immunohistochemical Profile of High-grade Urothelial Bladder Carcinoma and Prostate Adenocarcinoma. Hum Pathol. 2002; **33**: 1136–40.

Epstein JI, Kuhajda FP, Lieberman PH. Prostate-specific Acid Phosphatase Immunoreactivity in Adenocarcinomas of the Urinary Bladder. Hum Pathol. 1986; **17**: 939–42.

Lane Z, Hansel DE, Epstein JI. Immunohistochemical Expression of Prostatic Antigens in Adenocarcinoma and Villous Adenoma of the Urinary Bladder. Am J Surg Pathol. 2008; **32**: 1322–26.

Wang W, Epstein JI. Small Cell Carcinoma of the Prostate. A Morphologic and Immunohistochemical Study of 95 Cases. Am J Surg Pathol. 2008; **32**: 65–71.

Yao JL, Madeb R, Bourne P, et al. Small Cell Carcinoma of the Prostate: An Immunohistochemical Study. Am J Surg Pathol. 2006; **30**: 705–12.

Agoff SN, Lamps LW, Philip AT, et al. Thyroid Transcription Factor-1 is Expressed in Extrapulmonary Small Cell Carcinomas But Not in Other Extrapulmonary Neuroendocrine Tumors. Mod Pathol. 2000; **13**: 238–42.

Ordonez NG. Value of Thyroid Transcription Factor-1 Immunostaining in Distinguishing Small Cell Lung Carcinomas from Other Small Cell Carcinomas. Am J Surg Pathol. 2000; **24**: 1217–23.

Rubenstein JH, Katin MJ, Mangano MM, et al. Small Cell Anaplastic Carcinoma of the Prostate: Seven New Cases, Review of the Literature, and Discussion of a Therapeutic Strategy. Am J Clin Oncol. 1997; **20**: 376–80.

Aparicio AM, Harzstark AL, Corn PG, et al. Platinum-based Chemotherapy for Variant Castrate-resistant Prostate Cancer. Clin Cancer Res. 2013; **19**: 3621–30.

Han B, Mehra R, Lonigro RJ, et al. Fluorescence in Situ Hybridization Study Shows Association of PTEN Deletion with ERG Rearrangement During Prostate Cancer Progression. Mod Pathol. 2009; 22: 1083–93.

Williamson SR, Zhang S, Yao JL, et al. ERG-TMPRSS2 Rearrangement Is Shared by Concurrent Prostatic Adenocarcinoma and Prostatic Small Cell Carcinoma and Absent in Small Cell Carcinoma of the Urinary Bladder: Evidence Supporting Monoclonal Origin. Mod Pathol. 2011; 24: 1120–27.

Schelling LA, Williamson SR, Zhang S, et al. Frequent TMPRSS2-ERG Rearrangement in Prostatic Small Cell Carcinoma Detected by Fluorescence in Situ Hybridization: The Superiority of Fluorescence in Situ Hybridization over ERG Immunohistochemistry. Hum Pathol. 2013.

Bodey B, Bodey B, Jr, Kaiser HE. Immunocytochemical Detection of Prostate Specific Antigen Expression in Human Primary and Metastatic Melanomas. Anticancer Res. 1997; 17: 2343–46.

Fan CY, Wang J, Barnes EL. Expression of Androgen Receptor and Prostatic Specific Markers in Salivary Duct Carcinoma: An Immunohistochemical Analysis of 13 Cases and Review of the Literature. Am J Surg Pathol. 2000; 24: 579–86.

Gurel B, Ali TZ, Montgomery EA, et al. NKX3.1 as a Marker of Prostatic Origin in Metastatic Tumors. Am J Surg Pathol. 2010; 34: 1097–105.

Miettinen M, Wang ZF, Paetau A, et al. ERG Transcription Factor as an Immunohistochemical Marker for Vascular Endothelial Tumors and Prostatic Carcinoma. Am J Surg Pathol. 2011; 35: 432–41.

Sheridan T, Herawi M, Epstein JI, Illei PB. The role of P501S and PSA in the Diagnosis of Metastatic Adenocarcinoma of the Prostate. Am J Surg Pathol. 2007; 31: 1351–55.

Tazawa K, Kurihara Y, Kamoshida S, Tsukada K, Tsutsumi Y. Localization of Prostate-specific Antigen-like Immunoreactivity in Human Salivary Gland and Salivary Gland Tumors. Pathol Int. 1999; 49: 500–05.

Yin M, Dhir R, Parwani AV. Diagnostic Utility of p501s (Prostein) in Comparison to Prostate Specific Antigen (PSA) for the Detection of Metastatic Prostatic Adenocarcinoma. Diagn Pathol. 2007; 2: 41.

Paterson RF, Gleave ME, Jones EC, Zubovits JT, Goldenberg SL, Sullivan LD. Immunohistochemical Analysis of Radical Prostatectomy Specimens after 8 Months of Neoadjuvant Hormonal Therapy. Mol Urol. 1999; 3: 277–86.

Oppenheimer JR, Kahane H, Epstein JI. Granulomatous Prostatitis on Needle Biopsy. Arch Pathol Lab Med. 1997; 121: 724–29.

Chuang AY, Epstein JI. Xanthoma of the Prostate: A Mimicker of High-grade Prostate Adenocarcinoma. Am J Surg Pathol. 2007; 31: 1225–30.

Cheville JC, Dundore PA, Nascimento AG, et al. Leiomyosarcoma of the Prostate. Report of 23 Cases. Cancer. 1995; 76: 1422–27.

Westfall DE, Folpe AL, Paner GP, et al. Utility of a Comprehensive Immunohistochemical Panel in the Differential Diagnosis of Spindle Cell Lesions of the Urinary Bladder. Am J Surg Pathol. 2009; 33: 99–105.

Jo VY, Fletcher CD. p63 Immunohistochemical Staining is Limited in Soft Tissue Tumors. Am J Clin Pathol. 2011; 136: 762–66.

Hansel DE, Herawi M, Montgomery E, Epstein JI. Spindle Cell Lesions of the Adult Prostate. Mod Pathol. 2007; 20: 148–58.

Gaudin PB, Rosai J, Epstein JI. Sarcomas and Related Proliferative Lesions of Specialized Prostatic Stroma: A Clinicopathologic Study of 22 Cases. Am J Surg Pathol. 1998; 22: 148–62.

Herawi M, Epstein JI. Specialized Stromal Tumors of the Prostate: A Clinicopathologic Study of 50 Cases. Am J Surg Pathol. 2006; 30: 694–704.

Bostwick DG, Hossain D, Qian J, et al. Phyllodes Tumor of the Prostate: Long-term Followup Study of 23 Cases. J Urol. 2004; 172: 894–99.

Dundore PA, Cheville JC, Nascimento AG, Farrow GM, Bostwick DG. Carcinosarcoma of the Prostate. Report of 21 Cases. Cancer. 1995; 76: 1035–42.

Osunkoya AO, Netto GJ, Epstein JI. Colorectal Adenocarcinoma Involving the Prostate: Report of 9 Cases. Hum Pathol. 2007 38: 1836–41.

Owens CL, Epstein JI, Netto GJ. Distinguishing Prostatic from Colorectal Adenocarcinoma on Biopsy Samples: The Role of Morphology and Immunohistochemistry. Arch Pathol Lab Med. 2007; 131: 599–603.

Jaggi M, Johansson SL, Baker JJ, Smith LM, Galich A, Balaji KC. Aberrant Expression of E-cadherin and Beta-Catenin in Human Prostate Cancer. Urol Oncol. 2005; 23: 402–06.

Lazari P, Poulias H, Gakiopoulou H, Thomopoulou GH, Barbatis C, Lazaris AC. Differential Immunohistochemical Expression of CD44s, E-cadherin and Beta-Catenin among Hyperplastic and Neoplastic Lesions of the Prostate Gland. Urol Int. 2013; 90: 109–16.

Whitaker HC, Girling J, Warren AY, Leung H, Mills IG, Neal DE. Alterations in Beta-Catenin Expression and Localization in Prostate Cancer. Prostate. 2008; 68: 1196–205.

Aslan G, Irer B, Tuna B, Yorukoglu K, Saatcioglu F, Celebi I. Analysis of NKX3.1 Expression in Prostate Cancer Tissues and Correlation with Clinicopathologic Features. Pathol Res Pract. 2006; 202: 93–98.

Bauer JJ, Sesterhenn IA, Mostofi KF, McLeod DG, Srivastava S, Moul JW. P53 Nuclear Protein Expression is an Independent Prognostic Marker in Clinically Localized Prostate Cancer Patients Undergoing Radical Prostatectomy. Clin Cancer Res. 1995; **1**: 1295–300.

Bethel CR, Faith D, Li X, et al. Decreased NKX3.1 Protein Expression in Focal Prostatic Atrophy, Prostatic Intraepithelial Neoplasia, and Adenocarcinoma: Association with Gleason Score and Chromosome 8p Deletion. Cancer Res. 2006; **66**: 10683–90.

Brewster SF, Oxley JD, Trivella M, Abbott CD, Gillatt DA. Preoperative p53, bcl-2, CD44 and E-cadherin Immunohistochemistry as Predictors of Biochemical Relapse after Radical Prostatectomy. J Urol. 1999; **161**: 1238–43.

Cheng L, Pisansky TM, Sebo TJ, et al. Cell Proliferation in Prostate Cancer Patients with Lymph Node Metastasis: A Marker for Progression. Clin Cancer Res. 1999; **5**: 2820–23.

Gurel B, Iwata T, Koh CM, et al. Nuclear MYC Protein Overexpression Is an Early Alteration in Human Prostate Carcinogenesis. Mod Pathol. 2008; **21**: 1156–67.

Gurel B, Iwata T, Koh CM, Yegnasubramanian S, Nelson WG, De Marzo AM. Molecular Alterations in Prostate Cancer as Diagnostic, Prognostic, and Therapeutic Targets. Adv Anat Pathol. 2008; **15**: 319–31.

Kuczyk MA, Serth J, Bokemeyer C, et al. The Prognostic Value of p53 for Long-term and Recurrence-free Survival Following Radical Prostatectomy. Eur J Cancer. 1998; **34**: 679–86.

Lotan TL, Gurel B, Sutcliffe S, et al. PTEN Protein Loss by Immunostaining: Analytic Validation and Prognostic Indicator for a High Risk Surgical Cohort of Prostate Cancer Patients. Clin Cancer Res. 2011; **17**: 6563–73.

Moul JW, Bettencourt MC, Sesterhenn IA, et al. Protein Expression of p53, bcl-2, and KI-67 (MIB-1) as Prognostic Biomarkers in Patients with Surgically Treated, Clinically Localized Prostate Cancer. Surgery. 1996; **120**: 159–66. Discussion 166–67.

Sarker D, Reid AH, Yap TA, de Bono JS. Targeting the PI3 K/AKT Pathway for the Treatment of Prostate Cancer. Clin Cancer Res. 2009; **15**: 4799–805.

Stapleton AM, Zbell P, Kattan MW, et al. Assessment of the Biologic Markers p53, Ki-67, and Apoptotic Index as Predictive Indicators of Prostate Carcinoma Recurrence after Surgery. Cancer. 1998; **82**: 168–75.

Wang HL, Lu DW, Yerian LM, et al. Immunohistochemical Distinction between Primary Adenocarcinoma of the Bladder and Secondary Colorectal Adenocarcinoma. Am J Surg Pathol. 2001; **25**: 1380–87.

Mhawech-Fauceglia P, Zhang S, Terracciano L, et al. Prostate-specific Membrane Antigen (PSMA) Protein Expression in Normal and Neoplastic Tissues and Its Sensitivity and Specificity in Prostate Adenocarcinoma: An Immunohistochemical Study Using Multiple Tumour Tissue Microarray Technique. Histopathology. 2007; **50**: 472–83.

Herawi M, De Marzo AM, Kristiansen G, Epstein JI. Expression of CDX2 in Benign Tissue and Adenocarcinoma of the Prostate. Hum Pathol. 2007; **38**: 72–78.

Lopez-Beltran A, Cheng L, Prieto R, Ianca A, Montironi R. Lymphoepithelioma-like Carcinoma of the Prostate. Hum Pathol. 2009 Jul; **40**(7): 982–87.

Suh N, Yang XJ, Tretiakova MS, Humphrey PA, Wang HL. Value of CDX2, Villin, and Alpha-Methylacyl Coenzyme A Racemase Immunostains in the Distinction between Primary Adenocarcinoma of the Bladder and Secondary Colorectal Adenocarcinoma. Mod Pathol. 2005; **18**: 1217–22.

Index

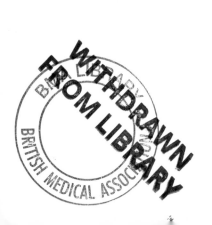

WITHDRAWN
FROM LIBRARY
BRITISH MEDICAL ASSOC